Introductory
Mental Health
Nursing

Introductory Mental Health Nursing

Donna M. Womble, RN, BS, MEd

Program Coordinator, Assistant Prof. of Nursing

Health Occupations—Vocational Nursing

South Plains College

Plainview, Texas

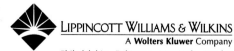

LIPPINCOTT WILLIAMS & WILKINS
A **Wolters Kluwer** Company

Philadelphia • Baltimore • New York • London
Buenos Aires • Hong Kong • Sydney • Tokyo

Acquisitions Editor: Elizabeth Nieginski
Managing Editor: Joseph Morita
Editorial Assistant: Joshua Levandoski
Project Management: Graphic World Publishing Services
Director of Nursing Production: Helen Ewan
Managing Editor/Production: Erika Kors
Art Director: Carolyn O'Brien
Senior Manufacturing Manager: William Alberti
Compositor: Graphic World, Inc.
Printer: R. R. Donnelly, Crawfordsville

9 8 7 6 5 4 3 2 1
ISBN: 0-7817-3685-4

Library of Congress Cataloging-in-Publication Data

Womble, Donna M.
  Introductory mental health nursing / Donna M. Womble.—1st ed.
    p. ; cm.
  Includes index.
  ISBN 0-7817-3685-4
    1. Psychiatric nursing.   I. Title.
  [DNLM: 1. Mental Disorders—nursing.   2. Psychiatric Nursing. WY 160 W872i 2004]
  RC440.W577 2004
  616.89'0231—dc22   2004048824

Care has been taken to confirm the accuracy of the information presented and to describe generally accepted practices. However, the authors, editors, and publisher are not responsible for errors or omissions or for any consequences from application of the information in this book and make no warranty, express or implied, with respect to the content of the publication.

The authors, editors, and publisher have exerted every effort to ensure that drug selection and dosage set forth in this text are in accordance with the current recommendations and practice at the time of publication. However, in view of ongoing research, changes in government regulations, and the constant flow of information relating to drug therapy and drug reactions, the reader is urged to check the package insert for each drug for any change in indications and dosage and for added warnings and precautions. This is particularly important when the recommended agent is a new or infrequently employed drug.

Some drugs and medical devices presented in this publication have Food and Drug Administration (FDA) clearance for limited use in restricted research settings. It is the responsibility of the health care provider to ascertain the FDA status of each drug or device planned for use in his or her clinical practice.

This book is dedicated to my beautiful
daughters,
Julie Kristine and Tanya Leigh
and
My late-husband, Charlie

Reviewers

Korbi Berryhill, RN, BA, CRRN
Program Coordinator/Assistant Professor
South Plains College
Lubbock, Texas

Sharon B. Bockus, RN, MS
Faculty/Coordinator
Columbus State Community College
Columbus, Ohio

Susan Boedeker, RN, MSN, FNP
PN and Nursing Instructor
Gateway Technical College
Kenosha, Wisconsin

Rose Corder, BSN, RN
Nursing Instructor
San Jacinto Community College North
Houston, Texas

Mary Ann Cosgarea, RN, BSN, BA
Coordinator/Nurse Administrator
Portage Lakes Career Center
Green, Ohio

Patricia Greer, RN
Intermediate Instructor of Practical Nursing
Tennessee Technology Center
Paris, Texas

Pamela Gwin, RNC
Director, Vocational Nursing Program
Brazosport College
Lake Jackson, Texas

Nancy T. Hatfield, BSN, RN, MA
Program Director/Department Chair
Health Occupations/Nursing
Career Enrichment Center
Albuquerque Public Schools
Albuquerque, New Mexico

Janet L. Joost, RN, BSN
Faculty
Front Range Community College
Longmont, Colorado

Linda S. King, RN, BSN
Instructor, Vocational Nursing
Montgomery College
Conroe, Texas

Sarah U. Lee, RN, BS, MA
Department Chair of Health Technologies
South Piedmont Community College
Polkten, North Carolina

Donna Lindblom, RN, Bed
Nursing Instructor
Northern Lakes College
Grand Prarie, Canada

Janell Sample, RN, MSN
Nursing Instructor
Del Mar Vocational
Corpus Christi, Texas

Bonnie J. Smith, RN, BSN
Coordinator, Practical Nurse Program
Sikeston Public Schools, Health Occupations
Hayti, Missouri

Beth M. Stone, RN, BSN, MSHPE
Coordinator Roper Hospital School
Roper St. Francis Healthcare
Charleston, South Carolina

Gale R. Woolley, EdD, ARNP
Professor
Miami-Dade Community College
Miami, Florida

Preface

After being asked to participate in this project, I began to ask myself about the inspiration to write this book. Having taught the subject of mental health and illness for many years, I saw a gap between what textbooks were available and what was needed. Some did not prepare the student adequately for the real world of mental issues, while others were much too complex for LPN/LVN students. Supplemental information was necessary year after year. Although this level of student nurse does not always have the opportunity for inpatient psychiatric unit experience, the majority of these graduates will encounter those with mental issues in a variety of healthcare settings. I attempted to integrate the demographics of LPN/LVN employment and functional roles into the text of this book. Regardless of the level of nursing credentials, it is essential for every nurse to have a basic understanding of how the mind and body work and influence the way we function as human beings.

Many times we do not realize that our perception of the environment is determined by the picture album of previous experiences in our mind. It is often difficult to understand our present situation and behavior unless we have some understanding of where we have been. Because students in the LPN/LVN programs do not typically have a theoretical foundation in psychology, it is difficult for them to conceptualize the basis for current psychotherapeutic treatment methods. To impose these concepts without a basic underpinning of how our thinking affects our behavior is unfair to the student. It is the aim of this text to provide a summarized overview of the theories integral in current treatment modalities. The presentation of human dynamics and the balance between adaptive and maladaptive responses to both internal and external stressors sets the climate for the presentation of the disorders.

This book presents the subject of mental health and illness by first establishing the essential groundwork. Unit I addresses the historical, ethical, and legal aspects of mental health nursing and acquaints the student with use of the nursing process in the psychiatric setting. Unit II provides the foundation concepts of anxiety and crisis, therapeutic communication methods, and theoretical models that give new perspective and meaning to human behavior. Building on these concepts, Unit III presents the mental disorders using a nursing process format. In Unit IV the special needs and disorder categories are presented as seen in the child and older adult. Unit V contains adjunctive material that is integral in all aspects of psychiatric/mental health care. Included in this unit are psychopharmacology, the treatment team, and specific treatment modalities. The last chapter addresses mental health care in nonpsychiatric settings, such as medical-surgical nursing units and correctional facilities.

Chapter objectives are written concisely and purposefully to anticipate learning outcomes. Specifically, they are intended to provide a mindset for the student to incorporate knowledge into application. Key terms are bold-faced in the manuscript to provide easy access to their meaning. Thought-provoking questions are posed throughout each chapter as Mind Joggers to encourage critical thinking. Important information is summarized or added in the form of Just the Facts margin supplements. At a Glance boxes are located throughout the book to give the student resource information in an easily viewed and compressed arrangement. Case studies are integrated into the text to provide opportunities for reflective thinking and content application.

Each chapter is followed by an integrated study guide, or worksheet, with various methods of assessing the subject content. These are written so that the answers are easily discernible after reading chapter content. Terminology and key terms are reinforced through completion and matching exercises. Scenarios present hypothetical situations in which the student can apply therapeutic interaction and communication concepts. Questions will also lead the student to utilize the nursing process in resolving identified problems. Critical thinking is anticipated as the student searches for incorrect information in the Seek and Find statements. This component is de-

signed to stimulate deductive thinking and reasoning. Multiple-choice questions are written using an NCLEX item-writing format to help prepare students for entry-level testing. An answer key is provided for all worksheets at the back of the textbook. Support references for content are provided at the end of each chapter.

It is my mission and hope that this textbook will help students to better understand the mental processes and how they are affected by factors in our everyday lives. It is my anticipated challenge that students will experience self-awareness and personal growth as they learn with a realization that to experience this energizes them to help others. Helping ourselves and recognizing how and why we think and act as we do is often the most beneficial side effect of this subject. By being willing to confront and change those things that can be changed and accept the unchangeable in our own life, we can open doors that allow us to role model this for our clients.

Acknowledgments

Reflection provides a full picture of how a book actually becomes a reality. Those who lend their support and expertise give texture to the project. The time and effort involved in completing the manuscript is extensive. As I look back over the timeframe invested in this book, I see the daily ongoing encouragement of my dear friends Nell, Amelia, Virginia, Suzanne, and Grady that have given me tenacity to the finish line. The faculty, staff, and administration of our college have given me a cheering section and much support. My students, both past and present, remind me of why this challenge has been a mission of caring and concern.

I was first contacted by Susan Rainey of LWW to work on this project. If it were not for her encouragement and believing in me when I didn't believe in myself, I may never have taken the leap forward. My thanks to Joe Morita, Managing Editor, for commanding this ship. He has provided direction and organization in seeing this venture to completion. I extend my most sincere thanks to Nancy Burnett, my Developmental Editor, for her vision, expertise, and commitment to structure in this manuscript. Through all of the working compromise between editor and author, her patience, support, and friendship have been priceless. Elizabeth Nieginski, Acquisitions Editor, came on board about midway through the project and has been very helpful through some very difficult situations. I would also like to thank the Production team at LWW.

And to my wonderful family, whose love and continued support have lifted me through many long hours of work on this project. Throughout this venture, they have been there with patience and understanding when threads wore thin. My heartfelt gratitude goes to Jimmy, Julie, Tanya, and Hagen for all your love and devotion. You are my greatest joy. I cannot close without mentioning my beloved late husband, Charlie, who died in 1999 from complications related to early-onset Alzheimer's disease. He was the love of my life and best friend for many years. Having worked with victims of this disease in my nursing experience, I was still ill-equipped for the role of care-giver throughout the journey of this devastating disease. Although the losses were so evident in his whole being, he often told me we needed to "write all this down for others." Was that an indication he wanted to give what he was experiencing to others? Although he has gone home to be with his Savior, perhaps his wish has been much of my inspiration for writing this book. I thank God for giving me this opportunity and for providing me with the strength and energy to fulfill this commitment.

Contents

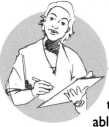

LEARNING OBJECTIVES

After learning the content in this chapter, the student will be able to:

1. Define mental health nursing as it relates to human behavior.
2. Identify those who have made contributions to the advancement of mental health.
3. Identify key factors that have changed the approach to treatment of mental illness.
4. Describe legislative actions that have influenced care of those with mental illness.
5. Discuss the shift of mental health care from institutional to community-based programs.

CHAPTER

1

Mental Health Nursing: A Historical Perspective

KEY TERMS

Americans with Disabilities Act (ADA)
Asylums
Institutionalized
Mental Health Act of 1983
National Mental Health Act of 1946
National Mental Health Parity Act
Omnibus Budget Reconciliation Act
Omnibus Budget Reform Act (OBRA)

The Advancement of Mental Health Care

Mental health nursing encompasses an identification and treatment of those problems that occur as a result of human responses to an actual or potential threat posed to a person's mental health. This branch of nursing has evolved into a specialized area of practice, employing the use of various theories about human behavior and the learned skill of therapeutic intervention. Mental health care providers have met numerous challenges in their effort to provide a vision of wellness for those with mental illness and to increase public awareness of its existence. Historically, the journey to provide this humane and therapeutic approach to those with mental alterations has been a difficult one.

Early Civilizations

Before the advent of psychotherapeutic drugs, which are now used extensively in the treatment of mental health issues, the available options for control of symptoms were few. Those with bizarre behavior were considered outcasts of society and harbored in asylums for the remainder of their lives. Many of the more violent clients were referred to as "lunatics," and they often became a spectacle for public viewing. The first institution for the mentally ill was opened in London as the Bethlehem Royal Hospital in 1247. The insane received cruel and inhumane treatment, and they were often required to wear metal arm and leg irons as they begged for food in the streets.

During the Renaissance, in the early 1400s, there was a growing interest in what led to various abnormal behaviors. An early classification of depression, neurosis, mania, and psychosis was developed by scholars and physicians according to the behaviors they saw. Despite the increased interest in what caused these situations, the care given to those with the mental disorders did not improve.

It was perhaps during the seventeenth century that conditions reached their lowest and most horrific point. Those with symptoms of insanity were locked in cells, starved, brutally beaten, and neglected. In the late 1700s, psychiatry emerged as a separate division of medical science. Those connected with the specialty began to question the way that those with mental problems were treated. Along with European countries, the U.S. colonies began to open **asylums** to house the insane along with prisoners and orphans. It was considered a place for the rejected of society. Care was provided by the poor and included such practices as blood-letting, purging, and confinement chairs. Although the study of psychiatry continued, the actual treatment of those with behavior problems remained unjust and cruel.

The Beginning of Change

An early nineteenth century physician by the name of Benjamin Rush (1745–1813) became the first American to advocate a change in the conditions for the mentally ill. A professor of chemistry and medicine, he theorized that there was a connection between blood circulation and diseases of the mind. He advocated that conditions for the mentally ill should include cleanliness, good air, lighting, and nutritious food. In addition, he felt that kindness and improved interaction between the client and care provider would have curative effects.

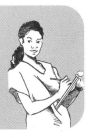

Just the Facts

In 1812, Benjamin Rush, referred to as the "Father of American Psychiatry," wrote the first American textbook of psychiatry.

Around the middle of the nineteenth century, we begin to see a change in perspective toward the care provided to those with mental illness. Dorothea Dix, a nineteenth-century schoolteacher, began to question the treatment of both prisoners and the mentally ill. She began a tireless effort to expose these conditions and provoke legislation to help in the construction of mental hospitals with standards for care.

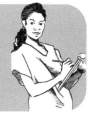

Just the Facts
Harriet Bailey wrote *Nursing Mental Diseases*, the first psychiatric nursing textbook, in 1920.

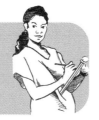

Just the Facts
Psychiatric-mental health nursing had its beginning in the late nineteenth century.

Mind Jogger
How does this early picture of nursing curricula reflect the holistic-centered approach to nursing today?

During the late nineteenth and early twentieth centuries, training programs for nurses were created and provided an option for those interested in caring for the sick. There was also an increasing social awareness of the problems that related to mental illness. Although the need for trained nurses was recognized, caring for the insane was not seen as a fit occupation for women. Linda Richards (1841–1930), a pioneer as the first trained nurse in America, was educated in psychiatric nursing at the New England Hospital in Boston. Several years later, she traveled to England to receive more training at St. Thomas's Hospital in London, the hospital established by Florence Nightingale in 1860. Here she met and trained under Florence Nightingale, who encouraged Richards to continue her studies in Europe. Upon her return to the United States, she established training curricula for schools of nursing. In 1882, Richards opened the Boston City Hospital Training School for Nurses, which specialized in training nurses to care for mentally ill clients. Although this was a beginning, it was not until 1913 that the first psychiatric content was included within the curriculum of a nursing school. Gradually as this was phased into all schools of nursing, the specialized training hospitals were closed.

Twentieth Century Progress

Slowly, a component of psychiatric nursing was included in all nursing curricula. The well-known **National Mental Health Act** of 1946 was the first legislation to provide funds for research, advanced nursing degree programs, and improved community service for the mentally ill. In 1955 the Joint Commission on Mental Illness and Health was established to conduct a study on the guidelines used by mental institutions to provide care for their clients. Funding became available for research and improved treatment programs. Funds were appropriated by Congress for the National Institute of Mental Health (NIMH), established in 1949, for its support and continued research in the field of mental illness.

These political and social changes were beginning to influence the present and future roles of psychiatric nurses. Although most clients with mental illness were still **institutionalized** in state mental hospitals, there was a growing trend toward the provision of community-based treatment at inpatient hospital units that specialized in the care of mental illness. This meant a growing need for trained nurses to fill both new and expanded roles. By the 1950s, many steps were taken toward improved conditions and treatment methods. In

1953, the National League for Nursing endorsed the inclusion of psychiatric nursing in all nursing programs.

It was during this period that the first psychotherapeutic drugs were introduced. These drugs provided relief of symptoms and put an end to the need for physical restraint in straightjackets and for lobotomies to remove portions of the brain to control behaviors. Sedatives were developed that quieted clients, and lithium carbonate was found to be effective in controlling mood swings. In 1956, the first antipsychotic drugs were introduced to control the bizarre behaviors seen in some disorders. Shortly thereafter, antidepressants and antianxiety drugs were developed.

As this new era of treatment emerged, the movement to deinstitutionalize clients with mental illness was in motion. Between 1950 and 1980, the number of institutionalized clients dropped from more than 500,000 to less than 100,000.

Just the Facts

Thorazine was the first antipsychotic drug to be used in the treatment of mental illness.

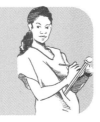

Community-Based Care

As the need for community-based mental health care gained recognition, federal legislation emerged to create funding for the establishment of centers that would offer these services. The Mental Retardation Facilities and Community Mental Health Centers Act of 1963 and the Community Health Centers Amendment of 1975 made it possible for clients to receive a variety of treatments designed to shorten hospital stays. Clients were returned to their homes with follow-up counseling and therapy on an outpatient basis. The trend toward improved and more compas-

sionate care for those with mental illness was under way. In 1982, the Omnibus Budget Reconciliation Act provided funds to support the treatment of those with drug addictions and other mental disorders. This bill was further legislated in 1987 when the **Omnibus Budget Reform Act** (OBRA) prevented the inappropriate placement of mentally ill clients into nursing homes. The **Mental Health Act of 1983** addressed the rights of people admitted to psychiatric hospitals, including their right to refuse being admitted to a psychiatric facility against their will and their rights while in treatment, following discharge, and during community follow-up.

The 1990s were declared the Decade of the Brain by President George H. W. Bush. In this proclamation, he specified the need for specialized studies to find ways of reducing the impact and prevalence of diseases affecting the brain. At the same time, the Americans with Disabilities Act (ADA) was signed; it was the first federal civil rights law to prohibit discrimination against persons with mental and physical disabilities. This legislation protects those persons with disabilities in the employment setting, while using public transportation or facilities, and in areas of mass communication. The **National Mental Health Parity Act** was signed into law in 1996 by President Bill Clinton; this law made it mandatory for insurance companies to provide annual and lifetime benefit limits for mental illnesses comparable to those allotted for physical illnesses. An amendment to expand this act was proposed in March of 1998 to prohibit limitations on cost-sharing applied to the cost of mental health care.

Throughout these legislative changes, modifications were made in the treatment of clients, both in hospital-based units providing inpatient care and those with outpatient services. The focus is on providing treatment and support systems to allow the client to return to a home setting or structured living situation. Integral to this approach was the need to define a logical and orderly way to fulfill the nurse's role in the treatment process. The expanded philosophy of mental health nursing was based on a scientific and systematic approach, later referred to as *the nursing process.* The work of Hildegard Peplau (1909–1999) laid the groundwork for the interpersonal and interactive processes so integral to the nurse-client relationship. When working with the psychiatric client, Peplau believed that the nurse acts as a resource person, counselor, role model, and support person for the client. In 1994 the American Nurses Association adopted standards of clinical practice for psychiatric-mental health nursing.

Mind Jogger
In what way does the nurse serve as a role model to those with mental illness?

to society as a whole. The co... tivity and income is paid by ... ing the public health care cor...

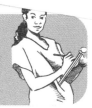

Just the Facts
The success rate for treating depression and other mental illness is approximately 80%.

Mind Jogger
How has the decrease in mental health services affected your community? What can we as nurses do to support legislation for change?

Present Issues

The access to care and the way in which mental health care is delivered has undergone many changes and reforms. However, as we begin the twenty-first century, there remains a stigma and lack of social awareness of the effects these disorders have on both those who have the illness and those who share the responsibility for their care. The impact of managed-care delivery of health care has been dramatic on mental health units. Many psychiatric units are closing owing to a lack of operational funds. The paradox of this trend is the growing population of those who need these services but are unable to secure them. Those living in community settings need ongoing management and support. Without these services, clients often become unstable and treatment becomes ineffective. The need for renewed interest and political attention to this issue is imperative. Legislation before the Congress in early 2004 has the potential to extend the Mental Health Parity Act of 1996, which is now expired. Lack of access to treatment has disastrous implications for the person with mental illness, their families, and

The role of nurses in mental health care continues to be as providers of a systematized method of care. Many psychiatric nurses are advanced-practitioners who provide counseling, prescribe medications, and facilitate therapy services. Nurses have a responsibility to provide mental health care in every aspect of the continuum. Clients with mental disorders and psychosocial needs are seen in every client-care setting. It is necessary to assess the need for and utilize therapeutic interventions in each client encounter. Nurses can and will continue to make a difference in the lives of those who share the pain and tragedy of mental illness.

Summary

The road to current treatment modalities for the client with mental illness has been long and rough. From the time of ancient civilizations, those with disorders of the mind have been pushed aside as if they are a subnormal gory of human beings. The inhumane and cruel treatment of people with inappropriate mental behaviors reached its lowest level during the seventeenth century.

The nineteenth century began to see some changes that would open doors for improved understanding of mental processes and the disturbances created by disorders of these processes. As this knowledge began to spread, pioneers emerged who were appalled by the conditions and treatment endured by the people with these disturbances. Included in these early advocates of change were nurses who exposed the neglect and worked to effect change, including the training of nurses in psychiatric care. The development of psychotropic and antipsychotic drugs allowed practitioners to control the symptoms of mental illness without restraints and other induced methods. Gradually, as these changes occurred, the political climate changed and legislation was passed to make care of the mentally ill mandatory, available, and standardized. Client rights were established to prevent hospitalization of people against their will and preserve their rights if treatment was carried out.

The need for improved access to care and available resources continues. Although the shift to community-based mental health services has deinstitutionalized the care of those with mental illness, there is still work to be done. The number of those needing treatment and continued care exceeds the resources available to pay for these services. Nurses can and will continue to play a part in addressing the needs of the mentally ill and their families. The interpersonal therapeutic relationship between the nurse and the client is perhaps one of the most fundamental of the healing arts for the person affected by puzzles of the mind.

Bibliography

Bee, S., & Gibson, M. J. (1998). Mental health parity: An overview of recent legislation, AARP research. Available at http://research.aarp.org/health/fs69_mental.html. Accessed July 1, 2004.

Boyd, M., & Nihart, M. (1998). *Psychiatric nursing—contemporary practice*. Philadelphia, PA: Lippincott.

Frisch, N. C., & Frisch, L. E. (2002). *Psychiatric mental health nursing* (2nd ed.). Albany, NY: Delmar.

National Mental Health Association. (2004). Congress must pass mental health parity now. Available at www.nmha.org/federal/parity. Accessed July 1, 2004.

Student Worksheet

FILL IN THE BLANK

Fill in the blank with the correct answer.

1. The _____ of 1946 was the first legislation to provide funds for research, advanced nursing programs, and improved community service for the mentally ill.

2. The development of _____ medications allowed behaviors and symptoms to be controlled without restraints and surgery.

3. _____ was the first trained nurse and first psychiatric nurse in the United States.

MATCHING

Match the following terms to the most appropriate phrase.

a. First antipsychotic drug developed.

b. Theorized a connection between blood circulation and mental diseases.

c. Prevented inappropriate placement of mentally ill in nursing homes.

d. Addressed client rights for admission to psychiatric units.

e. Wrote the first psychiatric nursing textbook.

1. _____ Omnibus Budget Reform Act

2. _____ Mental Health Act of 1983

3. _____ Benjamin Rush

4. _____ Harriet Bailey

5. _____ Thorazine (chlorpromazine)

MULTIPLE CHOICE

Select the best answer from the multiple-choice items.

1. Which of the following pioneers worked diligently to secure legislation to help in the construction of mental hospitals with standards for care?
   a. Dorothea Dix
   b. Linda Richards
   c. Florence Nightingale
   d. Harriet Bailey

2. The dynamics of interpersonal nurse-client interaction is largely credited to which of the following nurses?
   a. Harriet Bailey
   b. Linda Richards
   c. Hildegard Peplau
   d. Dorothea Dix

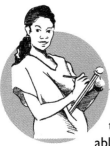

LEARNING OBJECTIVES

After learning the content in this chapter, the student will be able to:

1. Identify how client rights are preserved in mental health settings.
2. Differentiate between types of commitment to psychiatric treatment.
3. Discuss legal issues involved with client confidentiality.
4. Identify areas of nursing accountability in the mental health setting.
5. Define criteria for the use of seclusion and restraints.

Legal and Ethical Aspects of Mental Health Nursing

KEY TERMS

Accountability

Chemical restraint

Client advocate

Confidentiality

Ethics

Informed consent

Involuntary commitment

Physical restraint

Seclusion

Voluntary commitment

Legal and Ethical Responsibilities of the Nurse

Many decisions of health care professionals involve matters that include both legal and ethical issues. Like any other aspect of the system, the care of clients with mental disorders involves a certain standard of principles and values. The nurse must have knowledge of the laws and ethical governance of mental health care delivery. In addition, the nurse is responsible for maintaining standards within the nursing profession itself.

Ethics

The term **ethics** refers to a set of principles or values that provides dignity and respect to clients. Ethics also provides a guiding philosophy for the nursing profession and protects clients from unreasonable treatment. Nurses have an obligation to be familiar with the rights of clients and current laws concerning care. Integrating positive values into client care improves the self-esteem of clients and facilitates the therapeutic relationship.

Client Rights

All clients entering a treatment facility have certain rights that have been documented in the Patient Bill of Rights. Those that apply to the client with mental illness were declared in the Mental Health Systems Act Bill of Rights passed by the U.S. Congress in 1980. Clients are given the opportunity to read these rights at the time of admission. This document is usually displayed in a prominent area of the client service units so that it is available to clients and families. It is a nurse's responsibility to be familiar with these rights and to ensure that they are preserved and protected.

Right to Appropriate Treatment. Although the nurse is not directly responsible for deciding where or what treatment is provided, it is an integral part of the nurse's responsibility to ensure that the client receives appropriate care. All clients are entitled to receive care based on a current and individualized treatment plan that includes a description of the services that are available and those that are offered upon discharge. Clients have a right to:

- Know the qualifications of the professionals who will be involved in the treatment process.
- Receive explanations of treatment and be involved in the planning of their care.
- Refuse to be a part of experimental therapy or treatment methods.
- Understand the effects of prescribed medications along with any potential adverse effects.
- Be treated in the least restrictive setting— one that prevents excessive restraint within a confined atmosphere.
- Decide which treatment options are best for them.
- Refuse treatment unless there is a court order that dictates reasons for admission.

Mind Jogger

In addition to being a responsibility, how does a knowledge of client rights protect the nurse?

Just the Facts

Least restrictive environments can include locked or unlocked hospital units, community living centers, or outpatient treatment centers, depending on the individual needs of the client.

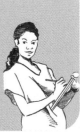

Informed Consent. Prior to admission to any health care setting, the client received an explanation of client rights and institutional policies from the agency. In the case of an incompetent or incoherent client, a family member or legal guardian should be given this information. The agency providing the services is protected by getting a signed statement of understanding from the client. At the same time, the client has the right to refuse any aspect of treatment and may elect not to sign the consent. At the time of admission to a mental health setting, the client receives an explanation of the unit policies regarding available services, visitation, phone usage, unit rules, and physician contact. The agency representative also explains insurance benefits or payment options, as well as the contracts between the treating professionals and third-party payment reimbursement. The full explanations give the client, or those who may have legal guardianship for the client, a choice of treatment.

Just the Facts

Informed consent consists of sufficient, accurate information for the client to voluntarily give consent within his or her legal capability.

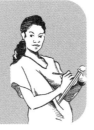

Confidentiality. Confidentiality refers to the client's right to prevent written or verbal communications from being disclosed to outside parties without authorization. To facilitate a client's trust, nursing students and licensed nurses must assure them that all communication is confidential and will not be communicated to anyone not participating in their care. The Nurse Practice Act of each state Board of Nursing requires nurses to protect the client's right to privacy by maintaining confidentiality. Every member of the treatment team has a duty to uphold this ethical standard. The privacy and confidentiality provisions of the Health Insurance Portability and Accountability Act (HIPAA) of 1996 went into effect in April of 2003. This law ensures that security procedures protect the privacy and confidentiality of this information. The client has the right to know what information is being disclosed for payment benefits or other treatment reasons, and to whom it is being given.

Mind Jogger

In what way might confidentiality raise more of a concern to the client in a psychiatric unit than the client on a medical or surgical hospital unit?

Protecting the client's record from unauthorized personnel is a nursing responsibility. Health care providers who are not consulted by the physician or providing direct client care do not have the privilege of observing the medical record without permission. Student nurses should be careful to disguise any clinical material that is used for education purposes. Situations that require disclosure of client information may include:

- Intent to commit a crime
- Duty to warn endangered persons
- Evidence of child abuse
- Initiation of involuntary hospitalization
- Infection by human immunodeficiency virus

Another way of providing privacy is to conduct the nursing report in a private area where other clients and uninvolved hospital staff cannot hear what is being said. Report sheets should be kept in a discreet place and shredded before leaving the nursing unit. At no time should the nurse discuss a client's problems or treatment with another client. Acknowledgment of a client admission should not occur via telephone to outside parties unless a policy and system exists that can be used to ensure confidentiality. Some psychiatric facilities have codes that are provided to persons that the client approves.

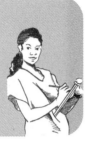

the clients and those rights that are legally afforded them.

Appeals and Complaints. Regardless of the setting in which clients receive mental health services, they have the right to receive information about how to channel complaints about their care or the professionals providing their treatment. This should be explained to clients at the time services are anticipated, whether in a hospital unit or an outpatient setting. Should the person wish to file a complaint to a professional board, the person should be advised of the procedure to do so. Some clients may wish to appeal decisions on payor systems and should be given the name and address of the appropriate contact.

Accountability

Student and licensed nurses are accountable for the care they provide, which means they must take responsibility for what they do. Each level of nursing is responsible for adhering to the standard of care that is acceptable for that particular level. The nurse practice act of each state identifies the scope and minimum standards of practice for both the LPN/LVN and RN. If a question arises with regard to a statute contained in the practice act, the nurse should contact the board of nursing for the state in which he or she is practicing. Nurses may be held accountable and liable to any client for an act of incompetence or negligence in the deliverance of care. All actions on the part of the nurse to facilitate appropriate treatment of the client should be documented to provide a written record of events. The nurse also has a legal and ethical responsibility to act as a **client advocate** to protect

Nurses have an obligation to maintain current licensure and educational requirements required by their board of nursing. In the area of psychiatric–mental health care, the nurse is also responsible for knowing institutional and governmental policies regarding client admission and rights. If uncertainty exists, the nurse is responsible for securing the correct information from other sources such as procedure manuals, textbooks, other health care professionals, or network resources.

Client Admissions

A client has the right to receive treatment in the least restrictive environment that would promote safety and therapeutic care. The type of facility and level of care provided depends on several factors. The client's history has a strong influence on the treatment methods that will be used. The circumstances that led to the current admission also contribute to the treatment and nursing care that will be needed. The physician or psychiatrist makes the determination whether the client will need to receive inpatient or outpatient treatment. Residential facilities are also available for clients who need to reside in a therapeutic environment for extended periods of time.

Many clients with mental health problems request admission to a psychiatric center for treatment. A **voluntary commitment** occurs when the client is admitted based on his or her chosen willingness to comply with the treatment program. In this situation, the physician writes the order for admission and the client signs and agrees to the terms of treatment. The person is then allowed to sign the appropriate documents and leave when treatment is complete. Policies may vary among facilities, but most states have an initial period (i.e., 72 hours) that allows the physician and other members of the treatment team the opportunity to assess the situation before the person can leave voluntarily. If the client leaves prior to this time or without a discharge order from the physician, he or she may be asked to sign an AMA (Against Medical Advice) form that releases the facility from any liability related to the person leaving treatment.

An **involuntary commitment** occurs when a person is admitted to a psychiatric unit against his or her will. The amount of time a person can be detained is determined by law, which varies from state to state. For an involuntary admission to occur, an evaluation statement that clearly indicates the person's mental state is a danger to self or others is necessary. This is a time-consuming and sometimes difficult process. The order for protective custody (OPC) is given by a court official. The client can be detained on an emergency status against his or her will for an interval of 48 to 72 hours. At the end of that period, the client must either be discharged, given voluntary admission status, or receive a court hearing to determine if there is a need for continued involuntary treatment. Laws may vary from state to state on these options. Involuntary commitment is most commonly used in an inpatient setting but can be ordered on an outpatient basis, such as in substance-abuse programs.

Seclusion and Restraints. The Joint Commission on Accreditation of Healthcare Organizations (JCAHO) and the federal government regulate the use of seclusion and restraints by health care workers. **Seclusion** refers to the placement of a client in a controlled environment in order to treat a clinical emergency. Many times this refers to placing a client inside a room with a locked door away from stimuli of the nursing unit. **Physical re-**

straint refers to the use of mechanical devices to provide limited movement by the client. Physical restraints are used to prevent harm to self or others and require careful monitoring. These may consist of padded leather or cloth devices for the wrist, ankles, waist, or fingers. **Chemical restraint** refers to the use of medication to calm a client and prevent the need for physical restraints. Chemical restraint is less restrictive and is generally the initial choice unless the situation warrants otherwise.

Just the Facts
Seclusion should never be used when a person is suicidal.

Just the Facts
Restraints are applied only with a physician's order and under the supervision of a registered nurse.

These methods are only used when verbal interventions or less restrictive methods of treatment have failed or are not available. It is essential that nurses attempt to de-escalate aggressive behaviors before these measures are necessary. Many times the environmental situation or other clients have provoked the behavior. In this case, removing the client to another area of the unit may allow the client to regain control without further intervention. If seclusion or restraints are employed, the client is usually given sedating medication to provide a calming effect and assist in behavior control. Continuous monitoring of the client in restraints or seclusion is mandatory. These methods are discontinued at any time they are seen as ineffective or at the earliest possible indication that the client has regained control. Time limits are a part of many state and institutional statutes.

Nurses should be familiar with the legal implications involved in the use of seclusion and restraint. It is important to know the qualifications and training of any person that is delegated the task of assisting with restraint. The nurse should know the facility rules and state laws regarding this procedure to avoid any probable cause of wrongful liability. Clients who are confined without justification or who are subject to inappropriate use of seclusion or restraint can be viewed in a civil court as having been falsely imprisoned. The restraint of clients with inappropriate use of force can be viewed as assault and battery. Having an awareness of how, when, and why to use confining methods will help the nurse avoid litigation for these circumstances.

Summary

All nurses are held to a standard of conduct that is outlined in a code of ethics for their particular level of nursing. This is usually referred to as *prudent behavior,* or actions that another person with the same level of education would do in the same situation. Nurses are accountable for their own actions. Within this accountability lies the responsibility to defend and uphold the rights of the client.

Nurses have an assigned role as a client advocate that requires them to monitor the treatment process and intervene if a presumed injustice is seen.

The Patient Bill of Rights provides any consumer of health care the opportunity of choice. This is no different for the client in need of mental health care. Because many clients may be compromised in their ability to understand the content of these statements, explanations are provided to both the client and others who may be responsible for their care. The efforts to protect and uphold the rights of those with mental illness are ongoing. Much lobbying is being done to secure funding and treatment options for a population that often falls between the cracks of the health care organization. Legislation to overhaul the benefit reimbursement system for psychiatric disorders is pending in the U.S. Congress as this text is being written.

Client rights for informed consent, confidentiality, and admission to a mental health treatment center have been given much attention by lawmakers and agencies responsible for the health care system. It is essential for the nurse to remain current and knowledgeable about laws and regulations that cover these aspects of care. Many litigated cases concern a violation of rights afforded the client by law. These situations are preventable but require knowledge and sound decision-making on the part of the nurse each and every time client contact occurs.

Bibliography
American Psychological Association. (1997). "Mental Health Patient's Bill of Rights." Available at www.apa.org/pubinfo/rights/rights.html. Accessed July 1, 2004.

Appelbaum, P. S. (1994). *Almost a revolution: Mental health law and the limits of change.* New York: Oxford University Press.

Simon, R. I. (2001). *Concise guide to psychiatry and the law for clinicians.* Washington, DC: American Psychiatric Publishing.

Stefan, S. (2001). *Unequal Rights: Discrimination against people with mental disabilities and the American Disabilities Act.* Washington, DC: American Psychological Association.

Student Worksheet

FILL IN THE BLANK

Fill in the blank with the correct answer.

1. _____ refers to a set of principles or values that provide dignity and respect to clients.

2. _____ _____ is a signed statement of understanding that provides protection for both the client and the agency providing the services.

3. _____ refers to the client's right to prevent written or verbal communications from being disclosed to outside parties without authorization.

MATCHING

Match the following terms to the most appropriate phrase.

a. Court ordered admission

b. Placement in controlled environment

c. Use of medication to control behavior

d. Taking responsibility for own actions

e. Client chooses admission for treatment

f. Defines the scope of nursing practice

1. _____ Accountability

2. _____ Nurse Practice Act

3. _____ Voluntary commitment

4. _____ Seclusion

5. _____ Involuntary commitment

6. _____ Chemical restraint

MULTIPLE CHOICE

Select the best answer from the multiple-choice items.

1. Under what circumstances can an order for protective custody be obtained?
   a. Client is hallucinating.
   b. Client is exhibiting sexually inappropriate behavior.
   c. Client's mental state is a danger to self or others.
   d. Client is angry and verbally hostile.

2. A student nurse who is not assigned to the psychiatric unit asks you about information regarding one of your clients. What would be your best response?
   a. Give the student the information.
   b. Ask the student why the information is needed.
   c. Inform the charge nurse of the information request.
   d. Remind the student that information cannot be disclosed.

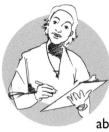

LEARNING OBJECTIVES

After learning the content of this chapter, the student will be able to:

1. Identify the five steps of delivering nursing care using the nursing process.
2. Describe types of information obtained in a psychosocial assessment.
3. Determine applicable nursing diagnoses for identified client problems.
4. Plan realistic expected outcomes for resolution of identified problems.
5. Evaluate client outcome of anticipated improvement in functioning and well-being.
6. Apply the nursing process to the care of the client in the psychiatric setting.

The Nursing Process in Mental Health Nursing

KEY TERMS

Assessment
Evaluation
NANDA
Nursing diagnosis
Nursing interventions
Nursing process
Objective data
Outcomes
Prioritize
Subjective data
Therapeutic milieu

Defining the Nursing Process

The **nursing process** is a scientific and systematic method for providing effective individualized nursing care and serves as an aid in resolving client problems. This problem-solving approach allows the nurse to help the client achieve a maximal level of functioning and well-being. The nursing process is accepted by the nursing profession as a standard for providing ongoing nursing care that is adapted to individual client needs. Accountability to the client and communication between members of the mental health care team is enhanced by the process (see Chapter 21, The Treatment Team). The use of the nursing process also allows nurses to share information that is important to the continuity of client care and treatment. The nurse can reevaluate each step of the nursing process to adjust, revise, or terminate the plan of care based on new or added information. It is important to remember that each client's response to therapy and treatment may be different. Adjustments can and will be made as the level of illness and dysfunction affects the independence and well-being of the client.

Vital to this process is the therapeutic climate of the interaction between the client and members of the mental health team. The nurse is often the first member of the team that is in contact with the client. It is at this point that a **therapeutic milieu** is established. The milieu is an environment or surroundings that are modified to create a setting in which the client feels safe, secure, and free to express feelings and thoughts without fear of rejection, retaliation, or punishment. The nurse can initiate this atmosphere and establish a sense of trust by approaching the client in an accepting and nonjudgmental manner. This trusting relationship is vital to the successful outcome of improved functioning and well-being of the client (see Chapter 5, The Therapeutic Relationship).

Steps of the Nursing Process

Integral to the nursing process approach to nursing care is an organized method of problem solving called the *care plan,* which is developed from the data that are gathered during the initial phase. It consists of five steps that provide planned actions for resolving the problem:

Nursing assessment
Nursing diagnosis
Expected outcome
Nursing interventions
Evaluation

Nursing Assessment

Assessment begins when the client is admitted or contact is made for the first time. Assessment continues as the cycle of the nursing process progresses and new information or changes occur in reference to the client. An assessment interview is usually conducted within the psychiatric setting; however, the psychosocial needs of a client are part of any nursing assessment, regardless of the setting, because symptoms seen in the mental health setting can also be seen in any area of health care. A standard assessment tool helps categorize the information received by the nurse. A basic psychosocial nursing assessment usually includes the client's history and mental or emotional status and encompasses both **subjective** and **objective data.**

Subjective Data. Subjective information is provided by the client. This information may need to be validated by other sources such as family, friends, law enforcement officers, or others who are involved. The client's information may be supported or contradicted by others. The data include the client's history and perception of the present situation or problem in addition to feelings, thoughts, symptoms, or emotions he or she may be experiencing.

When collecting subjective data it is important for the nurse to be as accurate and descriptive as possible. Citing a direct quote of a client statement is a way of describing what the client is saying without attempting to interpret the intended meaning. Using the client's own words to describe feelings or thoughts often provides insight into perceptual distortions or illogical thought processes.

Just the Facts

Input from the client's family can provide information about family dynamics, any present turmoil or disruption within the family, and how the client's problem may be affecting other members of the family.

At a Glance 3-1 Examples of Subjective Data

- Name and general information about the client
- Client's perception of current stressor or problem
- Current occupational or work situation
- Any recent difficulty in relationships
- Any somatic complaints
- Current or past substance use
- Interests or activities previously enjoyed
- Sexual activity or difficulties

The subjective information gathered during the initial assessment will allow the nurse to establish a baseline used to formulate the care plan. By asking direct leading questions, the nurse gets a clear picture of certain problems or issues concerning the client. Successful gathering of data is based on the ability of the nurse to listen to the client. When the nurse selects a climate that ensures privacy and confidentiality, the client feels free to openly communicate personal feelings. Following are examples of leading questions that can be used to obtain data from the client during the assessment interview:

- Tell me what brought you to the hospital today.
- Was there any situation that caused you to feel this way?
- How did you react to the situation?
- Tell me how you are feeling about being here.
- Where do you live?
- Who lives with you?
- What type of work do you do?
- Have you been able to work prior to admission?
- What causes the most stress in your life?
- What do you do to alleviate the stress?
- Do you blame yourself for bad things that happen to you?
- Tell me about things that overwhelm you each day.
- Are you currently taking medication to help you through the stressful times?

Objective Data. Objective information is observed by the nurse or provided by others who are familiar with the client or additional members of the health care team. The assessment includes the physical, emotional, intellectual, and social aspects of the client. A physical assessment includes medical history, past illnesses or surgeries, medication history, allergies, vital signs, height and weight, diet, and head-to-toe systems evaluation. Social issues may include relationships, family history of mental illness, religious and cultural beliefs, and specific health practices. The client's emotional state, behavior, and thinking processes are all part of the mental assessment.

Mind Jogger

How might a past medical and psychiatric history help to identify potential problems?

At a Glance 3-2 Examples of Objective Data

- Physical exam
- Behavior
- Mood and affect
- Awareness
- Thought processes
- Appearance
- Activity
- Judgment
- Response to environment
- Perceptual ability

A standard mental status examination tool is used to assess cognitive, emotional, and behavioral information. At a Glance 3-3 provides a summary of a basic mental exam. (The Mini-Mental Status Exam is found in Appendix B). It is most important to note both verbal communication and nonverbal mannerisms, expressions, and emotions. Look for congruency between what the client is saying and what is displayed in the accompanying behavior. It is also important to recognize if the client poses any immediate threat or danger to self or others, in which case safety becomes a priority and must be secured.

Nursing Diagnosis

Establishing a **nursing diagnosis** from collected data is the second step in the nursing process. The nurse analyzes all data gathered and compares it to normal functioning or values to find out if a problem or a potential problem exists. A nursing diagnosis is not a medical diagnosis but an identification of a client problem based on conclusions about the collected data. A nursing diagnosis may be an actual or potential health problem, depending on the situation. The most commonly used standard is that of the North American Nursing Diagnosis Association **(NANDA).** This is an approved list of problems that the nurse can legally address toward

At a Glance 3-3 Components of Mental Status Assessment

- Appearance (grooming, dress, hygiene, eye contact, skin markings, posture, facial expression)
- Motor activity (pacing, slow, rigid, relaxed, restless, combative, bizarre, gait, hyperactive, retarded, aggressive)
- Attitude (cooperative or uncooperative, friendly, hostile, apathetic, suspicious)
- Speech pattern (speed, volume, articulation, congruence, confabulation, slurring, dysphasia)
- Mood (intensity, depth, duration, anxious, sad, euphoric, labile, fearful, irritable, depressed)
- Affect (flat or absence of emotional expression, blunted, congruence with mood, appropriate or inappropriate)
- Level of awareness (level of consciousness, attention span, comprehension, processing)
- Orientation (time, place, person)
- Memory (recent and remote)
- Understanding of illness/insight (ability to perceive and understand illness—symptoms as related to illness)
- Ability to describe stressors (internal or psychologic/physical in nature, and external or actual loss)
- Thought processes (speed, content, organization, logical or illogical, delusions, abstract or concrete)
- Perceptual disturbances (hallucinations, illusions, depersonalization, distortions)
- Judgment (problem-solving and decision-making ability)
- Adaptive or maladaptive defense mechanisms
- Relationships (attainment and maintenance of satisfying interpersonal relationships)

a measurable outcome. A list of nursing diagnoses approved by NANDA is found in Appendix C.

Formulating a nursing diagnosis consists of three parts: (1) the actual or potential problem related to the client's condition, (2) the causative or contributing factors, and (3) a behavior or symptom that supports the problem. A nursing diagnosis is correctly written as follows: (problem) risk for injury, related to (contributing factor) marital breakup, evidenced by (behavior) suicidal ideation and gestures. Although a medical diagnosis is not used as the etiology of a nursing problem, signs and symptoms of the condition may be reflected in the cause. This is illustrated by a client who has sensory-perceptual alteration, related to auditory hallucinations, evidenced by talking to people who are not physically present. Determining the problem provides the groundwork for planning nursing interventions to meet the needs of the client for which the nurse is responsible.

Once applicable nursing diagnoses have been determined, they are **prioritized** according to the intensity and immediate urgency of the problem. Any health condition that endangers life will receive a high priority. Situations that are recurrent or chronic may be given a lower priority and will be addressed at a later time. A client with suicidal ideation or intent, for example, would have an immediate risk for self-injury. This problem would require the nurse's attention first. Based on Maslow's hierarchy of needs, basic physiologic needs such as oxygen, food, water, warmth, elimination, and sleep must be met before other needs of safety and security, love and belonging, self-esteem, and self-actualization can be achieved. This model can be seen as a staircase in which a client may vacillate between steps. Given that the client can move up and then back down, the nurse should understand that the priority given to a problem can change at any time during the treatment process. To illustrate this concept, a client who has begun to identify strengths and display positive self-talk (self-esteem level need) is told by another client that she is stupid and ugly. The client has now refused to eat for two meals. At this point the nutritional needs of the client become the priority.

Just the Facts

Maslow's hierarchy of needs is a based on the theory that one level of needs must be met before moving on to the next step.
- Self-actualization
- Self-esteem
- Love and belonging
- Safety and security
- Basic physiologic needs

It is also important to give priority to the problem that the client is currently experiencing (actual) over a problem that may happen (potential). An actual problem has priority over one that could possibly occur during the course of the illness. Acute withdrawal symptoms in the client with multiple substance abuse would have priority over the potential for social isolation in that individual.

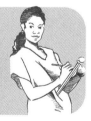

Just the Facts

Nursing diagnoses and care should be planned to include religious, cultural, and ethnic practices of the client.

Expected Outcomes

The next phase of the nursing process involves planning measurable and realistic **outcomes** that will anticipate the improvement or stabilization of the problem identified in the nursing diagnosis. These outcomes are defined in terms of short-term goals that address the immediate unmet needs of the client and long-term goals that achieve the maximal level of health that is realistic for the individual client at the time of discharge and as a member of society. These goals should be determined in collaboration with the client, so as to increase cooperation and compliance with therapeutic interventions.

Listed below are examples of both short-term and long-term outcome criteria for the nursing diagnosis, sensory/perceptual alteration, related to auditory hallucinations.

Short-Term Outcomes

- Client symptoms of auditory hallucinations will decrease within 48 hours.
- Client does not harm self or others in next 48 hours.
- Client identifies feelings associated with hallucinations with each episode.
- Client reports decrease in anxiety level within 24 hours.

Long-Term Outcomes

- Client demonstrates understanding of need for continued compliance with medication therapy by discharge.
- Client demonstrates awareness that hallucinations are the result of internal conflict within 1 week.
- Client identifies and demonstrates ways to maintain contact with reality at onset of symptoms by discharge.
- Client identifies environmental factors that precipitate the hallucinations by discharge.
- Client participates in activities that reinforce reality during hospitalization within 1 week.

Nursing Interventions

Nursing interventions are actions taken by the nurse to assist the client in achieving the anticipated outcomes. It is important to plan actions that are appropriate for the individual client and take into consideration the level of functioning that is realistic for that person. What may be realistic for one person may be unattainable for another. The written plan is a collaborative effort between all members of the health care team and is communicated to

each health care worker. This helps to ensure the continuity of care and consistency in the implementation of interventions by all personnel. Consistency is a vital component of the therapeutic milieu.

There are many clinical units that use standardized or computer-generated care plans or clinical pathways. In the current managed-care concept, these are designed to be cost-effective and improve the efficiency with which treatment is carried out. Regardless of the method used, the care plan identifies the outcomes and interventions that are to be addressed by each discipline of the care team. Specifically, the nursing care plan identifies those interventions for which the nurse has responsibility. It is imperative that the unique needs and problems of each client are retained as central to that person's plan of care.

Nursing interventions that focus on mental health care do not involve intensive physical care nursing skills. Rather, the nurse focuses on observing behaviors and symptoms, improving communication strategies, and assisting the client in problem-solving with improved overall functioning. Nursing interventions are implemented according to the nurse's level of practice (see Chapter 21, Mental Health Care in Nonpsychiatric Settings). Achievement of the anticipated outcomes is difficult for psychiatric clients. Many require extensive reinforcement and reassurance to change behaviors and understand the underlying emotional issues. At a Glance 3-4 provides a list of nursing intervention strategies for working with psychiatric clients.

Just the Facts

Nursing interventions are intended to encourage, maintain, and re-establish a level of mental and physical functioning that promotes the well-being of the client.

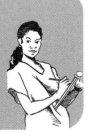

At a Glance 3-4 Nursing Strategies for Mental Health Nurses

- Respect and accept each client as he or she is.
- Allow client opportunity to set own pace in working with problems.
- Nursing interventions should center on the client as a person, not on control of the symptoms. Symptoms are important, but not as important as the person having them.
- Remember, *all behavior has meaning*—an attempt to prevent the occurrence or decrease the intensity of anxiety.
- Recognize your own feelings toward clients and deal with them.
- Go to the client who needs help the most.
- Do not allow a situation to develop or continue in which a client becomes the focus of attention in a negative manner.
- If client behavior is bizarre, base your decision to intervene on whether the client is endangering self or others.
- Ask for help—do not try to be a hero when dealing with a client who is out of control!
- Avoid highly competitive activities, that is, having one winner and a room full of losers.
- Make frequent contact with clients—it lets them know they are worth your time and effort.
- Remember to assess the physical needs of your client.
- Have patience! Move at the client's pace and ability.
- Suggesting, requesting, or asking works better than commanding.
- Therapeutic thinking is not thinking about or for, but *with* the client.
- Be honest so the client can rely on you.
- Make reality interesting enough that the client prefers it to his or her fantasy.
- Compliment, reassure, and model appropriate behavior.

Mind Jogger

How might client desire and motivation to participate in goal achievement influence the manner in which the care plan is implemented?

This step of the nursing process should focus on helping clients rechannel their energies in a constructive manner. The nursing interventions should be based on scientific principles for resolution of the identified problem and should be safe for the client and others involved. Other chapters in this text will include appropriate nursing actions for clients with the various categories of mental disorders. As strategies are implemented and documented, a picture of client progress evolves.

Data collection is continuous during the implementation phase. Client response to interventions provides valuable information that assists the nurse in determining whether the client is making progress toward the defined outcome criteria. Additional data also aid in the planning of ongoing nursing care.

Evaluation

During the evaluation phase of the nursing process, the nurse evaluates the success of the nursing interventions in meeting the criteria outlined in the expected outcomes. Either the goal has been achieved, some progress has been made toward the intended outcome, or no steps forward have been observed or documented. Specific client behaviors may be reviewed by the entire mental health care team to determine the overall success of the treatment plan. If a goal has been partially met, there may be supporting data to indicate continuance of the current plan of care. This approach recognizes that the client may need more time to make changes and adjust to them. A distinction must be made between a lack of client motivation and the need for continuance of the current plan to help the client achieve the outcomes. Some interventions may have been ineffective, and thus new strategies may be needed to help meet the needs of the client. It is also important to reevaluate the outcome criteria; the expected outcome may not actually be achievable for this client.

The evaluation phase is a form of validation for the entire nursing process in the delivery of care to the client. Continued data collection may indicate new problems or alterations in the original nursing diagnoses. Criteria are reevaluated to clarify realistic and measurable terms for the individual client. Nursing strategies are reevaluated for effectiveness. This persistence in maintaining a therapeutic approach toward resolution of client problems provides the continuity needed to expedite the treatment process.

Just the Facts

The nurse is the only member of the mental health team who can continuously evaluate client response to planned care.

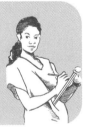

Mind Jogger

How is documentation vital to the process step of evaluation?

Application of the Nursing Process

As you study the various mental disorders and situations in this textbook, you will find a section in most chapters that reinforces the application of the nursing process. However, to facilitate your understanding of this process as it relates to the mental health setting, we need to apply this concept to an actual client situation. The following situation will demonstrate the application of the process for three applicable nursing diagnoses.

Sample Client Situation: End of the Road

Freda is a 47-year-old public school teacher who received word several days ago that her only child, 23-year-old Benjamin, was arrested for armed robbery. Benjamin is married and the father of two small children. Two months ago, Freda discovered that her husband of 26 years is having an affair. Freda blames herself for his indiscretion, stating that she is overweight and unattractive. She says that he would be better off without her anyway. She feels that she is a failure as both a mother and a wife. She is unable to concentrate in the classroom and has considered a leave of absence from her job. Last night Freda's husband told her he was leaving her and wanted a divorce. Freda is brought to the emergency room this morning after being found unresponsive by her daughter-in-law, Andrea. Andrea gives the nurse an empty bottle of Xanax (alprazolam). She also tells the nurse that Freda has been drinking a lot of wine in the past few months. After initial treatment, Freda is admitted to the psychiatric unit with a diagnosis of depressive episode: situational crisis with suicide attempt.

Nursing Assessment

The mental health nurse obtains the following data.

Objective Data

- Suicide attempt with Xanax and alcohol
- Was found unresponsive by daughter-in-law
- Is overweight and has unkempt appearance
- Son has been arrested for armed robbery
- Has two small grandchildren she loves
- Husband has asked for divorce after several months of infidelity
- Has been drinking more in past few months

Subjective Data

- "I don't blame him for finding someone else. I am so fat and ugly."
- "He would be better off without me anyway. I'm such a mess."
- "I must have done something wrong for my son to be in so much trouble. I can't do anything right."

CARE PLAN

Nursing Diagnoses	Expected Outcomes	Nursing Interventions	Evaluation
Risk for self-injury, related to suicide attempt, evidenced by suicide overdose with use of alcohol	Does not engage in self-destructive behavior while hospitalized Begins to explore reasons for substance abuse by 48 hours Expresses feelings of sadness and despair in 48 hours Signs contract that she will not harm herself in 24 hours	Monitor frequently for signs of oversedation Monitor vital signs every half-hour Assess for social withdrawal or isolation Assess for self-destructive thoughts Remove potentially dangerous items from room Provide quiet, soothing environment Monitor mood, affect, and behavior	Recovers from overdose without complications Expresses feelings about substance abuse Discusses harmful effects of substance use Participates in goal-planning sessions Identifies self-talk that is destructive Has not harmed self during hospitalization Develops supportive network of family, friends, and support group
Coping, ineffective individual, related to life events, as evidenced by drinking more and inability to meet role expectations	Performs activities of daily living in next 2 days Communicates feelings about current situation in next 2 days Participates in determining goals for improvement in 2 days Identifies at least two adaptive coping strategies in 2 days Implements one adaptive coping strategy by the end of 1 week Identifies support systems available to her by the end of 1 week	Help to perform activities of daily living Encourage to make decisions about self-care Encourage expression of feelings Help to identify internal factors of self-blame Teach and model adaptive coping strategies Encourage to use adaptive coping skills Praise efforts and successes in coping	Independently performs activities of daily living Makes independent decisions about self-care Openly discusses feelings and emotional response to life situations Identifies self-defeating thoughts and behaviors Demonstrates use of adaptive coping strategies

continues

CARE PLAN   (Continued)

Nursing Diagnoses	Expected Outcomes	Nursing Interventions	Evaluation
Self-esteem, situational low, related inability to handle life events, evidenced by feelings of self-blame and inadequacy	Refrains from self-blame and negative self-talk by end of 1 week Participates in self-care with interest in self-improvement in 2 days Identifies positive life accomplishments and personal strengths in 3 days Identifies internal factors that harm self-esteem in 1 week Participates in unit activities in 2 days Discusses realistic goals for self-improvement by discharge	Establish trusting relationship Provide safe and supportive environment Encourage to discuss life events Assist to distinguish between life situations over which she does and does not have control Help to recognize negative self-talk and self-defeating statements Encourage to keep journal of negative and defeating thoughts Encourage social interaction with others Assist to identify personal strengths and accomplishments Provide positive reinforcement for expression of positive feelings and thoughts	Demonstrates trust in mental health team Identifies realistic views of life events Demonstrates ability to recognize negative thought patterns Reframes negative self-talk with more realistic perspective Uses positive statements to describe self Identifies strengths and acknowledges accomplishments Interacts with others using positive approach

- "I can't even think clearly enough to teach my kids what I'm supposed to. I might as well quit."
- "The only good thing in my life are my little grandkids. They deserve better than me."

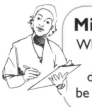

Mind Jogger

What other nursing diagnoses apply to Freda's assessment data? What outcomes might be expected?

Summary

The nursing process is a scientific, organized, problem-solving method of addressing those situations for which nursing can legally intervene. Nursing problems are often the result of medical conditions. The physician who treats psychiatric disorders is a psychiatrist. The psychiatrist is responsible for treating the medical or psychiatric disorder. As a member of the mental health team, the nurse is responsible for assessing and communicating information concerning the current status of the client to the physician and other members of the team.

Nursing problems or nursing diagnoses are formulated so that they are related to the cause or contributing factor for the symptoms. They are defined after relevant subjective and objective data from the client assessment have been reviewed. The nursing diagnosis statement is taken from a standardized list approved by the North American Nursing Diagnosis Association (NANDA). This statement includes the actual or potential nursing problem, the causative factor, and the supporting symptoms or behavior. Nursing diagnoses are prioritized according to the severity and immediacy of the problem. Basic physiologic needs such as oxygen, food, warmth, and sleep will obviously be met first. Maslow's hierarchy of needs is often used to provide a general guide for nurses in determining priorities for problem resolution.

Definition of the problem allows the nurse to determine what evidence will demonstrate the client's progress toward resolving the situation. This information is stated in an expected outcome with realistic and measurable criteria to decide when the goal has been accomplished. A description of the objective and subjective data provides evidence of whether the client is making progress and gives the nurse a blueprint to guide observation and contact with the client. Nursing interventions are planned and implemented to facilitate the effectiveness of the entire treatment process. Information is also shared with other team members to ensure the continuity and consistency of the approach that is being used to achieve client improvement.

Interventions are evaluated by determining whether the outcome criteria have been accomplished within the expected timeframe. If a goal is only partially achieved or has not been met, it is important to reevaluate the plan and develop new or additional actions to address the deficit. The nursing process is an ongoing continuum from admission to discharge and outpatient status. The problem-solving method used to approach client care can also be taught to clients as a way of dealing with the problems and situations of life in general. In this way, nurses have modeled one of the most effective and adaptive coping strategies available for clients with mental health disorders.

Bibliography

Doenges, M. E., Townsend, M. C., & Moorhouse, M. F. (1995). *Psychiatric care plans* (3rd ed.). Philadelphia, PA: F. A. Davis.

FILL IN THE BLANK

Fill in the blank with the correct answer.

1. The nursing process is a(n) _____ approach that assists the client in achieving a maximal level of functioning and well-being.

2. An environment that is modified to create a setting in which the client feels safe, secure, and free to openly express feelings and thoughts is a(n) _____.

3. Information that is provided by the client is _____ data.

4. Information that is observed by the nurse or provided by others who are familiar with the client situation is referred to as _____ data.

5. A nursing diagnosis consists of a problem that is related to a(n) _____, and behavior or symptoms that support the problem.

6. Goals and outcomes should be planned _____ with the client.

MATCHING

Match the following terms to the most appropriate phrase.

a. Actual or potential problem the nurse can legally address.

b. Measurable and realistic goal that anticipates the improvement or stabilization of the client.

c. Collection of subjective and objective data concerning the psychosocial needs of a client.

d. Defining immediacy or intensity of problems to determine the order in which they will be addressed.

e. Actions taken to assist client to achieve anticipated outcomes.

f. Determines success of strategies used in meeting anticipated criteria.

1. _____ Assessment

2. _____ Prioritize

3. _____ Nursing diagnosis

4. _____ Nursing interventions

5. _____ Evaluation

6. _____ Expected outcome

MULTIPLE CHOICE

Select the best answer from the multiple-choice items.

1. The nurse is assessing a client with chronic schizophrenia who has stopped taking medication and is being admitted with acute psychotic symptoms. The client's perception of the present problem would best be documented by the nurse:

   a. Using exact words in client statements.

   b. With information obtained from the family.

   c. By observing behavior for several hours.

   d. As interpreted from the client's words.

2. Which of the following is most important in establishing a trusting environment for the organized delivery of nursing care to a client?

   a. Cooperation of the client

   b. A completed psychosocial assessment

   c. The client's perception of the current situation

   d. Accepting and nonjudgmental attitude of the nurse

3. Which of the following is a component of the client's mental status nursing assessment?

   a. Past medical history

   b. Mood and affect

   c. Medical diagnosis

   d. Nursing diagnosis

4. When prioritizing nursing diagnoses to determine the order in which they should be addressed, which of the following would receive highest priority?

   a. Ineffective coping strategies

   b. Low self-esteem

   c. Suicidal ideation

   d. Social isolation

5. Which of the following terms would be descriptive of a client's attitude?

   a. Blunted

   b. Remote

   c. Retarded

   d. Apathetic

SCENARIO: ALONE AND LOST

Matthew is a 26-year-old carpenter who up until 5 days ago was employed by a building contractor. At the time of his termination, Matthew was told by his supervisor that his work had not been consistently satisfactory and to avoid legal problems, he was being fired. Matthew has been living with his girl-friend and her two children for the past 3 years. Two days after he lost his job, his girlfriend told him she was seeing someone else and wanted him to move out. Matthew is brought to the emergency room by the police who state he was wandering around a parking lot at 2:00 a.m., is disoriented, and is unable to tell them who he is or what he was doing in the parking lot. He told the police he is lost and doesn't know where he should go.

What subjective data should the nurse obtain from Matthew at the time of admission?

_____

_____

_____

What objective data is available from those who know about his situation?

_____

_____

_____

Complete the following nursing diagnosis statements for Matthew's situation:

Anxiety (severe), related to _____, evidenced by _____.

Coping, ineffective individual, related to _____, evidenced by _____.

Personal identity disturbance, related to _____, evidenced by _____.

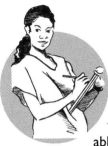

LEARNING OBJECTIVES

After learning the content in this chapter, the student will be able to:

1. Define stress and its relationship to anxiety.
2. Describe symptoms of four levels of anxiety.
3. Identify common etiologic factors contributing to stress and anxiety.
4. Differentiate between adaptive and maladaptive coping strategies.
5. Describe characteristics of a psychologic crisis situation.
6. Plan nursing strategies for crisis intervention related to anxiety.

CHAPTER

4

Understanding Stress, Anxiety, and Crisis

KEY TERMS

Adaptation

Adaptive coping

Anxiety

Crisis

Distress

Dysfunctional management

Eustress

External stressors

"Fight or flight" response

Internal stressors

Maladaptive coping

Palliative

Reframing

Stress

Stress reaction

Defining Stress

Stress is defined as the condition that results when a threat or challenge to one's well-being requires a person to adjust or adapt to the environment. According to the well-known stress researcher Hans Selye, there are two kinds of stress. **Distress** in response to a threat or challenge is actually harmful to one's health. This is a negative stress and demands an exhausting type of energy. **Eustress,** on the other hand, is positive and motivating, as shown by one's confidence in the ability to master a challenge or stressor. This type of stress may actually enhance the feeling of well-being.

Stress is further defined in terms of acute or chronic stress. Acute stress constitutes the reaction to an immediate threat, commonly called the **"fight or flight" response** when there is a surge of the adrenal hormone adrenalin into the bloodstream. It is referred to in this way because it provides the energy or instant strength to either fight or run away from a danger threat. This type of response can occur in situations where there is a sense of imminent danger, such as when in a parking lot or upon losing track of a child in a crowd. The response is usually reversed to a relaxation mode once the danger is past. Chronic stress occurs when the situation is ongoing or continuous, such as chronic illness of a family member or job-related responsibilities. It is important to recognize that most of us can relate to both of these situations, ones that we as health care workers share with our clients.

Mind Jogger

How can chronic stress be channeled into a productive outcome?

Signs and Symptoms of Stress

Common symptoms of stress generally fall into four categories. The physical response to the stressor, or the **stress reaction,** is triggered by the arousal of the autonomic nervous system. This response causes physiologic changes that include an increase in heart rate and blood pressure; faster breathing; increased mental alertness and sensitivity; and increased blood flow to the brain, heart, and muscles, with less blood going to the skin, digestive tract, kidneys, and liver. There is also a rise in blood sugar, fats, and cholesterol to provide additional energy, and an increase in clotting factors in the event of blood loss resulting from injury. Physical symptoms may include responses such as muscle aches, heart palpitations, abdominal cramping, headaches, or insomnia. Lack of concentration, loss of memory, inability to make decisions, forgetfulness, and confusion are among the mental symptoms that may occur. Emotional responses may include anxiety, nervousness, frustration, anger, irritability, or worry. The impact of stress also affects behavior as demonstrated by pacing, fidgety movements, nail-biting, smoking, drinking, yelling, swearing, or throwing things.

At a Glance 4-1 Common Signs and Symptoms of Stress

- Increased heart rate and blood pressure
- Heart palpitations
- Increased respirations
- Abdominal cramping, nausea, diarrhea
- Headaches
- Insomnia
- Lack of concentration and memory
- Inability to make decisions
- Forgetfulness
- Confusion
- Anxiety
- Nervousness
- Irritability
- Frustration and worry
- Fidgety movements
- Nail-biting
- Smoking and drinking
- Yelling, throwing things

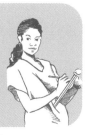

Defining Anxiety

Anxiety is such a natural occurrence that it is impossible to avoid. It is a built-in part of our instinctive response to an event that is a threat to our well-being. It is like a smoke detector that alerts our senses to the possibility of danger and prepares us to respond by either running or fighting. Anxiety is the mechanism that is triggered when the alarm sounds in our brain and actually prevents us from thinking logically about the situation. Therefore, anxiety may be present whether or not an actual danger exists. It can cause us to act impulsively not only when there is actual danger but also when we perceive the possibility of a threat. We cannot ignore the feeling of anxiety, but we often allow it to overshadow our logical and realistic thought processes.

Anxiety is an automatic and unconscious biologic response to a stressor that cannot be controlled by our conscious minds. It is the most basic of emotions seen in the statement that all behavior has meaning and purpose. Anxiety is defined as a feeling of apprehension, uneasiness, or uncertainty that occurs in response to a real or perceived threat whose source is not known. Anxiety occurs at a deeper level than fear, which is a reaction to a specific, defined danger. Normal anxiety is necessary for survival and provides the energy needed to manage daily life and pursue life goals. Acute anxiety may be experienced by a person who is about to undergo surgery or a series of diagnostic testing. When anxiety persists over a long period, the chronic feeling is demonstrated by a sense of apprehension and overreaction to all unanticipated environmental stimuli. This state may be shown through chronic fatigue, insomnia, poor concentration, or impairment in work and social functioning. If the feelings of anxiety become too overwhelming, they may be repressed out of conscious awareness and expressed through behavior.

Levels of Anxiety

The severity of the anxiety is expressed through the individual's perception and reaction to the stressor. This is usually exhibited in the person's physical, emotional, and mental behaviors. There are four levels at which anxiety may occur, each escalating to a level more severe than the previous one. As anxiety increases, the person experiences an internal need to try to relieve it as soon as possible.

Mild anxiety is natural and motivating toward productivity with an improved sense of well-being. Anxiety that increases to a moderate level becomes uncomfortable and difficult to tolerate for extended periods. If this level of anxiety is not relieved, it progresses to a severe state that is physically and emotionally exhausting. The individual is desperate for a way to relieve the mental and emotional turmoil. If steps are not taken to decrease this level of anxiety, the state of panic may develop, leading to hysteria, suicide attempts, or violence. The physical and psychologic symptoms for each level of anxiety are described in At a Glance 4-2.

Etiologic Factors That Contribute to Stress and Anxiety

An individual can experience both external and internal stressors. **External stressors** are those aspects of the environment that may be adverse, such as an abusive relationship or poverty-level living conditions. **Internal stressors** can be physical, such as a chronic illness

At a Glance 4-2 Common Signs and Symptoms of Anxiety

Level of Anxiety	Physical Symptoms	Psychologic Symptoms
Mild level	Increased awareness Increased energy Slight discomfort Restlessness Irritability Mild tension-relieving behaviors (fidgeting, nail-biting, foot tapping, lip chewing)	Sharp perception of reality Alert and aware of environment Able to identify things producing anxiety Motivated Preoccupied at times Good concentration Reasoning and logical thought processes Attentive
Moderate level	Voice tremors Muscle tension Rapid speech—change in pitch Difficulty concentrating Shakiness Repetitive questioning Misperception of stimuli Inability to complete tasks Autonomic response Headaches, insomnia Pacing Decreased eye contact	Reduced perceptual ability Decreased attentiveness Needs things repeated to grasp Still functional but decreased problem-solving ability (requires guidance) Decreased motivation and confidence Increased irritability Feeling of being tied in knots Bouts of crying and outbursts of anger Inability to learn or problem solve
Severe level	Feelings of impending doom Confusion Purposeless activity Increased somatic complaints Hyperventilation Palpitations Loud and rapid speech Threats and demands Increased pacing Diaphoresis Poor or no eye contact Insomnia Rapid speech Eye twitching Tremors	Distorted perception of reality Attention to details—loses sight of whole picture Focused totally on self and anxiety Defensiveness Oversensitive to comments from others Verbal threats Lacks reasoning or logical thought processes Unable to problem-solve

continues

At a Glance 4-2 Common Signs and Symptoms of Anxiety (Continued)

Level of Anxiety	Physical Symptoms	Psychologic Symptoms
Panic level	Hysteria	Out of touch with reality
	Incoherent	Irrational and disorganized
	Suicide attempts	thought processes
	Violent behavior	Absent perceptual ability
	Unintelligible speech	Unaware of reality
	Feelings of terror, extreme	Unable to perceive environ-
	fear	ment
	Immobility	Depersonalization
	Dilated pupils	Delusional thinking
	Withdrawal	Disorientation

or terminal condition, or psychologic as in continued worry about financial burdens or a disaster that may never happen. Research has also shown that heart disease tends to be more prevalent in people who are highly driven, competitive, ambitious, and success-oriented and have a chronic sense of time urgency and a chronic hostile personal style (referred to as Type A people) than in those who are more relaxed and easygoing (referred to as Type B people).

Both positive and negative aspects of life may include a fair amount of stress. For example, if you were experiencing an airplane takeoff for the first time, your heart might be pounding and your muscles tense. This short-term stress usually is of little consequence as adaptation occurs once the plane becomes airborne. In contrast, the everyday stress of marital discord or work demands may eventually impose a threat to one's health. It is important to recognize that many times we view external circumstances as the cause of our stress, but in reality, we create most of our own stress. We actually choose to make ourselves miserable and upset. When we monitor our anxiety-producing thoughts, our irrational thinking tends to overgeneralize and exaggerate things. This tends to give our thoughts an "all or none" frame of thinking. This type of thinking also leads to anticipating the worst possible outcome for situations. This is illustrated by a 45-year-old man whose wife makes a flattering comment about the young man next door. As the man thinks about the statement, he visualizes that his wife is looking for a younger man and will eventually leave him.

At a Glance 4-3 Internal and External Stressors

External Stressors

- Physical environment (noise, bright lights, weather, crowds)
- Major life events (death of a loved one, divorce, loss of a job, marriage)
- Work related (rules, deadlines, production pressures, gossip)
- Social (bossy or aggressive friends and associates, strained friendship, marital affairs)
- Everyday life (schedules, household duties, family conflict)

Internal Stressors

- Personality traits (perfectionist, workaholic, worrier, loner)
- Negative self-talk (pessimism, irrational thinking, self-criticism)
- Thinking snags (all-or-none approach, unrealistic and inflexible expectations)

He begins to quiz her about where she goes and who she meets. He watches her reaction as young men appear on a television show. He begins to view himself as inadequate and losing his masculine appeal.

Some events create more stress than others. A major factor in whether the stressor becomes a strain on the individual is the unpredictability of situations over which the person may have little or no control. A fireman, for example, faces uncertainty and ongoing threat of danger or injury with each call of duty. Another type of stress is the intermittent pressure experienced by students during final exams. Emotional triggers for higher levels of stress are those that are uncontrollable, repetitive, unexpected, and intense in nature. Stress is greater and damage more likely in these situations.

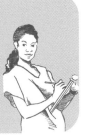

Just the Facts

Job-related "burnout" is a condition of mental, physical, and emotional exhaustion with a reduced sense of personal accomplishment and increased apathy toward one's work.

Mind Jogger

What types of stress might be more damaging than others?

Adapting to Stress and Anxiety

In most situations, the sense of control an individual feels over the particular stressor determines how he or she thinks about or perceives it. The first step in coping with a threatening situation is to assess if it really is what it seems to be. Once this has been determined, options can be reviewed to resolve the problem. The solution may be one of trying to deal with the situation itself, or one of controlling the emotional reaction that is felt in response to the stressor. A student who feels overwhelmed by requirements for taking a full semester course load with a fear of failing may decide to drop one or two classes to perform better in the remaining subjects. Another student with the same course load may decide to work out in the gym each day, along with budgeting time between the required subjects to deal with the stress.

The manner in which individuals manage their anxiety is referred to as **adaptation.** Coping strategies generally fall into four categories. When the problem is solved in a rational and productive way and the anxiety is reduced, it is said to be **adaptive.** If the solution temporarily relieves the anxiety but the problem still exists and must be dealt with again at a later time, coping is termed **palliative.** These two types of coping usually result in a positive outcome. For example, a drama student feels anxiety as time for a performance approaches and asks a classmate to review the script to refocus on the lines. A second student who feels anxious about the performance goes jogging with music to relieve the anxiety and increase his mental alertness to remember his lines.

On the other hand, if unsuccessful attempts are made to decrease the anxiety without attempting to solve the problem, coping strategies are **maladaptive** and the anxiety remains. The drama student might decide to ignore the anxiety and go to a movie the afternoon before the performance and rapidly look over the lines immediately before going on stage. During the performance, he forgets several of his lines and has to be prompted. The individual who does not attempt to reduce the anxiety or solve the problem is considered to have **dysfunctional management** of the stressor and the emotional response. Another student decides to get drunk the night before the performance and fails to show up for the performance until the second act, and is replaced by his understudy.

In managing and coping with the anxiety we experience in response to stress in our lives, it is important to accept the anxiety rather than fight it. Stress is a part of life. We have a choice to replace negative feelings with more positive ones. We can stand back and look realistically at the situation as we function along with the anxiety. We can expect the best. The outcome is rarely as bad as what we fear the most. Each time we are successful in dealing with an anxiety-producing situation, there is a better chance that we will manage to control the anxiety the next time.

Mind Jogger

Does avoidance of a conflict situation create or reduce anxiety?

Coping strategies are learned by observation of those who model them in our family and social environment. These can be either adaptive or maladaptive. We tend to use those skills that we know to deal with life stressors. Nurses have a major role in helping clients with anxiety to cope more effectively. We must recognize that to help our clients to deal with their levels of stress, we must learn to handle our own. Some of the most effective techniques for managing anxiety include:

- Positive self-talk and reframing irrational thinking
- Assertiveness training
- Problem-solving skills—view problems as opportunities for growth
- Communication skills
- Conflict resolution
- Relaxation techniques
- Meditation
- Support systems
- Practical attitude

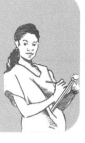

Just the Facts

Reframing is a way of restructuring our thinking about a stressful event into one that is less disturbing and over which we can have some control.

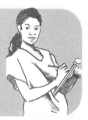

Just the Facts

A mental escape to a place of peaceful solitude will provide a temporary defense against anxiety.

At a Glance 4-4 Examples of Reframing Irrational Thoughts

Irrational Belief	Restructured Positive Thought
I always mess things up.	Even if things didn't turn out right this time I can do it differently next time.
He never does what I want him to do.	If I want him to do something, I need to communicate that to him.
She never pays any attention to me.	If I give her more attention, she might be more attentive to me.
I should have done better on the exam.	I can study harder and do better on the next one.
I can't be happy unless I am loved by the person I really care about.	If this person does not return my love, I can give my energy to finding someone better.

- Sense of humor
- Self-care (diet, exercise, sleep, leisure, avoiding things that increase stress such as caffeine and alcohol)
- Faith in spiritual power and in yourself

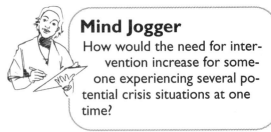

Mind Jogger

How would the need for intervention increase for someone experiencing several potential crisis situations at one time?

Crisis

Crisis differs from stress in that a state of disorganization and disarray occurs in the individual as usual coping strategies fail or are not available. The total inability to control the situation and to function in daily activities leads the person to seek a way out. The level of anxiety increases to a severe or panic level during which the individual feels helpless and lost. Attempts to cope may meet with little success. The state of dysfunction is usually receptive to the right intervention that can help the person stabilize and regain a sense of power and control over their being.

Crisis follows a typical sequence of events. First, a person is confronted by the threat or stressor that increases anxiety and mobilizes the defenses. If the first effort to resolve the issue fails, the threat continues and the person's functioning becomes disorganized as attempts to deal with the stressor are unsuccessful. As the attempts fail, the autonomic responses are engaged. At this point, the person may be able to make a temporary form of resolution that allows them to function and move on with daily activity. However, if this compromise is not made, the anxiety can overwhelm the individual, leading to serious disorganization of the mental defenses, confusion, fear, violence, or suicidal behaviors.

Crisis Intervention

The state of crisis is intolerable for more than a few weeks if help is not received. The dysfunctional state that continues without resolving the underlying problem will result in physical or mental symptoms. Resolution will usually allow the person to either emerge at a higher and more productive level of functioning, at the same level, or at a lower level of coping ability. The outcome depends on the actions taken by the individual to cope with the crisis and those taken by others to intervene. During a crisis, an individual is often more receptive to support from others and can learn adaptive coping strategies to assist in the resolution. Reassurance that the person is mentally healthy and has coped with crisis in the past often helps them to reinvest in their ability to face the current state of chaos.

Crisis intervention deals with the present situation and resolution of the immediate issue. Early intervention in assisting the individual to manage the current situation promotes the best chance for a positive outcome. Once the anxiety level is reduced to a tolerable level, the individual can be assisted in defining the problem, determining available support, and setting realistic goals for resolution of the issue.

The nurse is integral in providing support and returning control to the client. Listening to what the client says both verbally and nonverbally gives insight into the problem from the client's perspective. This allows the nurse to help the client identify alternative ways of reducing the anxiety and feelings of powerlessness. If the person is suicidal, protective measures must be initiated to provide a feeling of safety and security. This feeling will allow the

Just the Facts

Disorganization may result from an unrealistic perception of the threatening event, lack of a support system, or inadequate coping ability.

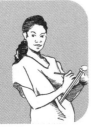

Case Study: Nathan in Trouble

Nathan feels that his world is coming to an end. Seventeen years ago, his fiancée was badly beaten by an intruder and left with multiple scars and a loss of vision in one eye. Last week, Nathan learned that the intruder was due to be released from prison and would be returning to the community. Nathan is so worried about further danger to the woman who is now his wife that he cannot sleep, eat, or function. Nathan feels that he will not be able to control his impulse to kill the man if he sees him.

How does Nathan's problem demonstrate a crisis situation?

_____

_____

What is the first step of the intervention to help Nathan?

_____

_____

Why is it so important to listen to what Nathan says both verbally and nonverbally?

_____

_____

_____

individual a temporary sanctuary in which the inner resources can be stabilized. Outcomes are aimed at promoting optimum psychologic and physiologic functioning. Therapeutic strategies are designed to assist in preventing future emotional states of dysfunction.

Summary

Stress and anxiety are considered a fact of life. There is no immunity to the reality that we will be confronted with both external and internal sources of stress in our everyday living. Some stress is motivating and actually allows us to perform at optimum levels of functioning toward success and accomplishment. Stress can also be a source of distress and threatening to our well-being. Acute stress comes in the form of a foreboding sense of danger or threat over which we temporarily feel a lack of control. Chronic stress can also occur in which the threat becomes an ongoing presence that must be dealt with on a continuous basis.

The stress reaction triggers the autonomic nervous system into action. The resulting symptoms of this response are both physiologic and psychologic. Anxiety is a natural occurrence included in this response. It is an automatic and unconscious feeling that cannot be controlled by our conscious minds. This feeling of uneasiness or uncertainty is uncomfortable. In its most basic state, it is the underlying current of survival that provides the energy we need to manage daily life. However, when levels of anxiety increase, the ability to manage decreases. Individuals then mobilize mental defenses to deal with anxiety and the underlying issues.

Anxiety can range from mild levels to those of panic. Both internal and external stressors can trigger the various responses. In some situations, there may be a very real source of danger or threat to one's well-being. There are also instances in which the issue is viewed from an irrational and unrealistic perspective. This type of thinking leads to an anticipation of the worst possible outcome. In most situations, the sense of control one feels over the stressor is a direct result of the thinking that occurs. The manner in which the individual responds may be adaptive or maladaptive based on this thinking. Coping strategies are learned behaviors. The situation can be dealt with more effectively if these behaviors have been used successfully in other times of stress.

If the stressful situation is not resolved, a state of crisis can develop in which the individual is in a state of emotional disorganization. The ability to function is impaired and intervention by a support system is required to reestablish a sense of homeostasis along with the ability to regain control. Nurses are often required to participate in the support team effort to effect stabilization in the client. The goal of intervention is to reduce the anxiety to a level that will allow the client to look at the situation realistically and develop a resolution to the problem.

Bibliography

Coon, D. (1994). *Essentials of psychology* (6th ed.). New York: West Publishing.

McCullough, C. J., & Mann, R. W. (1985). *Managing your anxiety.* New York: Putnam Publishers.

Posen, D. B. (1995). Stress management for patient and physician. *The Canadian Journal of Continuing Medical Education,* April, 1995. Available at www.mentalhealth.com/mag1/p51-str.html. Accessed July 1, 2004.

Sternberg, R. J. (1994). *In search of the human mind.* Orlando, FL: Harcourt Brace College.

Student Worksheet

FILL IN THE BLANK

Fill in the blank with the correct answer.

1. Acute stress is a response to an immediate threat, commonly called the _____ or _____ response in which there is a surge of adrenalin into the blood.

2. The physical response to the stressor that is triggered by the arousal of the autonomic nervous system is referred to as the _____.

3. When anxiety persists over a long period, its effect may be demonstrated by apprehension and _____ to all unexpected environmental stimuli.

4. The severity of anxiety is expressed through the individual _____ and _____ to the stressor.

5. A major factor in whether a stressor becomes a strain on an individual is the _____ of situations over which little or no control is possible.

MATCHING

Match the following terms to the most appropriate phrase.

a. Manner in which individuals manage their anxiety.

b. Positive and motivating stress.

c. Aspects of environment that may be adverse.

d. Feeling of apprehension, uneasiness, or uncertainty in response to a perceived threat.

e. Physical or psychologic situations causing discomfort.

f. State of emotional disorganization and loss of control.

g. Harmful response to a threat or challenge.

h. Condition that results when a threat or challenge to well-being requires a person to adapt.

1. _____ Anxiety

2. _____ Stress

3. _____ Eustress

4. _____ Crisis

5. _____ External stress

6. _____ Distress

7. _____ Internal stress

8. _____ Adaptation

MULTIPLE CHOICE

Select the best answer from the multiple-choice items.

1. Joan feels that she is going to be terminated from her job. She is having trouble concentrating and has to ask her supervisor to repeat directions several times. She is irritable and cries easily. Which of the following levels of anxiety is Joan experiencing?
   a. Mild
   b. Moderate
   c. Severe
   d. Panic

2. Elisha is an LPN/LVN who has worked in the dementia unit of a long-term care facility for the past 8 years. Recently, she has been calling in with various physical complaints and says she just doesn't care about the clients like she used to. It is most likely that Elisha is experiencing:

   a. Mental escape

   b. Crisis

   c. Burnout

   d. Dysfunctional stress

3. Which of the following statements reframes the irrational thought, "I will always be a failure," into a rational thought process?

   a. "I may fail at some things, but I am not always a failure."

   b. "I don't have to fail at anything."

   c. "I am my own worst enemy."

   d. "I usually fail because most things are just too difficult for me."

4. William owns a small business that has recently been experiencing reduced sales and profits. William obtained a bank loan to cover losses from the past few months and obtain merchandise for inventory. The bank loan will be due for repayment in 6 months. Which of the following describes William's solution to his anxiety over his financial situation?

   a. Adaptive coping strategy

   b. Palliative coping strategy

   c. Maladaptive coping method

   d. Dysfunctional management

SEEK AND FIND

Find the incorrect information in the following statements.

1. The first step in coping with a threatening situation is to think of a way to deal with the problem.

2. If a solution temporarily relieves anxiety but the problem still exists to be dealt with at a later time, coping is said to be adaptive.

3. Mental escape is a way of restructuring our thinking about a stressful event into a less disturbing issue over which we have some control.

4. In managing and coping with the anxiety we experience in life, it is important to fight the anxiety with our body defenses.

Communication and the Therapeutic Relationship

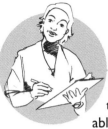

LEARNING OBJECTIVES

After learning the content in this chapter, the student will be able to:

1. Define what is meant by a therapeutic relationship.
2. Define phases and essential components of a therapeutic relationship.
3. Apply the concept of professional boundaries to the nurse–client relationship.
4. Identify effective tools used in a therapeutic nurse–client relationship.
5. Describe what is meant by self-awareness and its influence on behavior.
6. Differentiate between therapeutic and nontherapeutic communication techniques.
7. Identify appropriate therapeutic responses to difficult client behaviors.

KEY TERMS

Acceptance
Active listening
Blocking
Circumstantiality
Echolalia
Empathy
Flight of ideas
Focusing
Loose association
Neologism
Orientation phase
Reflection
Restating
Self-awareness
Termination phase
Validation
Verbigeration
Working stage

The Therapeutic Relationship

The concept of a holistic being views a person as the totality of biologic, psychologic, social, and spiritual functioning that result in a unique person. Integral to this concept is that each person is influenced by a different combination of genetic and environmental issues. The environment is viewed subjectively as it relates to past experiences and individual learning experiences. Each person learns to adapt to life and the environment by observing the world in which he or she exists. This complex nature of each person is a factor in the development of a therapeutic relationship. Because of the psychosocial differences between clients and nurses, there is no one effective model for establishing this relationship. Clients who have the same diagnosis may even have a different pattern of symptoms based on their past experiences, current situation, and individual needs. The external demands of the environment and the internal forces of each person will require an individual approach to the nurse–client relationship.

The therapeutic relationship is seen as a helping relationship in which one person assists in the personal growth and improved well-being of the other. In the nurse–client relationship, a series of interactions between the nurse and client provide information about the client's needs and problems. The nurse works in collaboration with other members of the mental health team toward a common goal of assisting the client toward adaptive and improved functioning within society.

Essential Components of the Nurse–Client Relationship

The establishment of a therapeutic nurse–client relationship is dependent on certain consistent behaviors by the nurse. One of the most important is that of **empathy.** The ability to hear what another person is saying, to have access to that person's feelings temporarily, and to perceive the situation from that person's perspective is vital to the establishment of trust. At the same time, it is important for nurses to maintain objectivity and remain in touch with their own feelings. To become sympathetic and meld into the client's problem is nontherapeutic.

The nurse's **acceptance** of the client as a person with worth and dignity who is not judged or labeled by the nurse's standards is necessary for the establishment of a trusting climate. It is the nurse's willingness to recognize the emotionally ill person as one who deserves respect and needs approval that helps the client to begin trusting the environment. The foundation of a therapeutic relationship is based on dependable interactions that demonstrate honesty, integrity, and consistency. Involved in this honesty is the establishment of boundaries and limit setting with predetermined consequences. This assists the client in self-control and management of behavior. The client needs constant reassurance to develop a sense of emotional security within the environment.

Self-awareness is a consciousness of one's own individuality and personality, or looking at oneself in the mirror. A knowledge of self as a whole person can become a reality only with a gradual awakening to oneself. We cannot have an understanding of others unless we learn about ourselves, how our lives are held together, and how we respond to our own insecurities and anxiety. This awareness of oneself as a whole person comes with an attitude of openness and wanting to come to an honest evaluation of behavior with a desire to make changes. We must listen to our daily record of self-talk and be willing to change the recurrent negative scripts. When we move beyond ourselves and see the world from the perspective of others, we open the door for growth. Insight into the connection between our "thinking" and our "behavior" provides the opportunity for us to change our behavior. The key is in our thinking! It is this same honesty and openness we try to elicit in our clients who have emotional and mental issues.

At a Glance 5-1 A Tool for Self-Assessment/Awareness

- How do I respond to the world around me?
- How do I respond to other people?
- Am I able to discuss issues with others?
- Do I have close relationships? With whom?
- How do I respond when I disagree with others?
- How do others respond to me in this situation?
- What type of stressors are most recurrent in my life?
- How do I respond to stress?
- Do I usually think of myself first, or do I consider others?
- What type of personal space is my comfort zone?
- How do I explain problems to myself?
- If I am threatened or scared, how do I respond?
- Do I recognize my own anxiety? What symptoms do I have?
- What coping mechanisms do I use to adapt? Do I use them frequently or occasionally?
- How do I respond to others who are withdrawn, anxious, or aggressive?
- Do I blame others for my problems and anxiety?
- What thoughts are on my mind most often? Do they focus on myself or others?
- What changes can I make to improve my interactions with others?

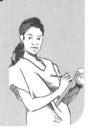

Just the Facts

Caring involves compassion, confidence in one's own abilities, a desire to do the right thing, and the courage to intervene as indicated.

Just the Facts

Preserving oneself when caring for others requires recognizing and accepting limits, liking what you do, being knowledgeable, taking pride in your accomplishments, and appreciating the joy in the "business" of each day.

At a Glance 5-2 Essential Components of a Therapeutic Relationship

- Empathy
- Caring
- Acceptance (unconditional positive regard)
- Mutual trust
- Honesty
- Integrity
- Consistency
- Genuineness
- Self-awareness
- Limit-setting
- Reassurance
- Explanations

Mind Jogger

How can self-awareness assist the nurse to help clients view themselves and their behavior more realistically?

Phases of a Therapeutic Relationship

Therapeutic relationships are dependent on the situation and needs of the individual client. The phases of this nurse–client relationship must focus on the client's ability to function in the process. The relationship may vary in intensity, length, and focus depending on the particular needs of the client.

Basic to the relationship are three phases of contact with the client. The **orientation phase** involves getting to know the client. It involves an explanation of the purpose for the nurse-client interaction as a means of establishing trust. The nurse and client contract a time and place for a meeting, during which the focus is the client's problems; the nurse's role is to be a facilitator. Confidentiality is explained in terms of information that is shared only with members of the treatment team as it applies to the client's well-being. Rules and boundaries are explained to provide structure with guidelines for behavior. It is important to assess the content of any negative feelings the client may be experiencing while reinforcing the limits for behavior. The nurse can also use this time to assess other client behaviors, immediate concerns and needs, and perceived reason for treatment. These initial data provide a baseline for the next phase of the relationship. It is essential for the nurse to convey a caring and honest concern for the client and to send a congruent message through both verbal and nonverbal communication. By showing a genuine interest and supportive attitude, the nurse helps the client to feel worthwhile, deserving of the nurse's time and respect.

client to develop an awareness of the problem and possible solutions to it. Through the use of problem-solving skills, the nurse assists the client to express feelings and thoughts about the present situation. It may be useful for the client to keep a journal of feelings and progress made between sessions. It is important for the nurse to model and teach appropriate coping skills. The client is encouraged to practice adaptive responses and evaluate the effectiveness of the changes. Every effort should be made to reinforce and support each small step of the client's progress toward change. Helping the client to set priorities provides a way of accomplishing short-term gains toward a bigger step or challenge.

The third phase or **termination** of the relationship is necessary to allow the client to depend on his or her own strengths while developing improved adaptive skills. The nurse should encourage the client to have increased social interaction and participate in all activities. This promotes independence in getting along with others in preparation for discharge and a return to the demands of society. It is important to discuss the termination with the client and respond to any feelings or concerns. It is not uncommon for nurses to feel like they are abandon-

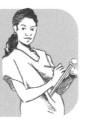

Just the Facts
Establishing rules and setting limits for behavior are consistent with patterns of law and order in society.

Mind Jogger
What behaviors might indicate the client's dependence on the nurse–client relationship?

The second phase is often referred to as the **working stage.** This is a period in which outcomes and interventions toward behavior change are planned and goals are developed to improve the well-being of the client. This involves work by both the nurse and the

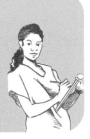

Just the Facts
When taken to extremes, traits found in good nurses such as commitment, selflessness, and responsibility can hinder progress toward client independence.

ing the client's trust as therapeutic closure occurs. The nurse should let the client know that the relationship was valued and purposeful in helping the client toward relying on his or her own ability to deal with their problems.

Professional Boundaries for Helping

It is essential for the nurse to remember that the needs of the nurse are distinctly different from those of the client. Some interventions are helpful and promote independence, but others actually allow the client to develop a dependence on the nurse–client relationship. As clients improve, they are expected to function independently. When nurses allow a need to "help" to overshadow a focus on the needs of the client, professional boundaries have been crossed. The nurse cannot let the relationship fulfill a personal need and remain objective about the client's needs at the same time. Anytime the nurse shows more concern for one client over another, he or she is at risk for becoming too involved. When focus on the client is maintained, it is less likely that the nurse will be manipulated into violating a professional boundary. The nurse–client relationship must not extend beyond the therapeutic termination phase. Any further contact by phone, mail, or socialization is in violation of the professional code of ethics. If a former client is seen outside of the mental health setting, it is important to avoid recognition or speaking to them unless they recognize and speak first. Detailed conversation or other interaction should be avoided.

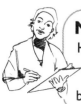

Mind Jogger

How might a nurse's strong sense of commitment lead to a violation of professional boundaries?

Therapeutic Communication

Communication between a sender and receiver is part of the holistic human component. This interaction occurs both verbally and nonverbally as we respond to an instinctive drive for connection to other human beings. Therapeutic communication is a purposeful and skilled language that is learned and requires practice. It is a combination of verbal and nonverbal techniques that are designed to help nurses and other members of the mental health team to focus on the needs of the client.

Before we discuss communication techniques, it is important to have an understanding of speech patterns that are common to the client with mental illness. Not all of these are exhibited by each client. As you progress to learn about the mental disorders, you will become familiar with those patterns that are more common to the individual disorders.

- **Blocking:** Unconscious block that results in loss of thought process; person stops speaking. (Example: "Then my father . . . . What was I saying?")
- **Circumstantiality:** Cannot be selective and describes in lengthy, great detail. (Example: When asked, "Do you have any physical illness?" replies: "My head hurts, but my nose has been leaking, my hair just won't stay in place, I have this cramping in my joints . . .")
- **Echolalia:** Repetitive response of last word heard. (Example: "Please wait here" is responded to with, "here, here, here, here . . .")
- **Flight of ideas:** Rapid shift between topics that are unrelated to each other. (Example: "My cat is gray. The food here is good. My hair needs a perm. My pants are too tight.")
- **Loose association:** Continuous speech with shifting between loosely related topics. (Example: "Martha married Jim. Jim is a good cook. I can cook. Cows are something we

can cook. The cook comes here before day-light. I get up in the daylight.")

- **Neologism:** Coins new words and definitions. (Example: "Hiptomites are real powerful people" in reference to a husky mental health technician on the unit.)
- **Verbigeration:** Repeating words, phrases, or sentences several times. (Example: Nurse: "It is time to take your pills." Client: "Take your pills, take your pills, take your pills, take your pills . . .")

Techniques to Facilitate Communication

Therapeutic interaction between the nurse or other mental health team member and the client is conducted with the specific goal of learning about the client and his or her problem. Although the focus is on the client, the exchange is planned and directed, in our case, by the nurse. The goal is to use techniques that guide the client to express the feelings and thoughts that are contributing to the present problem.

Nonverbal Communication. Nonverbal aspects of a therapeutic exchange must convey a sense of genuine caring and interest in what the client has to say. Body movements, such as hand gestures, facial expressions and movement, arm placement, and other mannerisms can invite the trust of the client or block further interaction. Some important aspects of body language to be aware of include the following:

- Intermittent eye contact will provide reassurance that you are interested and concentrating on what the client is saying.
- A facial expression that is congruent with other gestures assures the client of your interest and attention.
- Arms or legs that are not crossed convey a sense of openness to the client.
- Respect the physical or personal space between the client and yourself. Most people

have a personal space of 18 to 48 inches. This is a good guideline for nurses to maintain during times of communication.
- The use of touch is a given in the art of caring. However, when working with the client who has a mental problem, you must use caution and forethought about how the client might interpret your actions. A client who is suspicious, for example, might react with aggressive action toward a simple pat on the shoulder. Some cultures may also view personal touch as inappropriate except in certain circumstances.

Mind Jogger
What body posture would reflect an attitude of acceptance and genuineness?

Active Listening. The art of **active listening** is a learned skill. It includes observing nonverbal behaviors, giving critical attention to verbal comments, listening for inconsistencies that may need clarification, and attempting to understand the client's perception of the situation. This type of interaction allows the client to express feelings and thoughts without fear of being judged or criticized. Therapeutic techniques are tools that can be used to facilitate this involvement by the client. It is important to remember that some types of messages and behaviors can actually hinder and prevent progress of the therapeutic process. The nurse must constantly listen and cognitively review the comments and behaviors of the client before responding. Because clients tend to view the nurse as someone with power who cares and is available, the opportunities for interaction are more likely. Some responses by the nurse may not be effective or correct. The intended message can be misread by either the client or the nurse. It is important that both participants remain open to the possibility of error. Sometimes this actually allows the nurse to apologize and model appropriate behavior. This situation can also reinforce the genuineness of the nurse's efforts to help the client.

The perceived power of the nurse may at times relay a condescending attitude to the client. It is essential for the nurse to be constantly aware that manner of speech and actions are being observed and interpreted by the client. Many clients do not trust anyone and are especially suspicious of those in authority. Nurses are seen as authority figures. Keeping this in mind, the nurse must continuously monitor his or her own actions as well as the client's response to maintain a therapeutic climate within the relationship. It is important to be flexible and make the client physically and emotionally comfortable during the therapeutic interaction. Learn to anticipate the client's needs and meet them as completely and consistently as possible.

Therapeutic Verbal Communication. Communication is facilitated by allowing the client to lead the conversation with guidance by the nurse. Various techniques can be used to encourage the client to express feelings and thoughts. The nurse's response is chosen based on the content of the client's statements. At a Glance 5-3 provides some effective techniques and examples that can be used to improve communication with clients in the mental health setting.

Nontherapeutic Communication

In contrast to effective therapeutic communication, it is important to recognize that there are also ways that communication can be sidetracked and not accomplish the intended goal of helping the client. It is understood that closed body language with arms folded and appearing busy or uncomfortable with the conversation would send a message to the client that the relationship is superficial. If the nurse interjects opinions or personal values, or minimizes the client's feelings, he or she can present a condescending attitude that puts the client on the defensive. This type of approach will deny the client the chance to trust the nurse as a resource of help and hope. At a Glance 5-4 contains other blocks to therapeutic communication along with therapeutic alternatives.

At a Glance 5-3 Effective Verbal Communication Techniques

Effective Technique	Example	Therapeutic Effect
Clarification	**Nurse:** "Did I understand you correctly. . .?" "Let me see if I have this correct. . . ." "I seem to have missed something. Could you repeat that. . .?"	Clears up any possible misunderstanding and ensures that the message intended is the message received.
Validation	**Nurse:** "You seem anxious about something. . . ." "I get the feeling that something is bothering you. . . ." "You look down this morning. Would you like to talk about it?"	Attempts to verify the nurse's perception of feeling conveyed by either a verbal or nonverbal message of the client.

continues

At a Glance 5-3 Effective Verbal Communication Techniques *(Continued)*

Effective Technique	Example	Therapeutic Effect
Reflection (also called parroting)	**Client:** "I don't think my daughter will need me after she gets married." **Nurse:** "You are afraid you won't be needed after your daughter's marriage?" **Client:** "I am sick of all this mess." **Nurse:** "Sick of this mess?"	Shows nurse's perception of the client's message in both content and feeling—paraphrases the message client the has conveyed to nurse.
Restating	**Nurse:** "You have told me something about the problems between you and your wife. . . ."	Repeats to client the content of interaction and serves as a lead to encourage further discussion.
Focusing	**Nurse:** "Let's get back to the problem with your son . . ."	Helps client concentrate on a specific issue.
Using a general lead	**Nurse:** "Go on. . . ." "And then. . . ." "Continue. . . ."	Shows the nurse is listening and interested—encourages client to continue talking.
Giving information	**Nurse:** "The doctor has ordered a new medication for you. Let me go over this information with you."	Increases client involvement in plan of care—helps to demonstrate team effort to improve the client's well-being.
Using silence	Nurse remains silent with attentive manner.	Conveys willingness to continue listening—allows both the nurse and client time to collect thoughts.
Exploring alternatives	**Nurse:** "Have you considered taking a weekend for some time alone with your wife?"	Guides the client to possible options for problem solving.
Offering of oneself	**Nurse:** "I will be here awhile if you wish to talk. . . ."	Reassurance of interest and presence in client's problem.
Reinforcing reality	**Nurse:** "I know you hear the voices, but I do not hear them. You and I are the only ones in this room."	Provides reassurance that voices are symptoms of illness—helps client to trust the nurse as real.

Case Study: No Other Way Out

Olivia is a 27-year-old married mother of three children who is admitted to the psychiatric unit following a suicide attempt. She tells the nurse, "I never seem to do anything right. My family would be better off without me."

What would be an appropriate reflection response by the nurse to Olivia at this time?

_____

_____

How can the nurse validate Olivia's feelings at this time?

_____

_____

What technique would encourage Olivia to tell the nurse more about her feelings and thoughts leading up to her suicide attempt?

_____

_____

_____

At a Glance 5-4 Blocks to Therapeutic Communication

Ineffective Response	Example	Blocking Effect
Arguing/Disapproving	**Client:** "I want to try to get my girlfriend back." **Nurse:** "Why would you want to do that after what she did to you?" **Therapeutic Response:** "Tell me more about that. . . ."	Expresses opinions or interjects nurse's values of right and wrong on the client's actions—may prevent client from working through options in solving the problem.
Giving advice	**Nurse:** "You should not be so hard on your kids." "If I were you, I would do what the doctor says." **Therapeutic Response:** "It seems your kids are a problem for you. . . ." "Can you tell me what is bothering you about what the doctor has told you?"	Seemingly says that the nurse's values are correct. and devalues the client's actions.

continues

At a Glance 5-4 Blocks to Therapeutic Communication *(Continued)*

Ineffective Response	Example	Blocking Effect
False reassurance	**Nurse:** "You are going to be out of here before you know it." **Therapeutic Response:** "We are here to help you get stronger and feel better."	Minimizes the client's feelings and concerns—conveys superficial attitude.
Use of the word "Why"	**Nurse:** "Why did you act that way?" "Why are you getting so upset?" **Therapeutic Response:** "Can you tell me what you are feeling right now?" "You seem to be upset about something. Can you tell me about it?"	Puts client on the defensive—demands an answer. Invasive and direct probing of issue.
Closed-ended questions	**Nurse:** "Do you want to talk about it?" "Are you feeling better this morning?" "I don't think that's a good idea, do you?" **Therapeutic Response:** "Tell me about that. . . ." "Tell me how you are feeling this morning. . . ." "Let's talk about that. . . ."	Allows a "yes" or "no" response without encouraging further information from the client. (If client replies with a "yes" or "no," nurse can use a more effective response to elicit more conversation.)
Changing the subject	**Client:** "I really don't think I can handle going back home." **Nurse:** "Let's talk about the incident that occurred yesterday with you and Mike." **Therapeutic Response:** "Tell me what bothers you about going home. . . ."	Minimizes importance of client concerns—discourages further exploration of feelings and thoughts. May show nurse's insecurity in talking about the issue.
Agreeing or approving	**Nurse:** "You are absolutely correct." "I think that is a great idea." "You should do that." **Therapeutic Response:** "Tell me more about your idea. . . ." "Let's look at that again. . . ."	Can set client up for failure if idea doesn't work. Can be seen as judgmental.

continues

At a Glance 5-4 Blocks to Therapeutic Communication (Continued)

Ineffective Response	Example	Blocking Effect
Minimizing or belittling	**Nurse:** "That is how everyone feels when they are admitted." "We all resent being told what to do." **Therapeutic Response:** "I'm sure it is difficult for you to be told what to do. . . . tell me what you are feeling."	Conveys attitude that client's feelings are common, and devalues the uniqueness of the person.
Focusing on the nurse	**Client:** "I just broke up with my boyfriend a few weeks ago." **Nurse:** "That has happened to me several times. . . ." **Therapeutic Response:** "That must have been difficult . . . tell me about that time. . . ."	Pulls focus from client problem, and delays further exploration or information regarding client's feelings.
Stereotype statements	**Nurse:** "Tomorrow will be a better day." "Hang in there." **Therapeutic Response:** "You seem rather low today. Would you like to talk about it?"	Empty clichés close the client to further response.

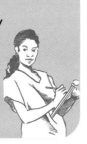

Mind Jogger
In what way is therapeutic communication between the nurse and client a matter of trial and error?

Just the Facts
Accept that as a nurse, you may have feelings of irritation and impatience toward a client. Looking at your own feelings and response to the client situation can help you to grow and be more effective.

Response to Difficult Client Behaviors

The nurse–client relationship may involve situations in which the nurse is challenged with brief periods of inappropriate or difficult client behaviors. It is important for the nurse to observe and anticipate behaviors that may require an immediate or directed response. These situations may include the following.

- **Manipulation for attention:** The nursing approach is to recognize what the client is attempting to do and reinforce limits. For example, a response to the client who is constantly asking the nurse to come to his or her room might be, "You seem to be uncomfortable being by yourself. Let's talk about what is frightening to you."

- **Violence:** It is not unusual for nurses to fear for their personal safety during an incident of client hostility or violence. If this should occur during a working session, it is important to take precautionary measures to protect both the client and yourself. For example:
  - Maintain at least two arms' length distance between you and the client.
  - Do not attempt to touch the client without his or her approval.
  - Call for assistance—many units have a code for this situation.
  - Do not provoke the behavior or threaten the client with action.
  - Do not enter a room alone when a client is out of control.
  - Offer the client time to regain control and stop the behavior.
  - Change the subject from the topic that is threatening to the client.
- **Altered thought processes (hallucinations, illusions, delusions):** Initially, if the client is seeing or hearing something that is not apparent to the nurse, the nurse should acknowledge and clarify the content. For example, if a client is seeing someone in the room who is not obviously present, the nurse can respond with, "I don't see anyone in the room except you and me. Tell me what the person is doing." If the client is hearing voices, a response of, "I don't hear anyone talking. Tell me what they are saying to you" is appropriate. Once the nurse has insight into the content, the focus should be diverted from the hallucination or delusional thought. It is nontherapeutic to allow the client to continue the description. It is ineffective to argue or tell the person what they are experiencing is not real. Remember that these are symptoms of the illness and are real to the person who is experiencing them. The nurse should reestablish the client's contact with reality and focus on the feelings the client is presently experiencing. For example, a client tells the nurse, "They are laughing at me and saying ugly things about me." Once the nurse has clarified the content, an appropriate reply might be, "I understand that is hard, but let's talk about the rejection you are feeling now." If the content of the altered thought process is threatening to the client, every effort should be made to protect the client and others from injury.

- **Sexually inappropriate behaviors:** Most clients will refrain from making suggestive or sexually oriented comments or advances once they are asked to do so. The nurse should be direct in letting the client know that the actions are disturbing and unacceptable. Once the limits have been established, the client has a choice to use self-control. The nurse can then proceed to discuss the underlying issue with the client. If the behavior continues, the nurse can terminate the session, citing the behavior as the reason: "I will not tolerate this behavior. I am going now. I will come back at a later time." This will allow the client time to reflect on the actions and leave open the option of discussing the behavior at a later time.

Summary

The therapeutic relationship is a helping, interactive exchange between a client and a mental health professional. This compact is formed with the goal of improved functioning and well-being of the client. The nurse–client relationship is based on trust with honest communication that focuses on the client's feelings and problems. An empathetic and accepting approach is necessary to see the client as a unique person with individual needs and issues. Empathy allows the nurse to use his or her experiences and present situation to view the problem from the client's perspective.

Self-awareness is a process of self-evaluation and an attempt to see oneself through the eyes of others. This provides insight into how we respond to our environment and how others react to our behavior. The willingness to see ourselves realistically can open the door for positive change and improved interpersonal relationships. This same awareness is encouraged in the client with mental health issues. Although it may be difficult for clients to identify problems related to their behavior, doing so can allow the them to take ownership of the problem and commit to a plan for change.

The therapeutic nurse–client relationship consists of an orientation phase, working sessions, and a termination point. The initial contact with the client identifies the purpose and guidelines for the interaction. In addition, it ensures a safe and trusting milieu designed to facilitate and encourage the client to express needs and problems without criticism or reprisal. A series of interactive sessions are conducted with therapeutic communication techniques designed to explore and identify client problems and possible options for reso-

lution. These sessions maintain a client focus to help set priorities for short-term goals that lead toward improved functioning. The relationship is terminated at a point when the client is seen as having adequate skills and emotional resources to function independently. This is an important step in helping the client move back into society in an adaptive manner.

Therapeutic communication encompasses both verbal and nonverbal techniques that facilitate the exchange of information. It is important to remember that no one model works for all clients. What may work for one client may work adversely with the next. The nurse often uses a trial-and-error approach when interacting with the client. Knowledge of both therapeutic and nontherapeutic interventions will assist the nurse to elicit the most effective and productive information exchange and help the client toward recovery.

Bibliography

Corey, G. (1986). *Theory and practice of counseling and psychotherapy* (3rd ed.). Belmont, CA: Brooks/Cole.

Horsfall, J. (1998). Structural impediments to effective communication, *Australian and New Zealand Journal of Mental Health Nursing, 7,* 74–80.

Varcarolis, E. M. (1998). *Foundations of psychiatric mental health nursing* (3rd ed.). Philadelphia: W. B. Saunders.

Wachtel, P. L. (1998). *Therapeutic communication: Knowing what to say when.* New York: Guilford Press.

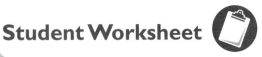
Student Worksheet

FILL IN THE BLANK

Fill in the blank with the correct answer.

1. The ability to hear what another person says and to borrow those feelings to perceive a situation from that person's viewpoint is referred to as _____.

2. _____ is a consciousness of our own personality and behavior in response to the world around us.

3. Therapeutic relationships are dependent on the _____ and _____ of the individual client.

4. It is important for the nurse to convey a _____ message through both verbal and nonverbal communication.

5. The termination phase of the therapeutic relationship promotes _____ for the client in getting along with others as preparation for discharge.

6. When nurses allow a need to "help" to overshadow a focus on the needs of the client, professional _____ have been crossed.

MATCHING

Match the following terms to the most appropriate phrase.

a. "Your hair is red—I have a red dress—I like red apples—apples, oranges, pears—you are shaped like a pear. . . ."

b. "Need a bath, need a bath, need a bath, need a bath. . . ."

c. "'Whymothig' is used to describe a puzzle."

d. "I like to go camping—that book is old—my necklace is broke—the sky is cloudy—fish are lucky. . . ."

e. "I have not seen my mother in 5 years . . . I need to go to the bathroom. . . ."

1. _____ Blocking

2. _____ Neologism

3. _____ Loose association

4. _____ Verbigeration

5. _____ Flight of ideas

MULTIPLE CHOICE

Select the best answer from the multiple-choice items.

1. A client tells the nurse, "The voices say that I am evil and I am going to be punished." Which of the following would be the most therapeutic response?

    a. "The voices are not real so why are you worrying about it?"

    b. "I don't hear the voices, but the words must be frightening for you."

    c. "You are imagining the worst when nothing is going to happen."

    d. "How can you hear voices when you and I are the only ones in this room?"

2. A client is admitted to the psychiatric unit in a hostile state. He continues to display anger toward the nurse, saying he does not need to be in this place. The nurse's best response would be:

   a. "You seem upset about being here. Can you tell me about that?"

   b. "All clients feel this way when they first come to the unit."

   c. "You obviously have a problem, or you wouldn't be here."

   d. "Why are you so angry about being here?"

3. The nurse is caring for a client who says, "I feel like I will never be able to leave this hospital." The nurse's most therapeutic reply would be:

   a. "You don't need to worry about that. We can only keep you for a certain length of time."

   b. "You keep working on your problem, and you will be out of here before you know it."

   c. "Everyone feels like it is hopeless, but we will discharge you when you are better."

   d. "You feel as though you will not get better and leave the unit?"

4. A client admitted with symptoms of hallucinations and delusional thinking says, "I can't eat because all the planet earth has been contaminated by the rain forest." To clarify what the client said, the nurse would use which of the following techniques?

   a. "Why in the world would that keep you from eating?"

   b. "You can't eat?"

   c. "Tell me again why you can't eat."

   d. "What did the rain forest do to the food?"

5. During a conversation a client tells the nurse, "My husband left me 6 months ago." The nurse notes that the client is repeatedly twisting strands of her hair. The most appropriate technique for the nurse to use at this time would be:

   a. Silence

   b. Verification

   c. Restating

   d. Focusing

6. Which of the following would be an open-ended question?

   a. "How would you describe what you are feeling today?"

   b. "Tell me about your family."

   c. "Do you always look at things in such a negative way?"

   d. "You are sad today because no one is talking to you."

SEEK AND FIND

Find the incorrect information in the following statements.

1. Reflection is a way of allowing the client to choose the topic for discussion.

2. "We have discussed the early years of your marriage . . . now we can discuss . . ." would demonstrate the technique of validation.

3. Clarification is a therapeutic technique that helps the client to concentrate on a specific issue.

4. A closed-ended question minimizes the client's feelings and concerns and conveys a superficial attitude.

5. "You will be feeling better in no time," is an example of giving advice.

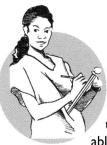

LEARNING OBJECTIVES

After learning the content in this chapter, the student will be able to:

1. Define the concept of the personality.
2. Describe the forces that shape personality development.
3. Define what is meant by temperament.
4. Discuss the basic relationship between behavior and the personality.
5. Identify the basic concepts of the various theories of personality development.
6. Explain the relationship between cognitive and moral development.
7. Describe the nursing model of interpersonal development as described by Peplau.
8. Discuss the Family System theory and how it applies to mental health.

Theoretical Concepts of Personality Development

KEY TERMS

Accommodation
Anal stage
Assimilation
Behaviorism
Central traits
Concrete operations
Conscious
Conventional
Defense mechanisms
Ego
Electra conflict
Equilibration
Formal operations
Genital stage
Hierarchy
Humanistic
Id
Interpersonal
Latency stage

Level of differentiation
Oedipal conflict
Oral stage
Personality traits
Phallic stage
Postconventional
Preconscious
Preconventional
Preoperational
Pseudoself
Psychosocial
Reinforcement
Secondary traits
Sensorimotor
Solid self
Superego
Temperament
Unconscious

Personality Development

Personality traits are defined as lasting patterns of perceiving, relating to, and thinking about the environment and oneself that are demonstrated in our social and personal interrelationships. Integrated into this personal portfolio are established characteristics and consistent behavioral responses that are unique to each person. This explains why everyone does not act the same in similar situations. **Central traits** are those general prominent features that are most often descriptive of the person, some of which are seen in all the behavior patterns. **Secondary traits** are those that may surface in some circumstances, such as in an anger-provoking situation.

From the moment of conception, our development is influenced by forces that ultimately shape the way in which we respond to the world around us. A person's natural tendencies are the result of a combined genetic transmission of personality traits from both parents. A unique blend of multigenerational family patterns is inherited through this genetic factor. There are also many societal and environmental forces that influence personality. Patterns of behavior are formed as one responds to the awareness and perception of the self as autonomous and capable of individual control. Abraham Maslow, a humanistic psychologist, theorized that one acts in response to a perceived internal or external force determined by certain needs that are unchanging and innate in origin. He defined these needs as a **hierarchy** in which some needs are more basic or more powerful than others, and as these needs are satisfied, we can move upward to meet other higher needs. It was his opinion that we cannot move to a higher level need unless the previous level of needs is satisfied. He believed that we have the unique ability to make conscious choices to seek certain things that provide value or meaning, which results in a personal identity. Life experiences may cause us to vacillate between levels and disrupt personal growth toward self-fulfillment.

Just the Facts

Abraham Maslow—Hierarchy of Needs
- Basic physiologic needs
- Comfort and safety, stability and security
- Love and belonging, relationships
- Self-esteem, self-respect, competence
- Self-actualization, growth and fulfillment

Humanistic theories view the developing person as a whole, a totality of the physical, emotional, spiritual, intellectual, and social aspects of life that influence us toward reaching our potential. This holistic view of human beings is the foundation of the nursing model of comprehensive health care delivery.

William Glasser, the founder of Reality Therapy and Control Theory, described four basic psychologic needs that determine our behavioral response in any given situation. He identified these as the need for love and belonging, power, freedom, and fun, which we must satisfy continually. The need to love and belong is internal, a hunger or void that may be filled by other people, pets, or even inanimate objects. Our drive for power often conflicts with our need for love as we seek to exert control over our world. Glasser asserts that we desire the freedom to exert this control over our lives and that when this drive is hampered, we respond or behave to regain the power that provides a psychologic homeostasis. He also theorizes that a measure of fun and playtime evens out the personality. In an effort to meet these needs, Dr. Glasser advocates that we have a choice regarding how to behave. From the moment of birth, we accumulate mental pictures from our experiences with the environment. This photo album provides the basis for our choices to behave in response to a given situation. Our behavior is a constant attempt to decrease the incongruence between what we want (pictures in our head) and what we have (our perception of the situation). Glasser asserted that we deny the reality of a situation instead of meeting our needs in a way that is responsible and within the boundaries of social norms and morality. He found that mental health is improved when we learn to meet our needs with responsible choices.

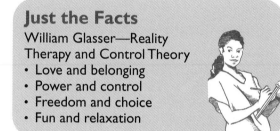

Just the Facts

William Glasser—Reality Therapy and Control Theory
- Love and belonging
- Power and control
- Freedom and choice
- Fun and relaxation

We might ask why one person would respond to a situation with anger but diffuse it quickly, while another may show a milder emotional reaction and others no reaction at all. Variances in character, including intensity and extent of feeling such as these are ones of **temperament,** which influences the development of personality and our interpersonal relationships. Studies describe three types of temperament in babies. *Easy* babies, who comprise the largest group, are seen as playful and adaptable. In contrast, a smaller number of babies are seen as *difficult* or irritable and unable to adapt well. A third group of *slow-to-warm-up* babies shows lower activity levels and slower adaptation to any new situation. The child develops in an environment that grows increasingly more complex as the basic family unit expands to include the influence of society and the culture of their world. The change and growth in personality have been the focus of much research from which theories have been developed to provide a basis for understanding of this process.

Just the Facts

Temperament
- Easy—playful and adaptable
- Difficult—irritable and unable to adapt well
- Slow-to-warm-up—slower adaptation

Mind Jogger

What adult behaviors might reflect a difficult temperament? A slow-to-warm-up?

Theories of Personality Development

Have you ever wondered why you think and behave in the way you do? This very issue leads to an integral concept in the study of psychology. Sigmund Freud was the first of many who studied and developed theories about the human mind and behavioral response to environmental forces. These theories are the foundation of therapeutic approaches to the treatment of mental illness.

Sigmund Freud (Psychoanalytic Theory)

Freud proposed that the psyche is made up of three components: the **conscious** or present awareness; the **preconscious** or that which is below current awareness but easily retrieved; and the unconscious; which he cites as the largest body of material. The **unconscious** includes past experiences and the related emotions that have been completely removed from the conscious level. This level is largely responsible for contributing to the

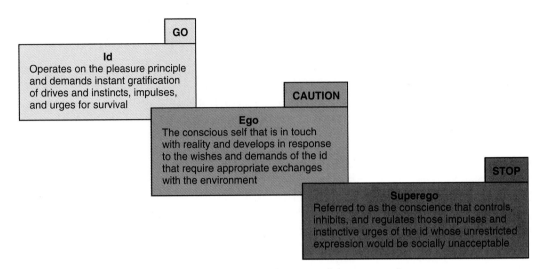

FIGURE 6-1. Freud's psychoanalytic theory: divisions of the personality.

emotional discomfort and disturbances that threaten us. Freudian theory also divides personality formation into three parts. The **id,** which operates on the pleasure principle and demands instant gratification of drives, is present at birth and contains the instincts, impulses, and urges for survival. These drives include hunger, aggression, sex, protection, and warmth. The **ego** begins to develop during the first 6 to 8 months and is fairly well developed by 2 years of age. This is the conscious self, which develops in response to the wishes and demands of the id that require appropriate exchanges with the environment. It is here that sensations, feelings, adjustments, solutions, and defenses are formed. The **superego,** often referred to as the conscience, starts developing at about 3 to 4 years of age and is fairly well developed by the age of 10 to 11 years. It controls, inhibits, and regulates those impulses and instinctive urges whose unrestricted expression would be socially unacceptable. The values and moral standards of parents are incorporated into this control along with the norms and moral codes of the society in which one lives and grows. The superego operates at both the conscious and unconscious

levels, decides right from wrong, and offers both critical self-evaluation and self-praise. The ego is the peacemaker and balance between the instinctual drives and societal demands.

Example:
Id—I want a piece of chocolate cake.
Superego—There are too many calories in that cake.
Ego—Be satisfied with a small piece.

The constant need for the ego to intercept the conflicts between the id and superego that are created in response to environmental stressors leads to increased anxiety. This anxiety creates a dilemma in which stability is needed to preserve our sense of self. Freud theorized that for the ego to remain in control, automatic psychologic processes called **defense mechanisms** are mobilized to protect us from anxiety and the awareness of internal or external stressors. (See At a Glance 6-1.) Most of these mechanisms are mobilized at the unconscious level. High levels of anxiety can disturb perception and performance, which compromises the ability to problem solve and learn. These unconscious defense tools provide us with protection from unacceptable thoughts and

At a Glance 6-1 Ego Defense Mechanisms—Freud

Mechanism	Description
Sublimation	Replacing a socially unacceptable behavior with one that is acceptable. Primitive impulses are not acceptable to the ego and are rechanneled into a constructive outlet. (Aggressive desire to attack another person is rechanneled into a sport activity such as football.)
Denial	Consciously rejecting reality or refusing to recognize facts of a situation. Ego refuses to see the truth because it causes severe mental pain. (Wife whose husband dies continues to set the table for two as if he will be present for dinner.)
Displacement	Transferring hostility or other strong feelings from the original cause of the feelings to another person or object. (Person who has a confrontation at his place of employment goes home and argues with his family.)
Fantasy	Consciously distorting unconscious wishes or needs by using imagination to solve problems. (Young child who sees father physically abuse mother may imagine he is attacking a wild animal and saves his mother from harm.)
Repression	Conscious distancing of events or thoughts that are too painful or unacceptable to one's ego into the unconscious level. These feelings can continue to influence behavior into adult years if unresolved. (Person who was sexually abused as a child is unable to achieve a meaningful intimate relationship as an adult.)
Regression	Returning to an earlier more comfortable and less stressful stage of behavior. (Child who is weaned returns to drinking from a bottle during hospitalization.)
Projection	Attributing or blaming emotionally unacceptable traits, feelings, or attitudes on something or someone else. Refusing to admit weakness or accept responsibility for own actions. (Person who drinks alcohol blames his wife for doing something to make him get drunk.)
Compensation	Emphasizing capabilities or strengths to make up for a lack or loss in personal characteristics. (Person who is not talented in athletics excels in scholastic achievement.)
Reaction-formation	Consciously attempting to make up for feelings or attitudes that are unacceptable to the ego by replacing them with the opposite feelings or beliefs. (Mother who secretly dislikes her child becomes overprotective and outwardly affectionate toward the child.)
Conversion	Transferring emotional conflicts into physical symptoms. (Person who dislikes her boss at work develops migraine headaches to avoid going to work.)

continues

At a Glance 6-1 Ego Defense Mechanisms—Freud (*Continued*)

Mechanism	Description
Undoing	Initiating a positive action to conceal a negative action or neutralizing a previously unacceptable action or wish. (Employer offers to take his secretary to lunch after verbally attacking her earlier in the day.)
Rationalization	Substituting false reasoning or justification for behavior that is unacceptable or threatening to the ego. Ignores the real reason for the behavior with falsehoods and avoids responsibility for the behavior. (Employee who is not given a promotion tells co-workers that he really did not want the position.)

impulses while continuing to meet personal and social needs in acceptable ways.

According to Freud, defenses are a major means of managing conflict and emotional response to environmental situations. These mechanisms differ from one another and may be adaptive as well as maladaptive. Maladaptive mechanisms may lead to distortion of reality and actual self-deception that can interfere with personal growth and interaction with society. For example, a person may continue to abuse alcohol using the mechanism of projection to blame his spouse and children for his behavior, while using denial to avoid self-blame and damage to his own ego. This maladaptive use of mechanisms interferes with an honest self-appraisal of reality and the detrimental effects of substance abuse. In contrast, a woman may temporarily deny her husband's extramarital affair by telling herself and others that he is just busy, yet project her feelings for her husband onto her children by punishing them for things they did not do. When she sees her husband with the other woman, she realizes the reality of the situation and apologizes to her children for blaming them for the way she feels toward their father. The determinant for the effective use of defense mechanisms is based on the frequency, intensity, and length of time they are used.

Human beings sometimes behave in ways that provide a means of escape from the realities and responsibilities of life. These patterns of adjustment are common to everyone and are used to resolve conflicts and provide relief from the anxiety and stress of everyday existence. Most of the time, we are not aware that a defense mechanism is being used to adapt to a situation. However, when this escape becomes habitual, it becomes a dangerous inability to deal with reality and constitutes a psychiatric problem.

Theory of Psychosexual Development. Freud believed that as the personality develops, there is an increasing self-identification and changing self-perception of sexuality and sexual identification. In his psychosexual theory, he proposed four major stages of development. The **oral stage** occurs during the first 2 years as the child seeks pleasure from sucking and oral gratification of hunger. The **anal stage** take place from 2 to 4 years of age, during which pleasure is achieved as the child develops an awareness and control of urination and defecation. In the **phallic stage,** around the age of 4 years, the child discovers pleasure in genital stimulation and also struggles to accept a sexual identity. According to Freud, this gives rise to the **Oedipal conflict** (boys) and the **Electra conflict**

(girls) in which the child begins to feel romantic feelings for the parent of the opposite sex but fears the wrath of the parent of the same sex. The child resolves the conflict by identifying with the parent of the same sex and redirects the feelings for the opposite-sex parent into developing this gender role. Freud believed these feelings are put into **latency** during the period of middle childhood in which the sexual desires remain subdued. The **genital stage** occurs as the child enters puberty and adolescence. It at this stage that Freud believed sexual feelings reemerge and become directed toward establishing a relationship with a person of the opposite sex. According to Freud, at any point during psychosexual development the child can become fixated and frustrated, resulting in exaggerated adult character traits that reflect the arrested growth. (See At a Glance 6-2.) Although it has been the subject of much controversy regarding its sexual orientation, Freudian theory laid the groundwork for future developmental theories.

Erik Erikson (Psychosocial Developmental Theory)

Erikson proposed that we develop in a pattern of eight **psychosocial** stages throughout our lifespan. Each stage consists of a developmental crisis that must be faced, indicating a period of vulnerability. Resolution of this critical period could enhance a healthy continuation of the process. If unresolved, the progression to subsequent stages of development could be adversely affected. Erikson's view demonstrates, however, that failures at one stage can be corrected by successes at a later stage.

Stage I: Trust versus Mistrust (Birth to 1 Year). A sense of trust results in a feeling of comfort and reassurance that the world is a safe

At a Glance 6-2 Adult Behaviors of Stage Theory Development

Stage	Signs of Successful Resolution	Indicators of Developmental Problem
Freud (Psychosexual)		
1. Oral	Satisfaction—gratification	Dependent on and easily influenced by others, manipulative cocky attitude, gullible
2. Anal	Giving, openness, self-control	Stinginess and orderliness; stubborn and rigid meticulousness
3. Phallic	Sexual identity accepted	Vanity and brashness, flirtatious
4. Latency	Sexual urges suppressed—expansion of social contacts beyond family	Unsuccessful attempts at expanding social relationships
5. Genital	Sexual energy channeled toward peers of opposite sex	Unconscious sexual conflict and inability to form intimate sexual relationship

continues

At a Glance 6-2 Adult Behaviors of Stage Theory Development (Continued)

Stage	Signs of Successful Resolution	Indicators of Developmental Problem
Erikson (Psychosocial)		
1. Trust versus mistrust	Hope	Suspicion and fear of people and relationships
		Extreme self-doubt and fear of independence
2. Autonomy versus shame and doubt	Will	Sense of inadequacy and defeat
3. Initiative versus guilt	Purpose	Inadequate problem-solving skills
4. Industry versus inferiority	Competence	Manipulation of others, no regard for the rights of others (such as in the workplace)
		Feelings of unworthiness, fear of failure
5. Identity versus role confusion	Fidelity	Uncertainty and loss of who one is in relationships with others
6. Intimacy versus isolation	Love and commitment	Emotional withdrawal into self
7. Generativity versus stagnation	Caring and giving	Inability to grow as an person
8. Integrity versus despair	Wisdom	Disillusionment with life and inability to view death as reality
Piaget (Cognitive)		
1. Sensorimotor	Growth of abilities related to senses and motor skill Goal-directed behaviors Egocentric thinking	Focus only on what one wants without regard to possible consequences of those actions
2. Preoperational	Exploration motivated by magical and imaginative thinking	Decisions based on intuition, fantasy, or superstition with inability to make choices rooted in reality
3. Concrete	Cognitive connections based on actual events or objects Logical thinking begins Thinking in terms of intentional moral response	Resistance to change with meager attempts at risk-taking strategies in which the outcome is an unknown
4. Formal operations	Abstract thinking Problem-solving ability Symbolic reasoning with conceptual theoretical thinking	Inability to visualize possibility or solution to a problem Unwillingness to formulate or accept reality-based decisions

continues

At a Glance 6-2 Adult Behaviors of Stage Theory Development *(Continued)*

Stage	Signs of Successful Resolution	Indicators of Developmental Problem
Sullivan (Interpersonal)		
1. Infant	Satisfaction of needs	Anxiety develops as a result of unmet physiologic needs Lack of bonding between infant and caregiver
2. Childhood	Self-control in gratification of needs	Increasing anxiety experienced with delay in gratification of own needs
3. Juvenile	Successful relationships with peer group	Difficulty relating to others and developing interpersonal group relationships/ workplace interaction
4. Preadolescence	Appropriate interactions with persons of opposite sex begins	Inability to relate in a meaningful way to persons of the opposite sex
5. Early adolescence	Sense of personal identity in heterosexual relationships	Fear and withdrawal of relationships with persons of the opposite sex
6. Late adolescence	Satisfying intimate relationship with another	Inability to form a long-term intimate relationship with another person

and pleasant place in which the child can live with a minimum of fear and apprehension. The emphasis in this stage is on the oral-sensory gratification received during feeding through which the infant develops a trusting relationship with the parent or caregiver. Consistency and responsiveness by the parent in providing for the infant's needs of nourishment, comfort,

and nurturing are essential to the development of trust. Babies who are not securely attached to their mothers are less responsive to the parent and show less effort in exploring the environment and world in which they exist.

Stage II: Autonomy versus Shame and Doubt (Ages 1 to 2). According to Erikson, children begin a period of increased self-confidence and independent striving to do more on their own. The most important event during this stage is toilet training. Children also try to do new things such as feeding or dressing themselves. It is essential that the parents positively reinforce these efforts while avoiding the urge to be overprotective and critical. Erickson believed that if parents do not show a consistent and reassuring attitude

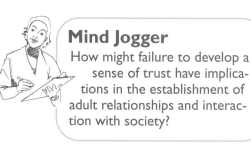

Mind Jogger

How might failure to develop a sense of trust have implications in the establishment of adult relationships and interaction with society?

during this stage, children would experience too much self-doubt and shame about their abilities, resulting in a lack of confidence that would persist throughout life.

Stage III: Initiative versus Guilt (2 to 6 Years).
During this period children are challenged with increasing responsibility to take care of their physical needs, their behavior, toys, and pets. This requires children to be assertive and creative in assuming this responsibility. Children in this stage are eager to do things, and it is essential that parents praise and recognize the child's efforts no matter how small they may be. On the other hand, children must also learn to accept that in their quest for independence there are some things that are not allowed or safe for them to do. It is important they be reassured that being imaginative and pretending to take on adult roles is okay. If they are not given the chance to do things on their own and to be responsible, a sense of guilt may result. The child will learn to believe that what they want to do is not good enough or is always wrong.

Stage IV: Industry versus Inferiority (6 to 12 Years).
In this stage of development, children are learning to be productive and to accomplish things on their own, both physically and mentally. This is a period when they master their ability to succeed in peer relationships, school, and activities. It is essential for children to receive encouragement and support in their drive for success from parents and others. Children learn by repeated efforts driven by self-confidence in their own ability. If children have difficulty relating to others outside of the home or in achievement of skills, a sense of inferiority and self-doubt may result.

Stage V: Identity versus Role Confusion (12 to 18 Years).
During the stage of adolescence, there is a search for identity and answers to questions concerning our purpose in life. Erikson believed that a basic sense of trust and self-confidence in ourselves was necessary to provide the foundation for ado-

lescents to make conscious choices about vocation, relationships, and life in general. Failure to resolve previous conflicts successfully would result in an inability to make these decisions and choices. As a result, adolescents may experience role confusion as to who they are and where they belong as they move into adulthood.

Stage VI: Intimacy versus Isolation (Ages 19 to 40 Years).
During young adulthood, the most important developmental goal is to form a committed relationship with another. A true intimate relationship requires sincerity and open sharing of feelings. Having a sexual relationship does not imply intimacy. A person can be sexually intimate without feelings for and commitment to the other person. Love relationships are strengthened by the ability of partners to relate on a deep personal level. The young adult who is unable to be open and committed to another may retreat into isolation and fear a giving and sharing relationship.

Stage VII: Generativity versus Stagnation (Ages 40 to 65 Years).
As we enter middle adulthood, the task is related to parenting and supportive involvement in providing for the next generation. This role includes being an active participant in issues that will make this world a safer and better place for the future. The inability to nurture and to give of whatever is ours to give in an attempt to ensure this progressive stability for our children may lead to stagnation and decreased meaning for one's life.

Stage VIII: Integrity versus Despair (Over 65 years).
The important event during these years is seen as a reflection on and acceptance of our life. According to Erikson, a positive outcome is demonstrated by a sense of fulfillment about a life lived and acceptance of death as an inevitable reality. This involves accepting responsibility for and being satisfied with choices that have been made over a lifetime. The older adult who has successfully reached this stage is

able to put the past in perspective and achieve a sense of self-satisfaction with the present. Those who are unable to reach this sense of fulfillment and wholeness will despair about life accomplishments and fear death.

Erikson maintained that if each developmental crisis was not resolved in sequence, the personality would continue to manifest this conflict into the adult years. (See At a Glance 6-2.) Although critics of the stage theory say that psychologic development may be influenced and altered by experiences throughout life, many have found Erikson's theory useful for continued study of personality development.

Just the Facts

Erik Erikson—Eight Stages of Psychosocial Development
1. Trust versus mistrust
2. Autonomy versus shame and doubt
3. Initiative versus guilt
4. Industry versus inferiority
5. Identity versus role confusion
6. Intimacy versus isolation
7. Generativity versus stagnation
8. Integrity versus despair

Jean Piaget (Cognitive Development Related to Personality)

Piaget proposed that personality is the result of increasing intellectual ability to organize and integrate experiences into behavior patterns. His observations led him to conclude that this organization tended to occur at certain age groups. Movement forward relies on four interdependent factors. Physical and psychologic growth or maturation occurs in the child during a specific stage as the child

thinks and *experiences* interaction with the environment. As the child begins to distinguish the self as a separate being, social experiences become a part of this learning. According to Piaget, **equilibration** occurs as the child brings all these factors together to build mental schema or connections that lead to a cognitive balance. Children are motivated to seek this balance by a perceived imbalance between what they already know (existing schema) and something new. Piaget refers to the ability to incorporate new ideas and experiences as **assimilation**, while **accommodation** is the ability to alter existing schema to incorporate the new information.

Piaget theorized that cognitive development occurs in four stages. In the first two years of life, the **sensorimotor** stage involves the growth of abilities related to the five senses and motor functions. Early responses are primarily reflexive in nature, with a gradual increase in skill as children adapt to their environment. These responses tend to reflect only a perception of that which is visible to the child. The perception that what is gone from view still exists (object permanence) begins to develop at about 9 months of age and is well developed by 1 year.

The **preoperational stage** of development occurs from 2 to 7 years. The mental schema developed during the earlier stage emerge into communication of thoughts that is largely egocentric without regard for another point of view. Language and actions reflect a focus on thinking that the world exists solely to meet the demands of the child's ego. As children grow, they explore and try out many new activities motivated by increasing magical and imaginative thinking.

From 7 to 12 years of age, Piaget saw children as able to perform **concrete mental operations** on their accumulated thoughts and memories. The phrase "seeing is believing" is descriptive of the child's need to base these cognitive connections on actual events or objects. Facts and routines with one way of doing things are a characteristic of this age group. The child begins to think logically, classify objects, and recognize that combinations are reversible. (For example: Daddy can also be a husband, brother, and uncle all at the same time.) Although they are capable of thinking more logically, children of this age still depend on concrete cues to develop these thoughts.

According to Piaget, the person moves into the stage of **formal operations** during the years of 11 to 12 and up. This period of growth involves abstract thought processes, problem solving, and systematic, purposeful mental relationships. The adolescent is capable of symbolic thinking and comprehension of theoretical concepts. They are able to visualize beyond what is known and formulate hypothetical reasoning.

Piaget maintains that once the child has entered a new stage, the process is irreversible, with each stage building on the previous level of development. (See At a Glance 6-2.)

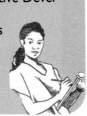

Just the Facts
Jean Piaget—Theory of Cognitive Development
Sensorimotor: Birth to 2 years
Preoperational: 2 to 7 years
Concrete: 7 to 11 years
Formal operations: 11 years and up

Lawerence Kohlberg (Theory of Moral Development)

In his research on cognitive development, Piaget concluded that changes in the child's level of thinking also affect the moral decisions the child makes. Motivated by Piaget's studies, Lawerence Kohlberg developed his own theory based on six stages of moral reasoning included in three levels. Basic to his theory is his belief that the choices one makes do not determine the stage of moral reasoning, but the reasons one gives to justify the behavior determine the moral stage. Like Piaget, he believed that the intellect and the child's emotional development occur in a parallel pattern of stages during which the child changes his or her concept of self in relation to interaction with others. The level of cognitive development determines how the child perceives a situation and what is learned from that experience. Each of the three levels builds on the previous with increasing complexity in the individual view of a moral issue.

Preconventional Level: Values indicate environmental pressure

> Stage 1: Acts or behaves to avoid punishment
> Stage 2: Is motivated by personal reward (What's in it for me?)

Conventional Level: Influenced by societal pressure

> Stage 3: Values and acts to meet the expectations of others (peer group)
> Stage 4: Is motivated by the laws of society/legal system

Postconventional Level: Influenced by standards and shared principles

> Stage 5: Acts for the good of society or the most people (e.g., U.S. Constitution)
> Stage 6: Bases actions on moral principles and ethical values (the right thing to do)

Mind Jogger
What do the stage theories have in common? How do they differ? What influence does each aspect of development have on the personality?

Harry S. Sullivan (Theory of Interpersonal Development)

Nurses in the mental health setting develop therapeutic relationships with clients in an attempt to help them develop the ability to interact successfully with others. Sullivan believed that behavior and personality developments are the direct result of these interpersonal relationships. Unlike Freud, who believed that all behavior is the result of unconscious drives and unfinished agendas, Sullivan believed that human behavior could be seen in the social interaction between people. The major concepts of his theory include:

Anxiety: A major force that develops as a result of unmet needs and interpersonal dissatisfaction.

Fulfillment of needs: All physiologic, comfort and security needs are met.

Concept of self: Incorporates those experiences and behaviors developed to protect the child against anxiety and provide security for the self. As a result, three images of self develop:

"Good-me" develops in response to positive feedback.

"Bad-me" develops in response to criticism from caregiver.

"Not-me" develops in response to intense anxiety and dread with resulting denial and repression of the situation to avoid the anxiety (this avoidance of emotions can result in mental disorders in the adult).

Sullivan divided development into six stages. During *infancy* (birth to 18 months), the child is concerned with oral satisfaction of needs. In *childhood* (18 months to 6 years), children learn to delay personal gratification with a minimum of anxiety. The *juvenile* (6 to 9 years) is learning to develop satisfaction in relationships with the peer group, while the *preadolescent* (9 to 12 years) is striving to develop successful interactions with persons of the same sex. During *early adolescence* (12 to 14 years) a sense of personal identity is formed as relationships with persons of the opposite sex are sought. In *late adolescence* (14 to 21 years) the person is working to develop satisfying and meaningful long-term relationships with others.

Sullivan believed that the attainment of successful interpersonal relationships was dependent on the formation of interaction skills at each level of development. (See At a Glance 6-2.)

Hildegard Peplau (Psychodynamic Nursing)

Peplau applied the interpersonal theory to nursing and the nurse–client relationship. She saw the stages of developmental growth as the basis for therapeutic interaction with clients, including many whose behaviors reflect a failure to understand their own feelings and actions, and the results of those actions.

Peplau's theory identified four stages of development. In *infancy,* the child is learning to count on others, while the *toddler* is learning to delay self-gratification. At the same time, the toddler derives much pleasure in a positive response from others to his or her actions. *Early childhood* is a time of developing the skill of behaving in a way that is acceptable to others, preceding *late childhood* in which the child learns to compromise, compete, and cooperate in participation and interactions with others. Learning to practice self-control and compromise in our relationships with others is a precedent to living successfully and interacting as a member of society.

Murray Bowen (Family Systems Theory)

The Family Systems theory asserts that a person is able to change behaviors based on an awareness of the impact that present and past family patterns of behavior have on the choices one makes. This awareness can lead

At a Glance 6-3 Other Theoretical Approaches to Personality and Behavior

Behavioristic Theory— B. F. Skinner	• **Behaviorism** is based on the concept that thinking, feeling, and interpersonal relationships are irrelevant and that all behavior is observable or learned behavior in response to a stimulus from the environment. • Behavior is the result of conditioning shaped by a system of reward, punishment, and **reinforcement.** • Human personality is formed in response to these stimulus-response situations. The personality may include both adaptive and maladaptive behavior as the result of reinforcement. • People show consistent patterns of behavior that will continue if the action is rewarded by a response. If no reinforcement is given, the behavior will decline. • Positive reinforcement of a negative behavior can lead to continuation of the very behavior we wish to negate. • Conditioning strengthens and weakens behaviors automatically without regard to the conscious thought processes.
Social Learning Theory— Albert Bandura	• Personality is largely shaped through learning by actively seeking out and processing information about the environment in response to a need for a positive outcome. • People can act to change their surroundings as a result of both internal and external forces that influence each other. • Social learning is based on observation and imitation of others. Both children and adults tend to imitate people they like or respect more than those whose persona is less appealing. • Models whose behavior leads to an approved outcome are also more likely to be copied. • Self-confidence develops as the belief that performance of behaviors should lead to the expected outcome becomes reality in the actions of that person.
Cognitive-Behavioral Theory—Aaron Beck	• Focus is on the person's abilities to think, analyze, and decide on certain behavior rather than acting on feelings. • Actions are the result of distorted perceptions, and thoughts that can be changed. This is unlike Freud who saw mental disturbances as being the result of childhood experiences. • Self-defeating behaviors are maintained because of irrational thoughts and erroneous beliefs. • Self-concept and evaluation of social image is affected by how people think others see them. Self-talk is used to praise or criticize and interpret situations. This is reflected in both normal behaviors and mental disorders as well. • Negative self-talk can be changed into more positive thoughts, leading to a more positive self-image and more productive outcomes.

to an intentional desire to make changes and a refusal to function in the way that has been perpetuated by members of the family.

Family is defined as the nuclear family of origin and extending to past relationships and family histories. Bowen saw this family as a single emotional unit composed of relationships that intermingle over several generations. He felt the dynamics of these family relationships held the key for understanding current behaviors. Integral in Bowen's theory is the recognition that there is a connection between biologic, genetic, psychologic, and sociologic factors in the determination of behavior. Actions are seen as preceded by feelings that to some degree can be controlled by the ability to think. People are able to predict their own patterns of response based on an awareness of the dynamics that are evident in the family system.

Bowen identifies two major variables that affect our behavior in terms of relationships. Anxiety is an individual reaction to stress that is seen as directly correlated to the person's **level of differentiation,** or the degree to which we define the self in terms of values and beliefs. The person whose behavior is based on internal convictions and principles is defined as a **solid self,** as opposed to the **pseudoself** whose behavior reflects an external locus of control. Persons described as a solid self are more adaptable, more flexible, and more effective in coping with stressful situations, while those defined as a pseudoself are less adaptable, less flexible, and less able to rely on internal sources of strength to cope with anxiety.

People tend to seek partners of similar differentiation levels, breeding relationships that are either open or closed systems. An open family system is made up of persons who are predominantly a solid self. This promotes flexibility and exchange of ideas within an accepting environment. They are comfortable with being visible and are free to clearly define themselves and their belief system. In contrast, those who are willing to compromise their values when pressured by external sources identify the closed family system. The result of these relationships is one of dys-

function, fusion, and rigid standards in which one person gains control and the other loses self. An increase in fusion increases the anxiety within the system. Families deal with this anxiety through emotional distancing and conflict, which eventually results in the dysfunction of one or more members of the family. Triangles are created that draw a third party into the conflict, further dismantling the homeostasis of the family unit. The differentiation of people within the system is projected onto other members of that family, creating a spiral effect as children marry and create another generation with similar characteristics and value systems.

> **Just the Facts**
>
> Murray Bowen—Family Systems Theory
> Level of differentiation: Degree to which one defines the self
> Solid self: Behavior based on internal convictions, values, and self-imposed beliefs
> Pseudoself: Behavior reflects external locus of control

This theory provides a way for us to understand how families function and how people are affected by the dynamics in this multigenerational process. Once clients are aware of how they are influenced by dysfunctional patterns of behavior, they can be supported in an effort to effect change and break the cycle.

Summary

The formation of our personality is essentially the formation of who we are over the continuum of a lifetime. Our drives, our thought processes, and our behavior are all integral parts of this holistic human system. The established theoretical models for the study of human cognition and behavior have provided current studies with an eclectic view of development. Research continues to uncover the many mysteries inherent in the human mind and personality.

Personality is a combination of characteristic patterns of how we perceive, relate to, and think about ourselves and the world in which we exist. These patterns are the result of genetics and the influence of social and environmental forces throughout the lifespan. The development of personality is most often described by stage theories that divide the lifespan into age-related periods. These theories provide an approach to personality and psychologic development that correlates with the physical growth and development.

Other theories have developed that reflect the various ways in which the human component can be studied and viewed. Since human behavior is most often seen as how we interact with one another and the social environment, it is most often studied within this context. Our patterns of behavior are established as a result of these interrelationships. The self-concept is developed as behaviors are reinforced or threatened by reprisal. As environmental situations confront us, we view them from the perspective of past encounters with similar occurrences. The way in which we respond is reflective of established patterns. It is also theorized that we have the ability to think, analyze, and decide on certain behaviors rather than just reacting to the environmental stimuli.

Family Systems theory asserts that we are able to change behaviors based on an awareness of the impact that present and past family patterns of behavior have on the choices we make. This awareness can lead to an intentional desire to make changes in the way we respond to environmental situations.

Knowledge of the various theories provides the basis for understanding the various therapeutic approaches to the treatment of mental illness. The dynamics that combine and develop over generations make us who we are. We cannot undo the past, but to understand it is an invitation to repair the present and the future.

Bibliography

American Psychiatric Association (2000). *Diagnostic and statistical manual of mental disorders text revision* (4th ed.). Washington, DC: American Psychiatric Association.

Johnson, B. S. (1993). *Psychiatric-mental health nursing* (3rd ed.). Philadelphia, PA: Lippincott.

Sternberg, R. J. (1995). *In search of the human mind.* Ft. Worth, TX: Harcourt Brace.

Weiten, W. (1995). *Psychology themes and variations* (3rd ed.). Boston, MA: Brooks/Cole.

Student Worksheet

FILL IN THE BLANK

Fill in the blank with the correct answer.

1. Patterns of perceiving, relating to, and thinking about ourselves and the world around us define the concept of _____.

2. _____ describes the variances in character that influence the development of personality and interpersonal relationships.

3. The process by which we bring factors together to build mental schema or connections that lead to a cognitive balance is called _____.

4. According to Piaget, _____ is the ability to incorporate new ideas and experiences into our existing mental schema.

5. Once new experiences are encountered, the ability to alter the existing schema to incorporate this new information is referred to as _____.

6. The concept that all behavior is observable or learned in response to a stimulus from the environment is the basis for the theory of _____.

7. The theory of development that states that the reasons we give to justify our choices and the behavior that results from those choices determine the level of moral development was the work of _____.

8. B. F. Skinner theorized that the human personality is formed in response to a conditioned stimulus-response of reward and punishment called _____.

9. The degree to which we define the self in terms of values and beliefs is referred to as the _____ of _____.

10. The person whose behavior is based on internal convictions and principles is defined as a _____ self.

MATCHING

Match the defense mechanism with the appropriate behavior.

a. Unhappy with her boss for his criticism, Clara turns around and takes her anger out on her husband.

b. David is unable to remember a boating accident in which his friend was killed.

c. After going to the movie the night before an exam, Molly states that she failed the exam because she did not study the right chapter.

d. An adolescent wants his mother to stay with him during a hospital stay.

e. Confined to a wheelchair, Jack becomes a computer specialist.

f. A young man who secretly desires to harm his wife appears on a television show against spousal abuse.

g. When Martha is confronted about her alcohol problem, she states she can quit anytime she chooses.

h. After taking funds out of their savings account to buy golf clubs, Hank tells his wife that the bank must have made a mistake.

1. _____ Rationalization

2. _____ Denial

3. _____ Repression

4. _____ Regression

5. _____ Projection

6. _____ Displacement

7. _____ Reaction-formation

8. _____ Sublimation

MULTIPLE CHOICE

Select the best answer from the multiple-choice items.

1. A 70-year-old client states to the nurse, "My life is a pile of shambles with nothing to show for it." The client is demonstrating what Erikson would term:

   a. Doubt

   b. Inferiority

   c. Despair

   d. Stagnation

2. A 4-year-old boy tells the nurse, "When I grow up I am going to marry Mommy." Which stage of psychosexual development is portrayed by this statement?

   a. Phallic

   b. Anal

   c. Latency

   d. Genital

3. According to Piaget, children who seek to control their world from a concentrated point of view would be in which stage of cognitive development?

   a. Sensorimotor

   b. Preoperational

   c. Concrete

   d. Formal operations

4. To avoid hurting his friend, John refrains from telling the truth to a friend whose partner is having an affair with a co-worker. According to Kohlberg, this demonstrates which level of moral development?

   a. Preconventional—stage 2

   b. Conventional—stage 3

   c. Postconventional—stage 5

5. Al has been arrested for physical assault. He has a history of previous aggressive offenses. Behavioral theory would explain this behavior as:

   a. Feelings of repressed hostility

   b. A diminished sense of self-esteem

   c. An innate impulsive drive for survival

   d. Reinforcement of early learning experiences

6. Surveys show that cigarette smoking and alcohol consumption are common among the adolescent population. These results reflect peer behavior and provide support for which of the following theories?

   a. Social learning theory

   b. Conditioning theory

   c. Psychosexual theory

   d. Human needs theory

7. Sue feels that her experiences have led her to a belief that she is responsible for most of the things that happen to her. According to Bowen, Sue tends to have:

   a. A strong superego

   b. An internal locus of control

   c. A strong pseudoself

   d. Strong unconscious drives

SEEK AND FIND

Find the incorrect information in the statements below.

1. The holistic view of human beings that serves as the foundation for the nursing model of comprehensive health care delivery is based on the theory of behaviorism, which views the developing person as a total person.

2. According to Freudian theory, the division of the personality that is most closely in touch with reality is the superego.

3. The theory of psychosexual development suggests that during the latency stage, the child is discovering pleasure in genital stimulation while struggling to accept a sexual identity.

4. According to Erikson, the child begins a period of increased self-confidence and striving to become more independent in the preschool years during the stage of initiative versus guilt.

5. The person who is unable to be open and committed to a giving and sharing relationship with another is said by Erikson to be stalled in the stage of identity versus role confusion.

Grief and Loss

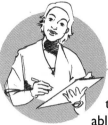

LEARNING OBJECTIVES

After learning the content in this chapter, the student will be able to:

1. Define grief as a process.
2. Describe the relationship between loss and grief.
3. Discuss adaptive versus maladaptive responses to grief and loss.
4. Identify factors that may contribute to dysfunctional grief.
5. Assess signs and symptoms that indicate unresolved grief.
6. Identify nursing diagnoses related to the grieving process.
7. Describe outcomes that demonstrate acceptance and resolution.
8. Plan interventions that the nurse can utilize to help clients cope during the grief process.

KEY TERMS

Acceptance
Anger
Anticipatory grief
Bargaining
Bereavement
Chronic sorrow
Conventional grief
Denial
Depression
Dysfunctional grief
Grief
Loss
Unresolved grief

Defining Grief and Loss

Grief is defined as the emotional process of coping with a loss. Instinctively, we associate this process with the death of a loved one, such as a spouse, parent, or child, or of any person who is important in our life. In a broader sense, the reality of loss can be applied to the absence of anything that is significant or meaningful to our existence. This can include a separation or divorce, loss of a body part, loss of a job or source of income, and losses that result from a natural or imposed disaster. All of these events or circumstances may leave the person with a sense of emptiness, hopelessness, and detachment from the meaning that previously was found in life. The extent to which emotional energy was previously invested in these objects, persons, and relationships will determine the intensity with which an individual responds to the absence of that object. Although a person may experience sadness or sorrow in response to making a mistake or doing something that is hurtful to another, the grief felt as the person adjusts to the absence of the endeared person or object is a deeper and longer lasting emotion that involves time and emotional energy.

Loss can be an actual or perceived change in the status of one's relationship to a valued object or person. This concept is easily associated with the death of a valued person or pet. There is also a major loss when losing a home to fire or natural disaster with a lifetime of memories suddenly gone from view and reality. The loss may be seen as the lack of certainty that a goal or desired outcome will be achieved, such as not receiving a job promotion or an academic failure. The attachment bond that is seen as strong and secure is suddenly shattered, making a person vulnerable to an unstable emotional response. Grief is the emotion encountered when an individual is confronted with a loss. It is a feeling of sadness and despondency centered on the experience itself. These feelings may lead to behaviors such as forgetfulness and crying at unpredictable times. It is helpful for the person to be reassured that this is a common reaction to grief. Tears are accepted as a part of the healing that takes place in the months after the loss.

Anticipatory grief may be seen in individuals and families who are expecting a major loss in the near future. This concept is helpful to nurses in understanding the reaction of the terminally ill client and the family who will be left to mourn the death of their loved one. In this case, death is inevitable and there is a time of preparation and closure that can ease the emotional pain at the actual time of death. This is the premise for hospice care, which provides palliative nursing and supportive interventions to assist the client and family members in coping with the imminent loss. The nurse can also apply this concept to those in the acute care setting who may be anticipating or facing the loss of a body part (e.g., amputation of a limb or a mastectomy) or change in body functioning (e.g., urinary or bowel diversion; chronic illness such as diabetes, emphysema, heart disease) that may inflict a major alteration in lifestyle.

Just the Facts

Anticipatory grieving: Entering the grieving process in anticipation of a loss
Conventional grieving: Feelings expected after a loss

Conventional grief is primarily associated with the grief that is experienced following a loss. This process of **bereavement** or adapting to loss may take days, weeks, or years, depending on the sense of loss for the person involved. Each person responds to loss in a personal and unique way and time. This response is based on the person's level of development, past experiences, and current coping strategies.

Children and adolescents respond according to the level at which they understand the concept of death or loss (see At a Glance 7-1). The response will reflect the age-related cognitive and psychologic development of the child. A toddler may respond to separation from a parent or attachment figure with anxiety but has no concept of loss. Should that attachment figure not return, the child will usually adapt to another attachment figure who is nurturing. The preschool child reacts with magical thinking, such as in a 5-year-old child who says, "Grandpa is sleeping. Will he wake up in time to take me to the park?" The concept of death as a finality is not yet understood. Associated with the growing moral concept of right and wrong, the school-age child may feel a sense of guilt or responsibility for a loss, such as when a parent is absent following a divorce. Although the adolescent understands the concept of death as finality, it is difficult for this age group to fit death or loss into their search for an identity.

Adults may view loss as temporary or permanent, and most are able to accept their losses and grow from these situations. Acceptance often opens the door of opportunity for new and expanded life experiences. It is important to remember that regardless of age, bereavement is a natural, healthy, and healing process that emerges in response to a significant loss.

At a Glance 7-1 Age-Related Concepts of Loss

Toddlers

- Egocentric and concerned with themselves
- Do not understand concept of loss

Preschool

- Use magical thinking, and may feel shame or guilt when thinking is associated with loss (i.e., belief that behavior is reason a parent is gone, such as in divorce)
- Primitive coping mechanisms result in more intense response
- Do not understand death as permanent

School Age

- Still feel guilt and responsibility in associating negative actions with loss
- Respond to concrete, simple, and logical explanation of death (often explained by death a pet)

Age 9 to 10

- Understand permanence of death and that some losses are temporary

Adolescent

- Able to understand the concept of death, but have difficulty accepting loss
- Perceive loss as a threat to their identity

Mind Jogger

How might failure to achieve one's ambition be seen as a positive experience?

Mind Jogger

How might environmental factors during childhood affect a person's ability to cope with loss?

Grief as a Process

The grieving process describes a series of occurrences in the resolution of loss. This process provides support as an individual works through the feelings of anger, hopelessness, and futility that accompany loss. It provides time to put things into perspective, to place into memory that which is gone, and to emerge with a newly developed embrace of life. Life is an evolving challenge of events that inevitably requires us to cope with disappointment and loss. Learning to deal with these situations in small increments better prepares us to deal effectively with a major loss. We can learn to accept loss as part of living, or we can choose to react with hostility, often suppressing the anger into hidden feelings that eventually may erupt in negative or maladaptive patterns of behavior such as substance abuse or suicide. Learning to cope or adapt to loss involves giving ourselves the right to grieve in whatever timeframe is needed to go through the process. It is important to recognize and accept the feelings, such as anger, fear, and guilt, that are normal and appropriately a part of grieving.

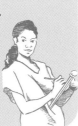

Just the Facts

Other Grief Reactions
Anxiety: Related to future without loved object
Panic: Related to inability to control the outcome
Blame: Self-blame for doing or not doing something to cause the loss

Growth occurs as the bereaved person comes to the point of letting go of the past. This does not reduce the importance of the loss but allows the person to continue living with new perspective. In time, the sadness and loneliness felt as a result of the void left by the cherished object are replaced with hopefulness as one is freed from the previous relationship. This acceptance indicates that the grief process is coming to a close.

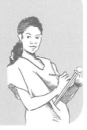

Just the Facts

Grief is a process of working through the emotional response to loss, reorganizing one's life, and accomplishing some degree of resolution or closure.

Stages of Grief

Perhaps the best known theory of bereavement is that of Dr. Elisabeth Kübler-Ross, a German psychiatrist, who described the stages that a person who is facing death, either their own or that of a loved one, encounters before coming to actual acceptance of death as a final stage of life. Dr. Kübler-Ross believed that the dying process is a lifelong process and that we repeat the stages each time we are confronted by loss.

Dr. Kübler-Ross identified five stages that we go through in reaction to loss or death. The first step is shock, disbelief, and **denial** that the event is happening. We want to avoid the reality of the loss and may act as if nothing has occurred, or as though the lost object or person is still present. Denial actually allows us an adjustment period in which to gather coping strategies for the grieving work ahead. As we realize that the loss is real, the denial gives way to feelings of bitterness, **anger,** and turmoil. Anger is expressed in many ways, often demonstrated openly in behaviors such as crying or expressions of self-blame and guilt. Some may turn the anger inward, resulting in physical illness and/or psychologic dysfunction.

Anger may be followed by **bargaining** as we attempt to postpone acceptance of the loss. As is often seen with terminal illness, this is a time when deals with God are attempted as a way to prolong the inevitable. Frequent labile moods are common and are often intermingled with continued anger and unwillingness to accept the loss. This period is gradually followed by a deep sense of loss as the reality of what has happened or is anticipated settles. At this point we may withdraw from social interaction, choosing to spend hours and days alone in the depth of loneliness for that which is gone. **Depression** is a normal response in this process as we adjust to life without the loved object and the full impact of the emptiness. For some people this period is overwhelming and recovery from the depth of sorrow felt is unlikely without professional support and guidance. The final stage is that of

acceptance when the person begins to experience peace and serenity. This is the time of letting go and allowing life to provide new experiences and relationships.

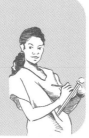

Mind Jogger

What objective signs might indicate a person has reached acceptance?

Just the Facts

Steps of Grieving
- Shock and denial
- Anger and pain
- Negotiation and bargaining
- Withdrawal and depression
- Acceptance and resolution

There are several theories that have evolved concerning the grief process, and while not absolute, the stages of grief supply a basis for understanding this process. A person may experience all stages in rapid succession or rally back and forth between stages, remaining in some longer than others. When the process of grieving becomes prolonged it may be seen as abnormal or maladaptive with symptoms of a major depressive episode such as extreme sadness, insomnia, anorexia, and weight loss. The person may consider these symptoms normal but may seek professional help for the insomnia or appetite loss. According to *DSM-IV-TR*, the diagnosis of major depressive disorder is not generally assigned unless the symptoms are still present 2 months after the loss.

Dysfunctional Grief

The psychologic process of grieving involves an emotional separation from the valued person or object. The loss is felt as a break in the continuity of the person's life and sense of se-curity. Even as life itself involves a series of separations in the search for autonomy and independence, the ability to cope with each loss poses a challenge in adaptive strategy. Coping skills are most often learned through observation of the social environment around us. If an individual has developed the psychologic tools to deal with loss and failure in an adaptive way, these resources will help the person to deal with a major loss in a similar way. However, if an individual has a lifelong pattern of inadequate coping skills, the chances are greater that a resolution to the grieving process will be delayed.

Dysfunctional grief is a failure to complete the grieving process and cope successfully with the loss. **Chronic sorrow** describes the feelings a person has while attempting to deal with the loss. Those factors that may contribute to **unresolved grief,** which then leads to the dysfunction, include:

- Socially unacceptable death such as suicide or homicide
- Missing person related to war or mysterious disappearance or abduction
- Multiple losses or losses in close succession (loss of several family members in short period with financial loss or disaster loss)
- Ambivalent feelings toward the lost person or object
- Unresolved grieving from a previous loss
- Guilt with regard to circumstances at or near the time of death
- Feelings of the survivor that he or she should have died with or instead of the deceased
- Consuming feelings of worthlessness with suicidal tendencies
- Physiologic response to the loss with marked decrease in functioning
- Delusional thinking or hallucinations of seeing the image or hearing the voice of the deceased

Because the intensity of feelings at this level is often desperate, it is essential that the person with prolonged bereavement receive clinical attention and treatment.

Application of the Nursing Process

Nursing Assessment

To deal effectively with the client experiencing grief, the nurse must first face the reality of his or her own mortality and concept of death. The nurse is conditioned by experience and by cultural and religious beliefs that develop a response pattern toward loss. Most people experiencing a crisis of major proportion require assistance and support to complete the grief process. The nurse needs to respect and attempt to understand the importance of grieving for oneself and for others.

During the initial client contact, open-ended statements can be used to determine at what point the person is in the grieving process. It is important to:

- Assess coping strategies that the client has used in the past to deal with individual or family loss.
- Determine what support system is now available to the client through family and friends. Identify the client's feelings related to the loss.
- Use leading statements to elicit any ambivalent feelings, guilt issues, anger, or hopelessness.
- Note if the person is having difficulty expressing feelings about the loss or is reliving the experience with no reduction in the intensity of those feelings.
- Observe the client's body language, noting any incongruence with verbal statements. Assess the potential for self-harm or suicide that may be inferred from the expressed feelings or statements of the grieving person.

Mind Jogger

How might body language indicate a sense of guilt or self-blame for the death or loss?

Nursing Diagnosis

Nursing diagnoses that may be applicable to clients with anticipatory or dysfunctional grieving associated with loss include:

- Grieving, anticipatory, related to actual or perceived loss
- Grieving, dysfunctional, related to lack of resolution to grief process
- Coping, individual ineffective, related to difficulty in expressing feelings
- Adjustment, impaired, related to ineffective attempts to reinvest in relationships
- Hopelessness, related to level of distress accompanying loss
- Sorrow, chronic, related to feelings of worthlessness
- Spiritual distress, related to feelings of despair
- Self-care deficit, related to loss of interest in self and others

Expected Outcomes

Once nursing diagnoses are determined to be relevant to the individual situation, the anticipated outcome can be addressed. Recognizing that the process of grieving is very individualized, it is important to consider the client's past patterns of resolution when setting the measurable criteria for outcome. Expected outcomes may include that the client will:

- Demonstrate progress in the stages of grief at own pace
- Verbalize an understanding of dysfunctional state
- Identify ambivalent feelings associated with the loss object
- Express feelings of sadness with diminishing intensity
- Participate in self-care activities toward independent functioning
- Verbalize belief in hope for the future
- Express interest in reinvesting in social relationships

Nursing Interventions

It is important for the nurse to use communication techniques that allow the grieving person to talk and to provide understanding and support through active listening. The nurse should meet clients' needs and requests as quickly as possible to reassure them of a caring attitude. Other interventions may include:

- Avoid reassuring clichés, such as "I know how hard it is" or "It was for the best." They only serve to decrease the genuineness of the support effort.
- Provide reassurance that feelings are acceptable and normal as the process follows its course.
- Provide referral to a grief support group, which may provide additional help for the grieving individual or family members.
- Encourage client to express feelings openly.
- Assist client to identify ambivalent feelings of guilt or anger toward loss object.
- Have client write letter to the deceased to bring closure to the past relationship.
- Help client to identify maladaptive coping behaviors.
- Assist in developing positive methods of coping with the loss.
- Provide positive feedback for use of effective coping strategies.
- Assist in setting realistic goals for progress in grieving process.
- Encourage client to utilize family, religious, or cultural supports that provide meaning for client.
- Encourage participation in group activities.

Evaluation

Once nursing strategies have been implemented, it is anticipated that the client will have shown progress in dealing with the loss that has occurred. Each person will advance at his or her own pace toward acceptance and resolution of the grief process. Success is determined as the client moves to establish new relationships and put the loss in perspective. Expressions of hope for the future and reinvestment in personal interests will demonstrate a positive self-image that is separated from the past relationship.

Summary

Grief is defined as the emotional process of coping with loss. Loss can occur with the death of a loved one or any person or object that is a needed and cherished entity in our lives. Loss of a job and income, a home, or other important parts of our lives are likely to elicit the same emotions of grief. Grief is the response that is experienced in anticipation of or as a result of a loss. Bereavement includes that process one goes through in adapting to life without the cherished object. Reaction to loss changes with the growth and maturation of cognitive ability. By the age of 9 or 10, the child is able to view death or termination with adult understanding of permanent or temporary loss.

Grief in itself is a process of mourning for the loss, coming to terms with the reality of the loss, and putting it into perspective as we move beyond the period of bereavement. Several theories have evolved that propose that this process involves stages. Dr. Elisabeth Kübler-Ross defined five stages of dying or grief that occur with loss: denial, anger, bargaining, depression, and acceptance. Once the loss is accepted, we are ready to adapt to a new period of growth without the esteemed object. If a person is not able to emerge from the grieving process and remains in a state of unresolved loss, it may fall into the category of maladaptive or dysfunctional grieving. Counseling and treatment may be required for the person with this level of grief.

Nursing interventions for the person who is grieving are centered around support and reassurance that this is a normal and healthy process of emotional response. Providing an atmosphere of open communication and active listening will give the person an outlet for the intense feelings of pain that are part of the healing involved in resolution. Grief support groups are especially helpful for some people who may need to know that they are not alone or that their feelings are not unique but are shared by others who have experienced loss.

Bibliography

American Psychiatric Association (2000). *Diagnostic and statistical manual of mental disorders text revision* (4th ed.). Washington, DC: American Psychiatric Association.

Barry, P. D. (1996). *Psychosocial nursing* (3rd ed.). Philadelphia, PA: Lippincott.

Milliken, M. E. (1998). *Understanding human behavior* (6th ed.). Albany, NY: Delmar.

Student Worksheet

FILL IN THE BLANK

Fill in the blank with the correct answer.

1. _____ is defined as the emotional process of coping with a loss.

2. Those who may be expecting a major loss in the near future will usually experience _____ grief.

3. The period of time involved in the process of adapting to loss is often referred to as _____.

4. Statements made to the person who is grieving that are seemingly appropriate but tend to be empty and show little support are termed _____.

5. _____ describes an actual or perceived change in a relationship between a person and a valued object or other person.

6. The 5-year-old child reacts to separation from a loved person or object with _____ thinking.

7. A lack of resolution to the grief process is referred to as _____.

MATCHING

Match the following stages of grief with the appropriate description.

a. Deep sense of loss with withdrawal from social interaction.

b. Adjustment period in which the reality of the loss is avoided.

c. Labile moods and attempts to make deals to postpone the loss.

d. Time of peaceful letting go and allowing life to move forward.

e. Feelings of bitterness, self-blame, guilt, and hostility.

1. _____ Denial

2. _____ Anger

3. _____ Bargaining

4. _____ Depression

5. _____ Acceptance

MULTIPLE CHOICE

1. Joan is scheduled for a radical mastectomy. As the nurse enters Joan's hospital room, the client says, "It would be easier if I just didn't wake up from the surgery." The best response for the nurse to make at this time is:

   a. "You are just afraid now. Everything will look different tomorrow."

   b. "You feel it would be easier to die than to face the loss of your breast?"

   c. "Some people feel the way you do, but this does not mean the end of your life."

   d. "Why do you think it would be easier to die than to wake up after surgery?"

2. Which of the following is Joan experiencing?

   a. Resolution

   b. Conventional grief

   c. Bargaining

   d. Anticipatory grief

3. Maria has been in a comatose state for the past 8 months as a result of an automobile accident. Although doctors have told her husband, Reuben, that there is no brain function, Reuben insists that she is showing purposeful response. Which of the following stages of grief is Reuben experiencing?

   a. Bargaining

   b. Anger

   c. Denial

   d. Depression

4. Which of the following describes how 9-year-old Jeremy would most likely respond to the death of his grandfather?

   a. Feels death happened because he went skating with a friend instead of visiting his sick grandfather.

   b. Sees the loss as interfering with his ability to determine a sense of who he is.

   c. Believes that angels took his grandfather in a chariot and went riding into the sky.

   d. Would not understand the concept of permanent loss.

SCENARIO: LOST AND ALONE

The clinic nurse is assessing Art, whose wife died 6 months ago. He describes himself as "lost, forgetful, and unable to concentrate." He also states, "I seem to cry at the most inconvenient moments, so I just stay to myself." What feelings might be responsible for Art's symptoms?

_____

_____

How should the nurse respond to Art?

_____

_____

_____

What stage of the grief process is Art most likely experiencing?

_____

_____

What referrals may be appropriate for Art?

_____

_____

_____

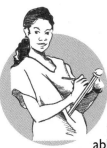

LEARNING OBJECTIVES

After learning the content in this chapter, the student will be able to:

1. Distinguish between common anxiety and anxiety as a symptom.
2. Identify precipitating factors in uncontrolled anxiety attacks.
3. Assess signs and symptoms characteristic of anxiety in each disorder.
4. Identify nursing diagnoses related to anxiety disorders.
5. Develop realistic anticipated outcomes for clients with anxiety disorders.
6. Plan appropriate nursing interventions toward client improvement.
7. Evaluate the effectiveness of planned nursing interventions toward goals.

CHAPTER

8

Anxiety Disorders

KEY TERMS

Agoraphobia
Anticipatory anxiety
Automatic relief behaviors
Compulsion
Cued
Emotional numbing
Free-floating anxiety
Generalized anxiety
Obsession
Panic attack
Social phobia
Specific phobia
Uncued

Anxiety as a Symptom

Anxiety is a vague, uneasy emotional feeling experienced by everyone in response to a perceived threat or danger. As the stimulus of a threatening situation is processed by the brain, the result is fear. Anxiety is felt as the fear is realized. It is when anxiety increases to the point of discomfort or distress that the person senses something is wrong. Sometimes the person can identify the stimulus that is causing the uncomfortable feeling. In other cases, a cause cannot be identified. **Free-floating anxiety** occurs when the person is unable to connect the anxiety to a stimulus. This factor in itself can create additional anxiety.

The manifestations of anxiety can take many forms. Experiences range from vague discomfort to extreme panic. Increased levels of anxiety can be experienced continuously or periodically. Thoughts, feelings, and behavior are all affected as anxiety increases. A person may act "out of character" or in a bizarre manner, such as counting continuously or shouting. This is illustrated by a person who is late for an appointment and delayed in traffic. When a police officer approaches, telling him there is an accident scene that will be cleared in about 30 minutes, the man starts shouting at the officer. In other situations, subtle anxiety behaviors such as clenching the jaws, tapping fingers on a table, fidgeting, and other behaviors may be evident. These automatic relief behaviors are aimed at relieving the anxiety. Although the person may be unaware of their actions, they may be annoying to other people. For example, the person sitting next to you at a conference is constantly clicking her ballpoint pen. After this continues for nearly 30 minutes, you ask her if she would mind laying her pen down as you cannot hear the speaker. Unaware of her behavior, she apologizes. She states that she is "very nervous in this room full of people." She goes on to say, "I was required to be here to keep my job." Both people in this example are experiencing anxiety, but the anxiety being experienced by the person who is uncomfortable in a crowded room will most likely continue to escalate unless she leaves the room. This situation illustrates how anxiety is created. Unless measures are taken to remove the cause, anxiety continues to grow. If it is unrelieved and continues over time, an underlying disorder may be identified.

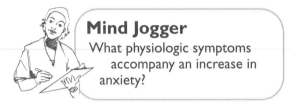

Mind Jogger
What physiologic symptoms accompany an increase in anxiety?

Anxiety Disorders

Anxiety disorders are described as a set of disorders that are characterized by uncontrolled anxiety that leads to impairment in social, interpersonal, and work functioning. Although signs and symptoms may vary from disorder to disorder, the common thread or feature of these conditions is overwhelming anxiety. Unlike anxiety felt briefly during a thunderstorm, the level of anxiety that leads to a disorder is disabling and progressive unless treatment is obtained. Anxiety that is out of control is the underlying cause of anxiety disorders.

Panic Disorder

A **panic attack** is described as an intense feeling of fear or terror that occurs suddenly and intermittently without warning. The person experiencing the panic is unable to determine when these attacks will occur or reoccur. When the person is unable to connect any particular stimulus with the panic attack, it is referred to as one that is **uncued.** It is said to be **cued** when an identified trigger can be associated with the attack. Some people may only experience a single attack, while others go on to develop a panic disorder.

A panic disorder is characterized by recurrent, unexpected panic attacks. The frequency and severity of these attacks may vary. Some people may be able to endure brief exposure to the situation that causes panic. Others may not be able to expose themselves to the situation at all. When this occurs, the consequences of the disorder are much greater, and the functional capacity of the person decreases significantly.

Mind Jogger

What type of life situations might trigger recurrent panic attacks?

Signs and Symptoms. A state of panic results in sympathetic nervous system symptoms of heart pounding, palpitations, dizziness, sweating, weakness, and numbness. The person may also feel shaky and chilled with accompanying nausea, chest pain, feelings of suffocation, and being out of control. Attacks may occur daily, weekly, or monthly. Attacks may also occur during the night. Most last only a few minutes, but they may last longer. People experiencing panic attacks often have a fear of "going crazy" or "losing it." Self-esteem may also be affected in varying degrees. Many seek frequent medical attention because of their fear of having a life-threatening illness. Fear of having the "next attack" can cause significant impairment in the person's overall functioning.

Just the Facts

Persons who become aware of their anxiety learn to identify specific fears that overwhelm them during a panic attack.

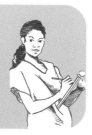

People with panic disorder often develop **agoraphobia,** or an avoidance of certain places or situations that tend to trigger the panic attacks. Because they fear a reoccurrence of the panic state, they often restrict their activities to avoid the possibility of this happening. Everyday activities such as shopping for groceries and attending church or family events may be avoided because of fear that escape from these situations might be difficult or embarrassing. They may have fears of being in a crowd or on a bridge, or traveling in a bus, airplane, or automobile. Should the person be entrapped in this situation, the anxiety experienced would lead to a feeling of helplessness and panic. By limiting the possibilities that this would happen, the person often becomes homebound or restricted to home surroundings.

At a Glance 8-1 Signs and Symptoms of Panic Disorder

- Heartbeat rapid and pounding
- Increased perspiration
- Chilling or flushing
- Tingling or numbness of hands
- Nausea
- Chest pain
- Feeling of being suffocated
- Fear of being out of control
- Fear of dying or having a heart attack
- Agoraphobia
- Depression

Incidence and Etiology. Although they can occur at any age, panic disorders typically have an onset between late adolescence and the mid-30s. First-generation biologic relatives are more likely to develop the disorder. Agoraphobia and panic disorders are also more prevalent in females than males. More than 95% of those diagnosed with agoraphobia have an accompanying diagnosis of panic disorder.

Case Study: Jack Goes to the Baseball Game

Jack is a 42-year-old male who loves baseball. However, Jack has a fear of crowded places from which there is no accessible exit. Jack usually has been able to secure a ticket for a seat close to the exit ramp. Once there, he discovers that his ticket is not for an aisle seat. He suddenly becomes very aware that the stadium is crowded and he will have to move between many people to get to his seat. He begins to feel his heart throb and has a general flushed feeling. Little beads of sweat begin to form on his scalp and down his back. Instead of going to his seat, he quickly goes back down the ramp toward the main entrance to the stadium. Thinking he will never get there, he has to weave around and in between people the entire trip. At this point, he panics and feels a sense of terror. He suddenly cannot think and feels nearly paralyzed. A stranger notices his distress and offers to drive him to the hospital. Jack manages to nod "yes" but is unable to verbalize which hospital. The stranger takes him to a nearby hospital to get help.

How does Jack's behavior support the presence of a panic disorder?

_____

_____

_____

In what way is Jack's behavior different from free-floating anxiety?

_____

_____

How is this problem impairing his ability to function in a social setting?

_____

_____

Mind Jogger

What impact would agoraphobia have on a person's lifestyle?

Specific Phobia

A specific phobia is characterized by an excessive and persistent irrational fear of specific objects or situations that actually pose little threat of danger. The common cate-

Unemployment and school drop-out is common. Decreased work functioning is evidenced by the inability to complete tasks, repeated absences, and difficulty interacting with others. Up to two thirds of those with this disorder also experience depression or engage in substance abuse to cope with the anxiety.

Just the Facts
Specific phobias usually cause little concern because the person can plan ahead to avoid the feared stimulus.

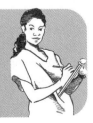

At a Glance 8-2 Examples of Specific Phobias

Fear of animals—zoophobia
Fear of fire—pyrophobia
Fear of riding in a car—amaxophobia
Fear of sleep—somniphobia
Fear of confined spaces—claustrophobia
Fear of spiders—arachnophobia
Fear of yellow color—xanthophobia
Fear of ghosts—phasmophobia
Fear of blood—hematophobia
Fear of the number 13—triskaidekaphobia
Fear of heights—acrophobia
Fear of crossing a bridge—gephyrophobia
Fear of germs—microphobia
Fear of pain—algophobia
Fear of thunder—brontophobia

gories of phobias include animals, height, water, storms, blood or needles, flying, elevators, or enclosed spaces. Others may have a fear of sensations such as choking or falling.

Signs and Symptoms. When a person comes in contact with the object or situation that causes the fear, the person usually experiences an immediate severe anxiety or panic attack. The distance between the person and the feared object will affect the level of response. A person who fears dogs will experience the most anxiety while in close proximity to the animal. Whether there is a way to escape from the feared stimulus also plays a role in the intensity of the anxiety the person feels. A person who has a fear of going over bridges, for example, will have the most anxiety if there is no way to avoid crossing the bridge. Although children may not be aware of the stimulus causing the anxiety, adolescents and adults are usually aware that their response is extreme and unrealistic. Those with intense fears may experience anxiety symptoms when just thinking about the precipitating factor.

Some people avoid the activities of everyday life because they experience discomfort or increased anxiety when faced with the feared stimulus. During times when there is no exposure to the feared object or situation, however, their anxiety level is no higher that it would normally be. It is when this avoidance significantly impairs the person's ability to continue functioning in social and work settings that the diagnosis of specific phobia is made.

At a Glance 8-3 Signs and Symptoms of Specific Phobia

- Irrational and persistent fear of object or situation
- Immediate anxiety on contact with feared object or situation
- Loss of control, fainting, or panic response
- Avoidance of activities involving feared stimulus
- Anxiety when thinking about stimulus
- Worry with anticipatory anxiety
- Possible impaired social or work functioning

Incidence and Etiology. Specific phobias affect over six million adult American people. They are twice as common in females as males. Although phobias are common, they are rarely severe enough to be diagnosed. Symptoms usually have an onset during childhood or adolescence and persist throughout adult life. The fear of a particular stimulus is usually present for some time before it is severe enough to be considered a disorder. Phobias following a traumatic event such as the fear of water after a near-drowning situation can develop at any age.

Social Phobia (Social Anxiety Disorder)

Social phobia is characterized by excessive fear of any social situation in which embarrassment is possible. The person with this disorder experiences intense discomfort when being watched or at risk of being judged or ridiculed by others.

Typical occasions where this occurs are social activities and occasions where the person will be speaking, dining, or writing in public. Although the person may recognize that the fear is extreme and unrealistic, they are helpless to stop it. Social anxiety may be related to one particular situation such as indoor activities or loud music, or it may be related to social occasions in general. Symptoms may be severe enough to interfere with the person's work or school functioning. Social isolation may result in which the person has few friends or contacts.

Mind Jogger

How might social phobia prevent a person from fulfilling goals in life?

Just the Facts

Persons with social phobia often try to decrease the overwhelming anxiety felt in the feared situation by using drugs and/or alcohol.

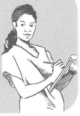

Signs and Symptoms. Physical symptoms of anxiety are usually experienced by the person with social phobia. These may include hyperventilation, trembling hands or voice, inability to speak correctly, blushing, sweating, muscle tension, or diarrhea. The person may be embarrassed by the symptoms, which adds to their discomfort. Most people will avoid the difficult situation altogether, while others will tolerate the activity but with intense anxiety.

Anticipatory anxiety occurs well in advance of a particular situation such as a public speech or social event. This leads to thoughts of dread leading up to the event. The

added anxiety results in actual or perceived failure in the situation, leading to embarrassment and further anxiety. This pattern sets up a vicious cycle of persistent discomfort that can be incapacitating. Many people who have social phobia are underachievers because of test anxiety, poor job performance, or poor communication skills. They may have few or no friends, a decreased support system, and poor interpersonal relationships.

At a Glance 8-4 Signs and Symptoms of Social Phobia

- Hyperventilation
- Sweating, cold, and clammy hands
- Blushing
- Palpitations
- Confusion
- Gastrointestinal symptoms
- Trembling hands and voice
- Urinary urgency
- Muscle tension
- Anticipatory anxiety
- Fear of embarrassment or ridicule

Incidence and Etiology. The incidence of social phobia tends to be equally distributed between men and women. The disorder usually has an onset in childhood or early adolescence. Onset may be abrupt, following an embarrassing event, or may be insidious or slow in onset. There is a tendency for this condition to run in families.

Obsessive-Compulsive Disorder

Obsessive-compulsive disorder (OCD) is characterized by **obsessions** or the reoccurrence of persistent unwanted thoughts or images that cause the person intense anxiety. **Compulsions** are the repetitive behaviors or rituals the person engages in to reduce the high level of anxiety. For diagnosis, the obsessions and compulsions have to be severe enough to cause a significant decline in the client's level of functioning with the actions consuming at least 1 hour of the person's day.

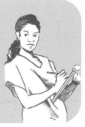

Signs and Symptoms. It is common for everyone to have some recurring uncomfortable thoughts or concern, for example, whether a car is locked or garage door closed. However, in OCD, the thoughts tend to be related to sexuality, violence, illness, death, or contamination. These thoughts are frequently invasive and inappropriate. The person may recognize the thoughts as unusual and self-generated but has no ability to control them. This lack of control leads to the extreme anxiety.

In an attempt to deal with the anxiety, the person performs repetitive acts that serve no purpose but to relieve the anxiety. The person who feels contaminated with sexual thoughts may wash his hair repeatedly until the scalp is bleeding. The person with violent thoughts of harming her family may check locks and gas knobs every few minutes. In the person with OCD, the symptoms severely interfere with social and occupational functioning. The ability to finish a task is impaired by lack of concentration, invasion of the obsessive thoughts, and need to perform the actions. Symptoms may be intermittent or get worse over time.

Mind Jogger

How would fear of riding in an automobile affect the quality of a person's life?

At a Glance 8-5 Common Types of Obsessive Thought Content

- Contamination—thoughts of being polluted with germs (e.g., by touching doorknobs or shaking hands with others).
- Repeated doubts—questioning thoughts as to whether one did or did not do something (e.g., turning off the stove or locking the door).
- Orderliness—thinking that one has to have everything in a particular order (e.g., placing things symmetrically on the desk or dresser, placing shoes in alphabetical order by color in a closet, or wearing clothes that always match perfectly with shoes and accessories). When the order is disrupted for any reason, the person experiences intense distress.
- Impulses that are aggressive or horrific in nature—recurring thoughts about doing actions that could bring great distress to others (e.g., hurting someone who is completely defenseless such as a baby or a person who is physically impaired).
- Sexual imagery—thoughts about sexually revealing images or pornography (e.g., a person sees all people of the opposite sex as wearing see-through clothing or a monogamous married person thinks about sexual activity with multiple partners).

At a Glance 8-6 Signs and Symptoms of Obsessive-Compulsive Disorder

- Recurrent unwanted thoughts referencing contamination, sexuality, aggression, need for perfection, or abnormal doubt
- Attempts to reduce the effect of the thoughts with other thoughts
- Repetitive acts, impulses, or rituals such as showering, washing hair or hands, checking, hoarding, rearranging things for perfect alignment, repeating words or phrases
- Recognition that the thoughts are produced in his or her own mind
- Lack of concentration and task completion
- Impaired social or work functioning

Case Study: Not Good Enough

Meredith is a 25-year-old college student who has OCD. She has an older brother, Vince, who is a practicing lawyer. Meredith's parents have told her that she "can't hold a candle to Vince." No matter what she does or how well she does in her college courses, she never does as well as her brother. Recently, Meredith has begun having recurring thoughts that if her brother were not here, maybe she could be "somebody" to her parents. She finds herself wishing he would be killed in an accident or struck by lightning. She realizes the extreme and unreasonable nature of these thoughts, but cannot control their continuous intrusion in her mind or the anxiety they create. She has begun calling Vince 20 to 30 times night and day to make sure he is okay. He cannot convince her there is nothing wrong with him. Meredith is having difficulty maintaining her concentration and has been skipping classes to make the phone calls. Vince does not understand what is wrong with Meredith but is becoming annoyed by the phone calls. He has his mobile and home phone numbers changed and asks his secretary to screen calls at his office. This action increases Meredith's anxiety. She has decided to drop out of her college classes and moves to a location adjacent to Vince's home.

How is Meredith's behavior characteristic of OCD?

_____

_____

What impact is this behavior having on her functioning? How does changing the phone numbers affect Meredith?

_____

_____

What psychologic factors may be causing her obsessive-compulsive behavior?

_____

_____

_____

_____

Incidence and Etiology. Occurrence of OCD is evenly distributed between males and females, although it tends to occur at an earlier age in males. Prevalence within the general population is less than 5%. Onset is usually in childhood or adolescence. Most adults with the disorder have experienced the symptoms since childhood. There tends to be an occurrence of the behavior pattern in families.

Posttraumatic Stress Disorder

Posttraumatic stress disorder (PTSD) is characteristically seen when a person has been subjected to a situation that involves an actual death or threat of severe injury. The trauma can be related to one's own personal physical well-being, observing someone else's death or severe injury, or receiving word that a close relative has been seriously injured or has died. In each situation, the person experiences an intense feeling of fear and dread with each recurring mental rerun of the event.

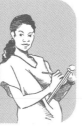

Just the Facts
Traumatic events may include military combat, terrorist attack, robbery, automobile accident, sexual assault, murder, kidnapping, or natural disaster.

Signs and Symptoms. The person with this disorder is plagued with increased anxiety that was not present before the precipitating event. Some people may feel extreme guilt for surviving when others did not survive. People, activities, or places that may be connected to the situation are avoided because of the **emotional numbing** that accompanies the exposure. This numbness is shown by an expression of little or no emotion soon after the event as an attempt to prevent future mental pain. The person may continue to show a lack of affect for the remainder of his or her life. It is common for the person to mentally reexperience the event or to reencounter the trauma in dreams. This may lead to insomnia, inability to concentrate, and impaired social or work functioning. The duration of symptoms must be longer than 1 month to be given the diagnosis of PTSD.

It is not uncommon for people experiencing the symptoms of PTSD to dissociate or depersonalize as a result of the mental anguish they experience. (For more information on dissociation, see Chapter 14.) Panic attacks, perceptual alterations or hallucinations, and depression may also result. Some people may resort to violence, drugs, or suicide to deal with the recurring disturbing mental pictures.

Exposure to similar events can also impose flashbacks or mental images that increase the chances of these complications.

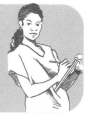

Just the Facts
During a flashback, the person feels as though he or she is reliving the traumatic experience.

Mind Jogger
Why do you think substance abuse tends to be more common in persons with PTSD?

At a Glance 8-7 **Signs and Symptoms of Posttraumatic Stress Disorder**

- Intense feeling or fear and dread following traumatic event
- Mental reruns of the event
- Emotional numbness following the event
- Avoidance of people, places, or things associated with event
- Insomnia
- Increased vigilance or watchfulness
- Startles easily
- Irritability and aggressiveness
- Depression
- Impaired social or work functioning
- Difficulty in interpersonal relationships

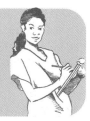

Just the Facts
Persons with PTSD may experience an general lack of trust that impairs their ability to interact with others.

Incidence and Etiology. Not everyone who is exposed to a traumatic experience develops a posttraumatic disorder. Factors that contribute to this disorder include the sudden occurrence of the event, such as a plane crash or fatal accident; the severity of the situation, such as the horror of the Oklahoma City bombing or the terrorist attack of 9-11; and the time of exposure, such as that seen in a kidnapping or hostage situation. PTSD is more common in females and can be seen in any age-group. When seen in children, the child may be unaware of the thoughts but demonstrates the trauma through repetitive play. There is evidence that PTSD is more common if there is a family history of the disorder.

Generalized Anxiety Disorder

In **generalized anxiety** disorder, the person experiences an increased level of anxiety and worry about various situations on most days over a period of at least 6 months. The person has difficulty controlling the anxiety, leading to considerable discomfort, lack of concentration, and impaired ability to function.

Signs and Symptoms. In addition to the excessive worry and anxiety over several different activities or events, the person also experiences at least three other symptoms that include restlessness, irritability, muscle tension, difficulty falling or staying asleep, and fatigue. Other somatic complaints may also be reported such as chest pain, hyperventilation, or gastrointestinal disturbances. The existence of continued tension and feeling on edge leads to a reduced quality of life and overall dissatisfaction with self and others. The occurrence of symptoms may be cyclical but tend to be chronic in nature.

> ### Mind Jogger
> What factors might contribute to the familial tendency of generalized anxiety disorder?

> **At a Glance 8-8** Signs and Symptoms of Generalized Anxiety Disorder
>
> - Chronic excessive worry and anxiety (no particular stimulus)
> - Negative self-talk
> - Fatigue
> - Difficulty falling or staying asleep
> - Increased startle reflex
> - Inability to relax
> - Muscle tension
> - Anticipating the "worst"
> - Inability to control the anxiety
> - Tremors
> - Irritability
> - Headaches
> - Breathing difficulties
> - Increased urinary frequency
> - Gastrointestinal disturbances

Incidence and Etiology. Most people who are diagnosed with generalized anxiety disorder have felt excessive worry and anxiety all of their life, although most do not request treatment until their mid-30s. Onset is usually in childhood or early adolescence and is often associated with stressful life situations. Anxiety tends to run in families and is more common in females. A coexisting diagnosis of depression is commonly seen with generalized anxiety disorder.

> ### Just the Facts
> Typical fears of the person with generalized anxiety disorder include physical injury, major illness or death, mental illness, loss of control, and rejection.
>
>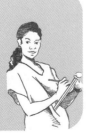

Application of the Nursing Process

When establishing a nurse–client relationship with the person experiencing excessive anxiety, it is important to initially take steps to lower the anxiety level. The person cannot identify the problem until this is accomplished. The nurse can best encourage trust by a calm and reassuring approach.

Nursing Assessment

During assessment of clients with high levels of anxiety, the nurse should make observations of basic characteristics such as thought processes, affect, communication, and psychomotor and physiologic responses. The nurse should use directive questions to elicit subjective information about how the client is currently feeling and what happened before the onset of symptoms. At a Glance 8-8 provides examples of leading statements the nurse can use to gain an understanding of the situation from the client's perspective. Ask the client about other somatic symptoms such as fatigue, muscle aches, eating patterns, bowel habits, sleeping patterns, and fatigue that might further indicate a psychologic origin for the complaints. Observe the client during activities of daily living and interaction with others to determine when symptoms are most obvious. Assessing the client during usual activities can also provide clues about the client's thought processes. Even though something may not mean much to others, it may be very meaningful to the client. For example, while sitting in the dayroom with peers watching a movie, a client leaves the room quietly and does not return. When assessing what just happened, the nurse finds out that part of the movie took place in a circus, similar to the circus where the client had been raped as a child. Although seeing a circus in a movie was insignificant to the other clients, it was very significant to that particular client. Withdrawing from the stimulus was an attempt to lower anxiety.

> **At a Glance 8-9** Leading Statements That Encourage Client Participation in Providing Information
>
> - Tell me what happened.
> - Tell me details of what happened.
> - How did you feel at that time?
> - What were you thinking when that happened?
> - What emotion were you feeling at that particular time?
> - Give me a specific example of what that was like for you.
> - Tell me more about that.
> - Go on . . . And . . .
> - Who was there?
> - Who were you there with?
> - What year did this occur?
> - What did friends and family say to you?
> - Can you describe your feeling?
> - How do you feel right now?
> - What emotion do you feel?
> - What are you doing to decrease that feeling?
> - What can you do to decrease that feeling when this situation happens outside this room?

When faced with a frightening situation, a person's anxiety levels increase and his or her thoughts can become more disorganized or extremely focused. The client may complain of not being able to collect his or her thoughts or not being able to control the thoughts. Either way, the client is unable to think, speak, or perform tasks as effectively as before. While taking a test, for example, a student knows the answer to a question but cannot recall it. The student can remember what page the answer is on and which paragraph it is in, but still cannot recall it. This is an example of increased anxiety affecting thought processes of memory. Thought blocking or inability to recall information is a common response when suddenly faced with increased anxiety. After relaxing at home later that evening, the student may be able to recall the answer without difficulty. When questioning clients, the nurse must remember that thought blocking may occur and further increase the client's anxiety. Clients may approach the staff at a later time stating the information asked of them earlier.

The nurse also needs to note the client's affect. Affect usually provides more meaningful insight into the client's feelings because it is harder to disguise facial expressions. A client may report that he is fine but has a facial grimace. The facial expression usually reflects true feelings before behavior does. The nurse may note a flat affect several times during the day when the client is unaware that she is being observed. The nurse should observe for congruence of nonverbal and verbal messages during each observation or contact with the client.

It is also important for the nurse to determine how well the client is able to communicate. When assessing for interactive skills, the nurse should take into consideration the client's level of education. For example, a client who has been in the hospital for 4 days consistently complains about the food and asks the staff to order something different for him. Noting that he selects food for the following day from a menu, the nurse observes him during the time he is making selections. The client is very anxious and unable to make decisions or direct thought processes long enough to mark the menu. Using a sensitive approach, the nurse determines that the client is illiterate and is unable to understand what food choices are available. Determining how well the client is able to communicate thoughts is also relevant. If the speech is choppy and pressured, the client may be experiencing anxiety and subsequent distress from impaired communication skills. During interaction with the client, the nurse must also be aware of his or her own verbal and nonverbal message. Anxiety is contagious and can contribute to the client's difficulty in communicating.

The client's ability to perform and complete tasks should be observed. Psychomotor responses can reach a hyperactive level and be counterproductive when anxiety is high. On the other hand, when anxiety is extremely high, psychomotor responses can become slowed and also decrease functional ability. The nurse needs to determine if the client's inability to perform tasks is the result of impaired thought processes or impaired motor responses. For example, when observing a depressed client attempting to get dressed, the nurse notes several articles of clothing lying on the bed. The client is across the room crying and wringing her fingers. At this point, the nurse concludes the client may be experiencing increased anxiety about making a decision between choices of what to wear.

Observation of the client with particular attention to specific anxiety-reducing behaviors should be part of the initial and ongoing assessment for each client. Sometimes symptoms are expressed in subtle ways, such as leaving group therapy to go to the bathroom or avoiding an activity where several clients are participating. It is important to note if behaviors are improving with the administration of antianxiety medications. Observation for side effects of these drugs is also a nursing responsibility.

Nursing Diagnosis

Once the assessment is made and data are collected, the information is reviewed and sorted into meaningful clusters. From this data, problems are identified to determine applicable nursing diagnoses. Relevant nursing diagnoses for the client with an anxiety disorder may include:

- Anxiety, related to feeling of actual or perceived threat
- Anxiety, related to intrusive thought processes
- Ineffective individual coping, related to unmet needs
- Fear, related to extreme and unrealistic perceptions
- Powerlessness, related to lack of control over anxiety

- Risk for violence directed at self or others, related to reoccurring intrusive thoughts
- Sleep pattern disturbance, related to excessive worry and anxiety
- Social isolation, related to feelings of guilt or emotional numbness
- Altered family processes, related to situational crisis
- Skin integrity, impaired, related to compulsive repetitive behaviors
- Self esteem disturbance, related to feelings of inadequacy

Expected Outcomes

Once the nursing diagnosis is made, appropriate outcomes for clients can be determined. Careful consideration should be given to a realistic time frame in which the outcomes can be achieved. Outcomes are always client centered and time limited. Examples of outcomes may include that within 7 days, the client will:

- Identify initial signs and symptoms of anxiety
- Identify effective coping methods to use when anxiety begins to occur
- Demonstrate effective strategies to lower anxiety
- Experience increased energy
- Identify alternative methods of coping that decrease social isolation
- Demonstrate decreased cleaning rituals
- Participate in small group discussions with decreased anxiety
- Look at pictures of a phobic stimulus without excessive anxiety
- Ventilate anxiety appropriately and safely to others
- Experience improved sleep pattern
- Demonstrate improved impulse control

Nursing Interventions

When dealing with anxiety in others, the nurse should take into consideration his or her own anxiety level and how it may affect nursing care. Subtle behaviors such as a change in the tone of voice, rushed movements, or spending less time with the client can communicate the nurse's anxiety to the client. This in turn can generate increased anxiety in the client. Establishing a sense of trust includes an ability to maintain a calm and supportive environment in which the client feels a sense of safety and security. It is important to use caution when touching or approaching the person having a panic attack This action by the nurse may pose an additional threat to the client or invasion of his or her personal space.

When planning interventions, the nurse must remember that interventions should be timely, client-centered, and realistic. The nurse should plan only what the client is able to do at that time. It may be difficult for the client to take more than small steps toward reaching expected outcomes. Overwhelming the client with unrealistic expectations may indicate increased anxiety in the nurse and counterproductive results in the client. Assessing the client's tolerance for change is essential for planning appropriate client-centered nursing interventions. Reassessment should occur to ensure the continuing relevance of the interventions. Every effort should be made to assist the client in identifying the issues that precipitate the feelings of anxiety. Linking the behavior exhibited by the client to a particular situation can help the client to develop an awareness of feelings that precede the anxiety attacks. The nurse can also model and help the client to try new, more adaptive coping strategies.

Additional nursing interventions include:

- Encourage participation in social interaction and exercise activities.
- Give positive reinforcement for the client's efforts to participate.
- Teach stress-management techniques (progressive relaxation, music therapy, deep-breathing).
- Give positive reinforcement for the client's efforts to participate.

- Assist the client with compulsive behaviors to find ways to set limits on the rituals.
- Acknowledge the behaviors but do not focus on them—it is important to express an empathetic response rather than criticize the behavior. For example, in response to a client who has shampooed her hair 4 times in 2 hours, the nurse might say, "I am sure your scalp is getting sore from washing your hair so much," rather than, "You only need to wash your hair once a day."
- Observe for automatic-relief behaviors.
- Encourage open discussion of feelings and thoughts.
- Monitor for indications of escalating anxiety.

At a Glance 8-10 Sources of Information on Anxiety Disorders

National Institute of Mental Health (NIMH)
6001 Executive Blvd., Room 8184, MSC 9663
Bethesda, MD 208922-9663
Phone: 301-443-4513 or 1-866-615-NIMH
(6464), toll-free
(www.nimh.nih.gov)
Anxiety Disorders Association of America
8730 Georgia Ave., Suite 600
Silver Springs, MD 20910
(www.adaa.org)
Obsessive Compulsive (OC) Foundation
227 Notch Hill Road
North Branford, CT 06471
(www.ocfoundation.org)
National Mental Health Association (NMHA)
2001 N. Beauregard St., 12th Floor
Alexandria, VA 22311
Phone: 1-800-969-6642
(www.nmha.org)
American Psychological Association
750 1st St., NE
Washington, DC 20002-4242
Phone: 1-888-357-7924
(www.psych.org/index.cfm)

- Encourage time-out for impulsive clients to regain self-control.
- Administer antianxiety medications.
- Provide explanations regarding medications and side effects to client and family.
- Avoid giving advice to client.
- Provide client education regarding anxiety and precipitating factors.

Evaluation

Evaluation of the plan of care occurs at the end of the time-frame that was set to reach client outcomes. Success is determined based on whether the outcome criteria were achieved. The plan of care is revised if outcomes were not met, the problem persists, or if a new problem has developed.

Effectiveness of planned interventions will be demonstrated in the client's ability to recognize and deal with the anxiety-producing factors. Once the client identifies the relationship between unreasonable thoughts and subsequent behaviors, it is more realistic to anticipate the use of more effective coping strategies to reduce his or her anxiety. It is important for the client to openly express feelings and thoughts related to the situation. The effectiveness of active listening by the nurse and learned coping skills are shown when the client reports that anxiety has been reduced to a manageable level. This can also be demonstrated as the client shows relaxed participation in unit activities and reports longer periods of restful sleep. Further indication of learned skills is shown as the impulsive client resolves conflict situations using improved self-control. It is anticipated that through learning what precipitating factors can be changed and steps that can be taken to lower anxiety for those that cannot be changed, the client will demonstrate more effective problem-solving methods to improve overall functioning and well-being.

Summary

Anxiety is an unconscious uneasy feeling that everyone experiences at some time. Although we are often unaware of what is causing this feeling, we exercise ways to cope with the situation and continue to manage everyday life. When the anxiety that accompanies events or situations that are perceived as threatening is increased to high levels, some people are unable to find an effective way to respond. The inability to associate a precipitating factor with the subsequent uncontrolled behavior is common to all people with anxiety disorders.

The level of anxiety that results in a disorder is intense and disabling. Unlike that experienced momentarily, the person with panic level of anxiety feels a sense of terror and fear that leaves them exhausted and emotionally drained. Some who have panic attacks develop agoraphobia and avoid places or events that tend to trigger the response. The excessive and persistent nature of the irrational fears is also demonstrated in those who experience intense anxiety when exposed to specific objects or situations. A social activity in which embarrassment is possible is also a contributing factor. Although the person may recognize that the fear is extreme and unreasonable, they are unable to control the symptoms. In other situations, the person may have reoccurring unwanted thoughts or images that produce intense anxiety. The person converts this anxiety into a compulsive action that provides a primary gain of reducing the anxiety. The actions are repetitive and ritualistic in nature and tend to have a crippling effect on the person's ability to carry out personal, work, and social responsibilities. The person is usually aware that the thoughts are psychologic but is unable to control them.

Experiencing or witnessing a horrific event can be emotional devastation. It is not uncommon for those who are subjected to an actual threat of death or severe injury to respond with a posttraumatic response. Whether the incident involves the person or someone close to them, the reaction is emotionally numbing and leaves continued mental images that intermittently plague the conscious mind. Without treatment, the person may resort to violence, drugs, or suicide to cope with the flashbacks that occur without warning.

Treatment of anxiety is focused on reducing the anxiety level to a point at which the person can identify the precipitating factors and their connection to the resulting behaviors. Antianxiety medications may be needed initially to reduce the anxiety to a level at which the client is able to review the present incident along with past incidents and previous methods of coping. Once ineffective skills are identified, improved methods of adapting and managing future situations can be taught and implemented. The nurse's role is important in assessing symptoms and client response to the therapeutic milieu. When interacting with clients, the nurse should learn to monitor his or her own anxiety level. Anxiety is contagious and easily transferred to the client. A calm and reassuring approach is necessary to give the client a sense of a safe and supportive environment. Explanations with an unhurried manner will go a long way in helping the client to trust others and participate in treatment.

Bibliography

American Psychiatric Association (2000). *Diagnostic and statistical manual of mental disorders text revision* (4th ed.). Washington DC: American Psychiatric Association.

Beck, A. T., & Emery, G. (1985). *Anxiety disorders and phobias: A cognitive perspective.* New York, NY: Harper Collins Publishers.

Doenges, M. E., Townsend, M. C., & Moorhouse, M. F. (1995). *Psychiatric care plans* (3rd ed.). Philadelphia, PA: F. A. Davis Co.

Leger, E., Ladouceur, R., Dugas, M. J., & Freeston, M. H. (2003). Cognitive-behavioral treatment of generalized anxiety disorder among adolescents: a case series, *Journal of the American*

Academy of Child and Adolescent Psychiatry, 42 (3), 327–330.

National Institute of Mental Health. (2004). Anxiety Disorders Research, NIH Publication No. 99–4504 (http://www.nimh.nih.gov/publicat/NIMHanxresfact.pdf). Accessed on July 6, 2004.

Nelson, J., & Harvey, A. G. (2003). An exploration or pre-sleep cognitive activity in insomnia: imagery and verbal thought, *British Journal of Clinical Psychology, 42,* 271–288.

Student Worksheet

FILL IN THE BLANK

Fill in the blank with the correct answer.

1. Free-floating anxiety occurs when the person is unable to _____ the anxiety to a(n) _____.

2. _____ are behaviors of which the person is unaware that are aimed at relieving anxiety.

3. People who develop agoraphobia with panic attacks often _____ certain places or situations that trigger the response.

4. An excessive and persistent irrational fear of objects or situations that actually pose little threat of danger is referred to as a(n) _____ _____.

5. Social phobia is characterized by excessive fear of any social situation in which _____ is possible.

6. _____ are recurrent persistent and unwanted thoughts or images that cause intense anxiety for the person experiencing them.

7. Repetitive behaviors or rituals performed to reduce high levels of anxiety are called _____.

MATCHING

Match the following terms to the most appropriate phrase.

a. Fear of crossing a bridge

b. Fear of spiders

c. Fear of confined spaces

d. Fear of riding in a car

e. Fear of germs

f. Fear of blood

g. Fear of animals

1. _____ Microphobia

2. _____ Hematophobia

3. _____ Amaxophobia

4. _____ Zoophobia

5. _____ Claustrophobia

6. _____ Arachnophobia

7. _____ Gephyrophobia

MULTIPLE CHOICE

Select the best answer from the choices provided.

1. Which of the following nursing interventions would be the most important to implement while the client is experiencing a panic attack?

   a. Administer a prn dose of antianxiety medication

   b. Provide a detailed explanation of what causes panic attacks

   c. Assure the client that you will remain until the panic attack subsides

   d. Hug the client to show empathy for the distress he or she is experiencing

2. A client with generalized anxiety disorder approaches the nurse and states he feels dizzy. Which of the following would be the best response for the nurse to make?

    a. "Don't worry. It is just one of the symptoms you can expect."

    b. "Stay right here. I will be back with some medication to help you."

    c. "I'll help you to your room so you can lie down and rest until you feel better."

    d. "Can you tell me what happened about the time you started feeling this way?"

3. Which of the following would be the most appropriate outcome for someone with posttraumatic stress disorder?

    a. Associates feelings with fearful stimuli

    b. Does not experience another panic attack

    c. Demonstrates ability to reduce repetitive actions

    d. Controls the recurring intrusive thoughts or images

4. A client has just been diagnosed with panic disorder. Which of the following symptoms would the nurse expect to observe?

    a. Hypotension

    b. Feelings of suffocation

    c. Constipation

    d. Logical thought processes

5. Which of the following nursing diagnoses is most applicable for a client with generalized anxiety disorder?

    a. Altered thought processes, related to delusional thinking

    b. Impaired skin integrity, related to excessive handwashing

    c. Powerlessness, related to lack of control over anxiety

    d. Social isolation, related to emotional numbness

6. Which of the following would be the most appropriate direct statement for the nurse to use during an initial interview with a client who has just experienced a panic attack?

    a. "Does anyone else in your family have these feelings?"

    b. "Have you ever felt this way before?"

    c. "Tell me what you are feeling now."

    d. "Tell me about what causes you to feel this way."

7. Which of the following is the most appropriate initial outcome for the nurse to set for the client experiencing a panic level of anxiety?

    a. Will develop a trusting relationship with the nurse

    b. Will demonstrate insight into cause of anxiety

    c. Will identify alternate methods of coping

    d. Will reduce anxiety at least one level

8. Which of the following chart entries by the nurse would demonstrate progress in the client who experiences agoraphobia?

    a. Attends group therapy sessions four out of five times a week

    b. Conversing with two other clients during mealtime

    c. Participated in outing to park this afternoon

    d. Has showered and shampooed hair once today

9. Initially, which nursing intervention would receive the highest priority for the client with obsessive-compulsive disorder?

    a. Confront the client about the ridiculous nature of the behavior

    b. Isolate the client to reduce proximity to others

    c. Set limits for client to conform to unit schedule

    d. Allow extra time for client to perform rituals

10. The person who has a specific phobia diagnosis of acrophobia would be most likely to experience panic in which of the following situations?

    a. Sustains a severe cut while slicing bread

    b. Stopped at a scenic spot on the top of a mountain

    c. Fishing by a lake when rain storm arises

    d. In a room without windows when the door closes and locks

SEEK AND FIND

Find the incorrect information in the following statements.

1. For the person with obsessive-compulsive disorder, the repetitive acts serve to provide a secondary gain as the anxiety from intrusive thoughts is relieved.

2. In social phobia, anticipatory anxiety occurs immediately before a particular situation such as a public speech or social event.

3. An excessive display of emotions is often seen soon after the traumatic event in the person with posttraumatic stress disorder.

4. It is reassuring for the nurse to touch or hug the person who is having a panic attack.

SCENARIO I: EVERYONE IS LOOKING

JoAnn is a 28-year-old female who has just been admitted to treatment with a diagnosis of social phobic disorder. She has difficulty participating in group activities with other clients. Her family reports that she has been very withdrawn for the past week prior to admission. She feels that everyone will laugh at her and criticize her for the way she looks and talks. Her family states she has not been eating well and seems to have no interest in anything she previously enjoyed. JoAnn is unable to maintain employment because of her fears. The nurse notes that JoAnn's hands are trembling as she is approached. She is also hyperventilating and immediately asks to be excused to use the bathroom.

How should the nurse approach JoAnn?

_____

_____

Why is JoAnn at risk for substance abuse?

_____

Identify three nursing diagnoses that would apply to JoAnn's situation:

_____

_____

_____

SCENARIO 2: EVERYTHING IS A MESS

Josephine is a 46-year-old female who is admitted with a diagnosis of generalized anxiety disorder after the loss of her job has left her very despondent. She states, "I don't blame my boss—I could not concentrate or get anything done. I did not want to make any decisions because I was afraid any decision I made would hurt someone's feelings." Josephine is tearful, jumpy, and on edge during the assessment interview. She states, "I just don't know what I'm going to do. I have to pay the bills because my husband can't work. The kids need clothes for school. I must be the most terrible mother and wife on earth. I can't sleep. Everything I try to do is a disaster." You notice her speech is rapid and she has dark circles under her eyes. She is constantly fidgeting with a Kleenex in her hand.

What objective and subjective symptoms indicate Josephine's level of anxiety?

_____

_____

_____

What is most important when initiating nursing interventions for this client?

_____

_____

_____

What outcomes might Josephine be expected to achieve?

_____

_____

_____

Mood Disorders

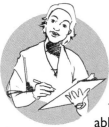

LEARNING OBJECTIVES

After learning the content in this chapter, the student will be able to:

1. Define mood as it relates to an abnormal state.
2. Identify four levels of suicidal tendencies and intent.
3. Perform a nursing assessment of clients with a mood disorder.
4. Develop appropriate nursing diagnoses related to mood disorders.
5. Plan expected outcomes for categories of mood disorders.
6. Select appropriate nursing interventions for clients with mood disorders.
7. Evaluate the effectiveness of planned nursing strategies toward outcomes.

KEY TERMS

Affect
Anergia
Anhedonia
Bipolar
Clang association
Depression
Euphoria
Grandiosity
Hypomania
Mania
Mood
Mood disorder
Negativism
Persecution
Rapid-cycling
Suicidal erosion
Suicidal gesture
Suicidal ideation
Suicidal threat
Suicide attempt
Unipolar

The Nature of Mood and Mood Disorders

Life involves everyday situations that trigger our emotions. Most people feel a sense of sadness in response to such disappointments as not winning a ballgame or not receiving an anticipated job promotion. This feeling is also felt by some on holidays or occasions on which a loss occurred. Sadness is seen as a normal state of depression, often referred to as feeling "down" or "blue." In most people, this sadness is limited, and they are able to return to a normal state of functioning. On the other end of the emotional spectrum are the feelings of happiness and joy. Elation is a normal feeling of well-being experienced with success and momentous occasions. The variance between these two emotions in most people is mild and congruent with the situation that triggers the feeling.

Mood is an emotion that is prolonged to the point that it colors the entire psychologic thinking of an individual. The feelings are changeable depending on the person's perception of sensory stimuli. **Affect** describes the facial expression that is displayed in association with the mood. Alterations in mood can range from mild to severe. When the mood alterations are mild, the person may experience minor changes in daily routine with minimal impairment in functioning. Severe mood alterations, however, can result in significant impairment of the person's ability to function; a prolonged inability to regain a sense of emotional balance is considered abnormal. A depressed mood is one in which sadness is intensified and continues longer than would normally be expected in a particular situation. In contrast, an excessive feeling of happiness or elation is seen in **euphoria.** This euphoric state can escalate to a frenzied unstable mood of **mania** in which the person may be out of touch with reality.

Mood disorder refers to a condition in which the person experiences a prolonged alteration in mood. These disorders are classified as depressive disorders and bipolar disorders. Those with a depressive disorder experience only symptoms of depression. When a person experiences symptoms of both mania and depression, that person is considered to have **bipolar** features. The symptoms of these disorders tend to reoccur in mood episodes and cause significant impairment in social, physical, and occupational functioning.

Suicide

Each year there are many people who end their lives because of the need for relief from agonizing emotional pain. People of all ages, races, and socioeconomic status may be included in these statistics. Although some people are at a greater risk for suicide, no one is excluded.

Some identifiable factors put a person in a mindset leading to the actual decision to end his or her life. A person may distance himself or herself from others with a feeling of hopelessness and worthlessness. This despondency may be related to loss of a love object, loss of health, or an escape from the realities of life. Others may be related to substance abuse or loss of control over situations that seem hopeless. Any kind of loss has the potential to precipitate depressive symptoms. In a person who is depressed, the symptoms may go undetected by family members or friends. A long-term accumulation of negative experiences throughout a person's lifetime can lead to **suicidal erosion.** Suicidal erosion occurs not as a result of a single factor that leads to suicidal thoughts, but because of a combination of situations over time. At a Glance 9-1 provides a list of warning signs, "flashing lights" that indicate the person may be considering suicide as a way out.

There are four levels of risk that apply to the person who may be contemplating suicide. A verbalized thought or idea that indicates the person's desire to do self-harm or destruction is **suicidal ideation.** This person may have recurrent thought processes that center around death as a means of ending

At a Glance 9-1 Suicide Warning Signs

- Talks about suicide
- Difficulty eating and sleeping
- Increased substance use
- Social withdrawal
- Loss of interest in school, work, or pleasure activities
- Giving away possessions
- Previous suicide attempt
- Unnecessary risk-taking
- Recent major loss
- Preoccupation with death and dying
- Lack of attention to personal hygiene

mental and physical anguish. A further step is taken if the person has devised a plan for ending his or her life. A statement of intent is considered a **suicidal threat** and is usually accompanied by behavior changes that indicate the person has defined their plan. Action that indicates the person may be about ready to carry out the plan is considered a **suicidal gesture.** If the person actually carries out a **suicide attempt,** the possibility of success is a reality. This is often the last desperate cry for help by a person who sees no other alternative.

Just the Facts

To the person who is unable to see any other way of improving the present situation, suicide seems to be a logical and rational solution.

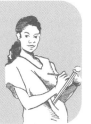

Depressive Disorders

Depression is described as a persistent and prolonged mood of sadness that extends beyond 2 weeks' duration. This state can occur in a single episode or in a recurring pattern over time. Depressive disorders are often referred to as **unipolar,** indicating that the person does not experience episodes of mania or hypomania.

Major Depressive Disorder (Unipolar Depression)

A major depressive disorder occurs when a person experiences a depressed mood or loss of interest in most activities. Depression that occurs without a precipitating event is often associated with decreased neurotransmitter availability in the brain and usually responds to antidepressant medication. Depression may also have a precipitating circumstance, such as chronic pain, loss of a job, lack of a support system, financial difficulties, or conflict with a friend or loved one. Seasonal depression is associated with decreased daylight hours during the winter months. An episode of major depression is usually severe enough to require treatment.

Just the Facts

The average person with major depressive disorder experiences four episodes over a lifetime.

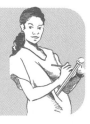

Mind Jogger

What impact would the symptoms of major depression have on the person's family, work environment, and social life?

Common Signs and Symptoms. People who are timid and anxious tend to have more difficulty adapting to loss and the increased pressures of life. Recovery from the impact of these situations may precipitate depression in those whose coping skills are inadequate. Indications of depression include feelings of hopelessness, guilt and self-blame, melancholy, fatigue, loss of appetite, weight changes, and a decreased libido or sex drive. In addition, the person may experience crying episodes, irritability, excessive worry, anxiety, and increased somatic complaints. The person may have lapses of memory, a lack of concentration, and difficulty making decisions. Even small tasks may seem overwhelming, leading to decreased efficiency and productivity. For example, a mother who previously had no problem shopping for groceries to feed her family now is unable to make decisions in the supermarket. Instead of selecting items, she feels defeated and leaves the store with nothing. **Anergia,** or a marked decrease in energy level, may make the person depend on others for even basic needs.

Many experience sleep disturbances such as waking too early or having difficulty falling asleep. Others may wake in the middle of the night and be unable to return to sleep, while others may sleep for prolonged periods. The person may require a longer time to complete basic tasks such as bathing and dressing. Hygiene is often neglected in response to the poor self-image and worthlessness felt by the person. Often **anhedonia,** or a lack of pleasure in things an individual previously enjoyed, accompanies the depressed state. This is illustrated by a person who previously had enjoyed reading to children at the library and now avoids the sessions because he no longer feels worthy of the children's attention. The affect of the depressed person is one of sadness and misery, with a lack of eye contact and apathy. Dwelling on exaggerated and perceived failures, the person is unable to see strengths and successes. Recurring thoughts of death and suicide are common.

Incidence and Etiology. Depression is more common in females and those who have a familial tendency for the disorder. Adolescents between the ages of 14 to 16 and adults older than age 65 have a higher incidence of major depression. At least one fourth of the population will experience depression in their lifetime. Approximately 15% of those with major depressive disorder will attempt suicide. A major depressive episode may develop over days or weeks and last for several months. Some may experience a single episode, while others have a recurrent pattern of symptoms. A major episode can occur at any age; the average age of onset is the mid-20s. Studies show that approximately half of those experiencing a major depressive episode will have another.

There are various theories about the cause of depression. Perhaps the most common is related to functional deficits of serotonin in the brain that lead to a chemical imbalance. This theory supports the successful use of antidepressant drugs in the treatment process. In addition to genetic and biologic predisposition, medication effects, viruses, thyroid deficiencies, and endocrine disturbances are all cited as possible factors.

At a Glance 9-2 Signs and Symptoms of Depression

The following symptoms are common manifestations in the client with an acute and severe indication of depression. This acute episode may occur as a single event or in recurring patterns. Severe depressive episodes are also seen in bipolar illness.

- Worry and anxiety
- Hopelessness and worthlessness
- Guilt and self-blame
- Crying episodes
- Fatigue, anergia
- Sleep disturbances
- Weight and appetite change
- Decreased sex drive
- Poor concentration and memory lapse
- Difficult decision-making
- Decreased productivity
- Irritability
- Extreme sadness with sad affect
- Physical complaints
- Anhedonia
- Thoughts of death and suicide

Dysthymic Disorder

The person with dysthymia experiences a recurrent state of depression over a period of at least 2 years. Depressive symptoms become a part of the person's day-to-day experience, never disappearing for more than 2 months at a time. The client with this disorder has never had a major depressive episode and does not exhibit any symptoms of manic behavior. The symptoms of dysthymia are less severe than those of major depression, but the disorder tends to be more chronic.

Common Signs and Symptoms. People with this disorder tend to struggle with the symptoms of depression over a lifetime. Life experiences have taught the person that he or she is ineffective and inadequate at coping with loss. The feelings of inadequacy, failure, and emptiness often result in a pessimistic attitude toward most aspects of the person's existence. **Negativism** is a learned sense of helplessness. Ill-equipped to cope with these continued feelings of despair, the person may resort to substance use, spending sprees, sexual promiscuity, or acting-out behaviors to escape the mental pain. The person may experience sleep difficulties, changes in eating habits, fatigue, low self-esteem, feelings of hopelessness, and decreased concentration and decision-making ability.

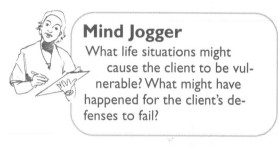

Just the Facts

The depressed person feels an on-going sense that something considered essential for happiness is missing from their life.

Mind Jogger

What life situations might cause the client to be vulnerable? What might have happened for the client's defenses to fail?

Incidence and Etiology. Dysthymia occurs two to three times more frequently in women than men. The disorder is more likely to occur in first-degree biologic relatives with depressive disorders. There is usually an early onset beginning anytime from childhood through early adulthood. Some of those who first experience depressive episodes will eventually develop bipolar disorder. In most cases where this occurs, there is a family history of bipolar illness.

Mind Jogger

Why do you think dysthymia and depression are more common in women?

Bipolar Disorder (Manic Depression)

In bipolar disorders there is a brain dysfunction that causes abnormal and erratic shifts in mood, energy, and functional ability. There are alternate changes between extreme moods, ranging from high manic episodes to low depressive periods that are often related to increased stress in the person's life. Other times,

---

At a Glance 9-3 Signs and Symptoms of Dysthymia

- Chronic depression symptoms
- Feelings of inadequacy, failure, emptiness
- Hopelessness
- Negativism
- Maladaptive coping skills
- Sleep difficulties
- Increased or decreased appetite
- Fatigue
- Low self-esteem
- Difficulty in concentration
- Decreased decision-making ability

there is no explanation for the mood shift. The frequency of the mood swings between the two states is unpredictable and varies from person to person. The severity of the symptoms may vary from mild to severe. Typically, severe recurrent episodes are referred to as bipolar I disorder. If the person does not develop severe mania but has periods of hypomania that alternate with the depression, it is referred to as bipolar II disorder. If the person has four or more mood shifts within a year, the person is said to be **rapid-cycling.** This feature is more common in later stages of the illness.

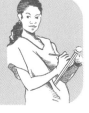

Just the Facts
Bipolar disorder typically begins with depression and there is at least one manic episode.

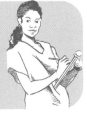

Just the Facts
Bipolar disorder has a younger age of onset and shorter cycles than major depressive disorder.

Signs and Symptoms. Although the disorder may not be recognized in its early onset, the first indications may be a state of mild to moderate mania called **hypomania** that lasts for a period of at least 4 days. The person is unusually cheerful with excessive energy and the ability to keep going long after others are exhausted. The need for sleep may decrease to 3 or 4 hours. This level of acceleration may feel good to the person, who may deny anything is wrong. There is an obvious inflated self-esteem or feeling of **grandiosity** during this time. The person may demonstrate an increase in goal-directed activity but with increased irritability and moodiness. The person usually talks incessantly with flight of ideas or jumping from one subject to another, and may describe thoughts as racing or pressured. Attention is easily distracted to things in the environment that are insignificant.

Irresponsible and impulsive behavior may accompany the increased moodiness and irritability. It is common for the person to spend large amounts of money on unneeded items or make senseless business deals. A preoccupation with seductive thoughts often leads to sexual promiscuity. The changes in mood are obvious to others, but not usually severe enough to require hospitalization. The person in hypomania does not experience psychotic symptoms of delusions or hallucinations.

Mind Jogger
There are artists and actors who have created some of their best work while in a state of hypomania. What characteristics of the mood might account for this?

When the person experiences periods of severe highs, or full-blown manic episodes, the symptoms are more extreme and pronounced. The elevated mood lasts for at least a week and causes disruption in the person's ability to function. The person's lack of insight and excessive level of activity predispose him or her to a dangerous and volatile psychotic state. The person may be offensive and violate the rights of others. When his or her wishes are not fulfilled, the mood may shift from extreme euphoria to extreme aggressive irritability. During these interpersonal conflicts, the person may perceive injustice and have delusional thoughts of **persecution** that a threat of harm exists. The constant shift in attention from one thought to another is seen in flight of ideas. Words may be strung together in rhyming phrases or **clang associations** that have no connected meaning (i.e., "Hair is bare and bear is a scare, scare is a fair, fair is there, you are a pear. . .."). The person projects an expansive thought pattern of grandiosity with false beliefs of wealth, power, and identity. Auditory and visual hallucinations may occur during the height of the manic episode. The female may dress bizarrely with bright flamboyant colors, excessive jewelry, and inappropriate makeup. Hygiene is often neglected as the thought processes escalate and activity accelerates. Items such as magazine pictures, containers, and food may be collected and stockpiled as the frenzied activity absorbs the person's time.

Just the Facts

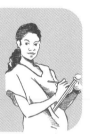

During a state of mania, the person has a continued mental flood of overly confident self-expectations that lead to frenzied psychomotor activity.

At a Glance 9-4 Signs and Symptoms of Hypomania/Mania

The following symptoms are typical manifestations in an acute episode of the "high" or manic phase in bipolar illness:

- Extreme euphoria
- Inflated self-esteem or grandiosity
- Talkative with rapid, racing speech
- Flight of ideas
- Excessive energy
- Decreased need for sleep
- Easily distracted
- Extreme irritability and moodiness
- Reckless and impulsive behaviors
- Lack of judgment
- Increased motor activity
- Irresponsible buying sprees or business deals
- Sexual indiscretions
- Delusions of grandeur or persecution (mania)
- Auditory and visual hallucinations (mania)
- Bizarre dress and accessories
- Poor hygiene

Incidence and Etiology. In many cases of bipolar disorder, there seems to be a genetic factor that is shown by the familial pattern of the illness. There are studies that show an increase in the severity in future generations. Environmental factors are also cited as a cause since not all cases have a family history of the disorder. Despite these theories, we do not know exactly what causes this condition. Evidence has linked bipolar symptoms to changes in the chemical neurotransmitters in the brain. Substance abuse and stressful life events have also been linked to the episodes.

Women are at greater risk than men for developing manic episodes, which can occur at any time. The average age of onset for a first manic episode is in the early 20s, but it can be as early as adolescence and as late as age 50. Manic episodes that occur in adolescence may lead to school failure, behavioral problems, and substance abuse. Manic episodes can also occur during postpartum periods in women.

Mind Jogger

What factors related to the postpartum period might contribute to a psychotic state of mania or depression? How might this lead to a dangerous situation?

Cyclothymic Disorder

Cyclothymic disorder is characterized by mood disturbances, which involve periods of hypomanic symptoms and periods of depression. The hypomanic symptoms are not as severe as those seen in a manic episode, and the depressive symptoms are not as severe as in a major depressive episode.

Common Signs and Symptoms. The symptoms of cyclothymia include recurrent episodes of hypomania and dysthymia. These alternating periods are recurrent with short periods of normalcy that usually do not last longer than 2 months. Delusional thinking and hallucinations are not present. The person's functioning is not severely impaired and hospitalization is usually not necessary.

Case Study: Out of Control

Mr. Karnes was admitted to the hospital while experiencing a manic episode of bipolar I disorder. Over the past 4 days, he has become increasingly loud and animated. He became very aggressive today with another client while playing cards. Now he is in the day room with family members of another client and is asking very personal questions of a sexual nature and touching one of them when he talks.

What actions should the nurse take at this time?

_____

_____

_____

What other symptoms can be anticipated in Mr. Karnes behavior?

_____

_____

Two days later, Mr. Karnes approaches the nurse and says he has to leave because he has a meeting with other national leaders from around the world this evening. He goes on to say that since he has been elected president of the country, he has hardly any time anymore. How should the nurse respond to Mr. Karne's delusional thinking?

_____

_____

_____

_____

At a Glance 9-5 Signs and Symptoms of Cyclothymia

- Recurrent episodes of hypomania and dysthymia
- States not as severe as in bipolar
- Short periods of normalcy
- No psychotic symptoms
- Functioning not severely impaired

Incidence and Etiology. Cyclothymic disorder occurs equally in men and women and begins in adolescence or early adulthood. It is usually chronic with an insidious onset. Most people do not realize the disorder is present until many symptoms have existed over

years. There is a greater risk for the person with this disorder to develop bipolar disorder.

Application of the Nursing Process

Nursing Assessment

When doing an assessment of the person with a mood disorder, the nurse should include mood and affect, thinking and perceptual ability, somatic complaints, sleep disturbances, changes in energy level, and the character of speech patterns. Mood and affect should be assessed for congruency. For example, when observed crying, a client should report feeling sad or down. A client who says he is sad but is laughing is not showing this consistency. Since mood is a subjective experience, it is important for the nurse to ask the client what feeling or emotion he or she is experiencing. Clients experiencing a manic episode will likely display a bright or happy affect, while a person with depression will usually display a flat affect with a lack of eye contact.

During mania, thought processes become faster and may become fragmented, leading to disorganized patterns of speech. The person may not be able to complete one thought process before the next one begins. Complaints of "racing thoughts" are common in people experiencing a manic episode. The person may be preoccupied with delusional thinking. Some things the nurse might do when working with a client with mania include the following:

- Determine whether the client can understand what is being said.
- Note whether the client is able to verbalize thoughts and feelings.
- Observe behavioral clues for what the client may be thinking if the client does not respond verbally.
- Determine the level of orientation. In depressive states, thought processes are retarded or slowed; concentration may be difficult for either the manic or depressed client.
- Assess for any suicidal ideation and whether a plan has been devised.
- Monitor patterns of verbal speech. The tone of voice, pace at which thoughts are processed and communicated, and the rate at which words are spoken are all relevant. Changes in the tone and rate can provide clues to mood and energy level. Clients in a manic state have very pressured or loud and forceful speech. Some clients may be unable to verbally communicate feelings, but may do so in drawings or written text.
- Ask the client about any somatic complaints. During depression, the tolerance

for pain may decrease, giving rise to generalized body aches, headaches, and gastrointestinal disturbances.
- Assess for clues that indicate increased or decreased sleep patterns. Persons going into a manic episode often go 2 to 3 days without sleep. Depressed people often have insomnia with difficulty falling asleep and staying asleep. Others may have hypersomnia and sleep for prolonged periods of time.
- Assess the client's energy level. Those with mania will usually report a drastic increase in energy, while the depressed client usually reports anergia or decreased energy levels.
- Assess appetite, recent eating patterns, and weight changes. Clients with depression may have little appetite or overeat as a coping tool. A loss of weight may be seen during a manic phase as the excessive activity minimizes the perceived need for food. The person does not take time to eat or is unable to remain seated long enough to eat.
- Determine the amount of assistance required for personal hygiene, dressing, and elimination needs. Both the manic and depressed person may lack attention to hygiene and bowel habits.

Nursing Diagnosis

Once data have been collected, the nurse identifies the individual needs of the client. The needs of the depressed person may be very different from those of one experiencing a manic episode. To differentiate the planning process for the individual client, the nurse needs to define the problems for each state.

Nursing diagnoses for the client in a state of depression may include:

- Activity intolerance, related to fatigue and anhedonia
- Anxiety, related to psychologic conflict
- Coping, individual, ineffective, related to situational crisis and ineffective skills
- Hopelessness, related to stress or lack of support system

- Violence, self-directed, risk for, related to suicidal thoughts
- Powerlessness, related to negativism and past failures
- Social isolation, related to feelings of worthlessness
- Sleep pattern disturbance, related to insomnia or hypersomnia
- Self-esteem, chronic low, related to perceived unmet needs
- Sexuality patterns altered, related to decreased sex drive
- Altered family processes, related to changes in role
- Nutrition, altered (less than body requirements), related to loss of appetite and feelings of worthlessness
- Self care deficit, related to feelings of hopelessness and helplessness

Nursing diagnoses for the client in a state of hypomania or mania may include:

- Anxiety, related to threats to self-concept
- Communication impaired, related to pressured speech
- Coping, individual, ineffective, related to delusional ideas
- Thought processes altered, related to delusions of grandiosity or persecution
- Sensory/perceptual alteration, related to bizarre thinking and overload
- Family processes, altered, related to manipulation and irresponsibility of family member
- Nutrition altered (less than body requirements), related to inadequate food intake and excessive activity
- Personal identity disturbance, related to delusional thinking
- Sleep pattern disturbance, related to inability to recognize fatigue and hyperactivity
- Violence, self-directed or directed at others, risk for, related to irritability and delusional thinking
- Injury, risk for, related to increased substance use
- Self-care deficit, related to hyperactivity and delusional thoughts

Expected Outcomes

Once problems have been identified, anticipated outcomes that are realistic in terms of the individual client should be formulated. Clients are often in a severe mood state when admitted to a psychiatric facility. Stabilization is necessary before the person is able to recognize and deal with the underlying issues. Outcomes should be determined as related to the type and level of mood alteration that is exhibited.

Expected Outcomes for the Client in a Depressed State
- Has increased energy level
- Identifies personal strengths
- Demonstrates improved skills to deal with loss
- Experiences decreased feelings of self-blame and doubt
- Openly expresses feelings
- Resumes sexual functioning with partner
- Demonstrates increased interaction with others
- Participates in at least two unit activities per day
- Consumes at least 75% of each meal
- Reports feeling well rested with 4 to 6 hours of sleep before awakening
- Reframes thoughts into positive statements
- Performs activities of daily living (ADLs) independently

Expected Outcomes for the Client in a State of Hypomania or Mania
- Demonstrates self-control with decreased agitation
- Verbalizes feelings in a appropriate manner
- Demonstrates decreased activity level
- Consumes at least 75% of each meal and nutritional supplements
- Performs ADLs independently within level of ability
- Receives 4 to 6 hours of uninterrupted sleep
- Demonstrates ability to complete simple tasks to completion
- Participates appropriately in unit activities

- Interacts appropriately with others
- Verbalizes realistic expectations of self
- Experiences family participation in planning process
- Channels psychologic energy into productive activity
- Maintains accurate perception of reality

Nursing Interventions

Nursing interventions should be planned individually for each client. All clients with an alteration in mood states may be very sensitive to behaviors and verbal statements of others. It is important for the nurse to plan actions that allow the person to make progress toward improved functioning and a sense of well-being. Interventions should be implemented according to priority of need.

Interventions will differ depending on the mood state the client is experiencing. The client with depression is often withdrawn and avoidant, making interaction more challenging. The nurse should employ methods that assist the client in meeting needs until he or she is psychologically and physically able to do so independently.

Nursing Interventions
for the Depressed Client

- Establish and maintain a therapeutic relationship with the client.
- Monitor for changes in current depressive symptoms or development of new ones.
- Ask the client about any suicidal thoughts indicating a plan of how, when, or where the client might harm or kill self.
- Assess the client's energy level—as energy increases, the ability to carry out a plan for suicide increases.
- Encourage the client to participate in unit activities.
- Provide positive feedback when the client makes efforts toward goals.
- Assess the client's ability to perform ADLs, and assist as needed.
- Provide a safe environment by removing potentially dangerous items.

- Educate client regarding depression and treatment.
- Stress the importance of taking medications as ordered.
- Assist in request for referral for spiritual needs.
- Encourage the client to explore feelings and communicate them in a safe manner.
- Assist the client to express anger and other negative feelings appropriately.
- Help client to recognize situations he or she can control and explore alternatives for those that cannot be controlled.
- Encourage the client to recognize negative thoughts and teach reframing techniques.
- Teach alternative methods of coping that are constructive and safe.
- Focus on client's strengths and positive attributes.
- Assist the client in establishing realistic goals.

When planning nursing interventions for a client with symptoms of mania, the nurse must remember that because of the nature of the client's illness, implementation may be difficult. The nurse should refrain from becoming emotionally reactive to the client's acting-out behaviors. Treatment modalities during the manic episode include various types of psychotherapies and the use of psychopharmacologic drugs. The most common drug used to treat mania is lithium carbonate, which assists in stabilizing the mood swings. (For more on this drug, see Chapter 20.)

Nursing Interventions for the Manic Client
- Create a safe environment.
- Decrease environmental stimuli.
- Observe the client frequently.
- Assess risk for accidents to self or others.
- Monitor own anxiety level and convey messages with a soothing tone of voice.
- Refrain from becoming angry with clients who are hostile or behaving in an inappropriate manner.
- Avoid arguing with or being charmed by clients.

- Convey a "matter-of-fact" or nonreactive attitude when the client displays bizarre or sexually inappropriate behavior.
- Educate client regarding medications and other treatment methods.
- Encourage noncompetitive activities to prevent escalating anxiety and anger.
- Provide nutritional finger foods when the client is unable to sit long enough to eat.
- Monitor intake and output—prevent dehydration by providing water and juices in containers client can carry.
- Monitor for escalating anxiety that may lead to explosive behavior.
- Set and maintain limits such as unit rules and policies.
- Spend time with the client—if the client is unable to sit, walk with him or her.
- Provide positive feedback when appropriate.
- Encourage client to dress appropriately and redirect the client when acting out in a sexual manner.

Other Treatment Modalities for Depressive Disorders. The treatment of depression usually involves a combination of treatment modalities.

- Psychotherapy involves assisting the client in exploring how negative thoughts and feelings are affecting his or her behavior. Once the underlying thoughts and feelings are understood, the client can identify more effective ways of coping. The client must be willing to explore and discuss painful thoughts for improvement to occur. Individual, group, and family psychotherapy may be needed. The type of psychotherapy needed depends on the circumstances and severity of the client's illness. Support or self-help groups are very useful for long-term management of depression.

Electroconvulsive therapy (ECT) involves passing an electric current through the brain. The client is given a muscle-relaxing agent and an anesthetizing medication before the treatment. Electrodes are placed against one or both sides of the head, releasing an electric current that mimics a generalized clonic seizure. Because the client has received medication before the treatment, only twitching of the toes or clenching of the fists may be seen. The nurse should monitor the client continuously and record vital signs as ordered.

- The actual mechanism by which ECT works is not known. It is thought that changes in neurotransmitter systems lead to the expected mood elevation. Unfortunately, because of the many changes in the brain, memory deficits occur. Depending on whether unilateral or bilateral ECT is used, the person may have either short-term or long-term memory deficits. ECT is used in cases where the client has experienced several episodes of severe depression and nothing else has worked. This type of depression is usually the result of a long period of events and losses that eventually lead to depression. When there is one incident that leads to depression, it is usually a more acute type of depression.

Psychotherapeutic drug agents are used very successfully in managing depression. The nurse should provide patient education regarding antidepressant medication and the importance of complying with the medication regimen prescribed by the physician. It is important to stress that medication effects are often not recognized for 3 to 4 weeks. Encourage the client to continue taking the medication during this time. When the medication becomes effective, the client's mood and energy level usually will improve. For more information on antidepressants, see Chapter 20.

Specific Interventions for a Suicidal Client. On admission, the client should be assessed for current risk factors that indicate suicide may be a possibility. Determine the content of any suicidal thoughts or ideations. If the client has a plan, this usually indicates that the client is more serious about committing suicide. Determine the lethality of the method. A more lethal method usually indicates increased likelihood of an attempt. It is also important to ask when the client intends to carry out the plan. The longer a client takes to carry out an attempt, the more time the client is willing to take to find another solution. If the client has decided on a location to do the act, determine how easy or difficult it will be to access this location.

Suicide precautions are usually initiated on admission to a psychiatric unit for those who are at risk of self-harm. These precautions may vary from one unit to another and are often implemented by levels. If the client has recently attempted suicide, continuous monitoring of the client with one-to-one observation may be indicated. Sharp and potentially dangerous items (e.g., scarves, belts, shoelaces, nail files, scissors, electric appliance cords) are removed from the client's room and personal effects. A "no-harm" contract may be established with the client every shift and renewed at a specific time. The contract should include a statement that the client will not kill or injure himself or herself and will notify the staff when suicidal thoughts first occur. Random client checks are done to avoid possible anticipation of time intervals that the checks are done. Clients often carry out incidents of self-harm during times when nurses are busiest, such as shift changes. Watch for "cheeking" behaviors in which the client holds medication in the pouch of the cheek to avoid swallowing it. The client can stockpile medication for use to overdose at a later time.

It is especially important to spend time with the client who is considering suicide as the only option. By using active listening and being present, the nurse conveys a sense of caring and appreciation for the worth of the client who is unable to find that feeling within his or her own self.

Evaluation

Evaluation will focus on determining whether improvement has occurred in the client's thought processes, behavior, and overall functioning. The effectiveness of interventions related to anxiety and coping ability will be demonstrated as the client appropriately verbalizes feelings and thoughts. Behavior changes indicate an improvement in self-control and application of more effective coping skills. Interest and participation in self-care and hygiene show an elevation in self-appreciation. Increased hope and worth relieves the acute need for self-destruction, although an increased risk may exist for those who are energized enough to carry out a preconceived plan.

As anxiety and excessive mood states are reduced, the client is able to eat and sleep with less disturbance. Improved communication and social interaction will result as thought processes become more rational and reality oriented. Hopefully, the client can return to a state of productivity and independent living. The maintenance of a continued state of mood stability will depend on compliance with the medication and follow-up treatment plan.

Summary

Mood disorders involve an array of emotions and can significantly impair a person's ability to function. The symptoms can range from hardly noticeable to extremely bizarre. The alterations in mood levels can have a ripple effect on every aspect of a client's life. The problems and results of behaviors are devastating to the person experiencing them and to those around them.

Depression can occur as a single episode or in a recurring pattern. There may be a precipitating cause such as a loss, or it may occur without an identified reason. Clients with major depression do not exhibit any signs of euphoric states. The sadness and melancholy are severe enough to require treatment. Functioning in all areas of the person's personal, social, and work activities are usually impaired. A lower level of depression is demonstrated in the client with dysthymia. A recurring cycle of the depressed state is demonstrated over a 2-year period. The person has feelings of hopelessness and despair combined with a negativistic attitude and indulgence in self-pity.

Bipolar disorders are characterized by a shift between elevated moods and depression. These swings produce dramatic behavior changes with underlying distorted thought processes. During the manic phase, the person's unrealistic inflated self-image leads to actions that bring regret and hurt to those around them. Thought processes thunder through the mind and demand the person's attention. These thoughts are often expressed in chains of phrases that have no meaningful connection. The impetuous and reckless actions exhibited by the person suffering from mania are irritating and destructive in relationships with family, friends, and co-workers.

As the person with bipolar disorder sinks to the bottom of the polar scale, the depression is painful and severe. The statistics of suicide attempts and lives ended during the barrenness of feelings during the plunge are alarming. Although drug therapy can level out the brain chemistry to minimize the highs and lows, many clients do not comply with treatment. This is in part related to the grandiose thinking in hypomania that they are fine and do not need medication. Once the blood levels of the drug decline, a vicious cycle is begun.

It is important for the nurse to know of the symptoms of both mood states. Many clients with these disorders are not seen in a psychiatric unit, but are part of the general population. Some may be seen in other health care agencies or admitted to extended areas of hospital care. Recognition of signs that might indicate a state of depression can help that person receive appropriate treatment. Some people are unaware that the signs of depression are present in themselves or others. By learning about these disorders, nurses can teach and assist in curbing the devastating impact these disorders can have on those affected by them.

Bibliography

American Psychiatric Association (2000). *Diagnostic and statistical manual of mental disorders text revision* (4th ed.). Washington, DC: American Psychiatric Association.

Berkow, R., & Fletcher, A. J. (2002). Mood disorders. *The Merck manual* (18th ed., Section 15, Chapter 189). Rahway, NJ: Merck & Co.

Goldberg, J. & Harrow, M. (1999). *Bipolar disorders: Clinical course and outcome.* Washington, DC: American Psychiatric Press.

Koukopoulos, A., Sani, G., Minnai, G. P., et al. (2003). Rapid cycling may predict bipolar prognosis. *Journal of Affective Disorders, 73,* 75–85.

Mitchell, P. (2003). Stressful life events effect differs in depression subtypes. *Journal of Affective Disorders, 73,* 245–252.

Peterson, T. (2001). Depressed patients share personality characteristics. *Comprehensive Psychiatry, 42,* 488–493.

Spearing, M. (2001). Bipolar disorder, NIH Publication No. 02-3679, September, 2001. Available at http://www.nimh.nih.gov/publicat/bipolar.cfm. Accessed on July 7, 2004.

Zarate, C. A. Jr., Tohen, M., & Fletcher, K.(2001). Cycling into depression from a first episode of mania: a case-comparison study, *American Journal of Psychiatry, 158,* 8.

Student Worksheet

FILL IN THE BLANK

Fill in the blank with the correct answer.

1. When combinations of negative experiences or loss accumulate over a period of time, it can lead to _____ _____.

2. A verbalized thought or idea that indicates a person's desire to do self-harm or destruction is a(n) _____ _____.

3. Depressive disorders in which the person does not experience hypomania or manic episodes are referred to as _____.

4. _____ is a recurrent state of depression over a period of at least 2 years.

5. The average person with depression experiences _____ episodes over a lifetime.

6. Delusions of _____ occur during interpersonal conflicts where a perceived injustice is viewed as a threat of harm.

7. Less severe cyclic symptoms of hypomania and dysthymia are seen in the client with _____.

8. _____ is the most common antimanic drug agent used in the treatment of bipolar illness.

9. Antidepressant drug agents require _____ weeks of continuous blood levels to produce significant mood elevation.

10. Clients on suicide precautions should be monitored at _____ time intervals to prevent anticipated checks.

MATCHING

Match the following terms to the most appropriate phrase.

a. Being tired with decreased energy.

b. Learned sense of helplessness.

c. Depressive episode without hypomania or mania.

d. Strings of words in rhyming phrases.

e. Action that indicates self-harm may be imminent.

f. Lack of pleasure in previously enjoyed activities.

g. Holding medication in the mouth without swallowing.

h. Four or more mood shifts within 1 year.

i. Thinking of self as excessively important.

j. Excessive feelings of happiness.

1. _____ Euphoria

2. _____ Anhedonia

3. _____ Clang association

4. _____ Cheeking

5. _____ Anergia

6. _____ Negativism

7. _____ Rapid-cycling

8. _____ Grandiosity

9. _____ Suicidal gesture

10. _____ Unipolar

MULTIPLE CHOICE

Select the best answer from the multiple-choice items.

1. The nurse is monitoring a client with mania who is constantly pacing the hallway and unable to be seated when the other clients are eating. Which of the following nursing interventions would best meet the needs of the client at this time?

   a. Keep the meal at the nurse's station until the client asks for something to eat.

   b. Allow the client to eat in a separate area to avoid distraction.

   c. Provide finger sandwiches and juice for client during the activity.

   d. Teach the client the importance of nutrition in providing energy.

2. The nurse is documenting observations of a client experiencing a manic episode who is very talkative, extremely happy, and laughing. Which of the following would be most appropriate to include regarding this client?

   a. Euphoric with appropriate affect

   b. Dysthymic with inappropriate affect

   c. Bright affect with dysphoric mood

   d. Flat affect with elated mood

3. A client admitted to the psychiatric unit with depression states she feels "life just isn't worth living anymore. My kids don't care about me. I'm all alone." She has remained in bed for the past 2 days. Which of the following statements best describes this client's present situation?

   a. Energy level is too low for her to carry out a suicide plan.

   b. Thought processes do not indicate that suicide is a threat.

   c. Most likely will not commit suicide because she has a family.

   d. Increased suicide risk because of despondent and worthless feelings.

4. When caring for a client with a manic episode, which of the following nursing interventions would convey a therapeutic attitude of acceptance?

   a. Tell the client to remain isolated until impulsive actions are controlled.

   b. Allow the client to describe delusional thoughts as long as needed.

   c. Walk alongside the client at intervals as long as pacing continues.

   d. Reprimand the client for inappropriate sexual hand gestures.

5. After 2 weeks of sexually inappropriate behavior during a manic episode, a client is now apologetic and embarrassed by his actions. When he returns to his job, he makes numerous attempts to make amends for his behavior. Which of the following statements would best describe what is occurring with the client at this time?

   a. He has developed delusions of persecution.

   b. He has improved insight into his behavior.

   c. His need for attention is escalating.

   d. This is an attempt to manipulate others.

6. Which of the following would the nurse document if describing a statement made by a client having a manic episode?

   a. "I am really worried about my family."

   b. "The puzzles are my favorite activity."

   c. "I built the tallest building in New York."

   d. "I have a hard time waking up in the morning."

7. When assessing a client for indication that suicide might be a possibility, which of the following would pose the most risk?

   a. Suicidal threat

   b. Suicidal gesture

   c. Suicidal ideation

   d. Suicidal plan

8. A client is admitted to the psychiatric unit with major depression. He has anorexia with a 10-pound weight loss in the last month. He moves slowly with a slouched posture. His mood is sad with a flat affect. Which of the following problems should receive first priority?

   a. Nutritional deficit

   b. Fatigue and anergia

   c. Sense of worthlessness

   d. Sad mood and affect

9. The nurse is caring for a client who does not want to get up to attend activities today. She states that she did not sleep well last night and just wants to get some rest. Which of the following would be the most appropriate response for the nurse?

   a. "You need to get up and get involved in some activities."

   b. "I will ask the physician to order you something to help you sleep."

   c. "It must be difficult to get up this morning. I will help you get dressed."

   d. "You agreed to the rules that state that you are to attend all activities."

SCENARIO: SAD AND LONELY

Mrs. Lopez is being admitted from the emergency department today. When she arrives on the unit, you immediately notice a flat affect, slumped posture, and an unkempt appearance. During your admission intake, Mrs. Lopez cries frequently and does not provide eye contact. She states, "My husband not only left me alone in this world, but left me all of the bills too." She begins to sob and states, "I just don't think it is worth it anymore."

The nurse's best response at this point would be

_____

_____

You finish your admission intake, and Mrs. Lopez is in the day room talking to her family and saying her good-byes. The physician has an order to implement suicide precautions for Mrs. Lopez. What are some objects you should remove from her room?

_____

_____

You escort Mrs. Lopez to her room after having made the room as safe as possible. You are going to implement a no-harm contract with her before leaving her room. What is the rationale for this intervention?

_____

_____

Mrs. Lopez is taking an antidepressant and has been receiving psychotherapy for nearly 3 weeks. She has been participating in all unit activities and socializes with everyone on the unit. Discharge plans are being discussed with her and her family. She tells the nurse, "Maybe now I can do things that I had planned to do before I came in here." How should the nurse respond to this statement?

_____

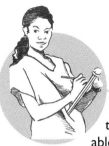

LEARNING OBJECTIVES

After learning the content in this chapter, the student will be able to:

1. Define what is meant by a maladaptive pattern of personality traits.
2. Describe characteristic behaviors of each personality disorder.
3. Perform a nursing assessment of the client with a personality disorder.
4. Formulate appropriate nursing diagnoses for a person with a personality disorder.
5. Plan realistic outcomes for the client with a personality disorder.
6. Identify nursing interventions for a person exhibiting a personality disorder.
7. Evaluate the effectiveness of planned nursing care.

Personality Disorders

KEY TERMS

Entitlement
Ideas of reference
Magical thinking
Passive-aggressive
Personality disorders
Personality traits
Self-mutilation
Splitting

Defining Personality Disorders

Each of us is born with a set of traits, temperament, and patterns of behavior that are a unique blend of characteristics that make us who we are. Our thoughts, feelings, and attitudes toward ourselves and the world around us are the distinguishing aspects of our personality. Personality traits are persistent ways in which we view and relate to other people and to society as a whole. Those with healthy personalities are able to adapt to life stressors and form interpersonal relationships with reasonable expectations.

Personality disorders are deeply ingrained, persistent, inflexible, and maladaptive patterns of behavior that are in conflict with a cultural norm. Because the behavior does not usually conform to the expectations of society, it leads to distress and impairment in all aspects of a person's life. Behavior characteristics are demonstrated in the person's thinking processes, emotional reactivity, interpersonal relationships, and self-control. Unless they become frustrated with their life pattern or peer relationships, most of these people are oblivious to the problem. They are usually annoying and aggravating to those around them because of their egocentric and demanding behaviors. Most people with these disorders have established the deviant patterns of behavior by adolescence or early adult life. Unlike many other mental disorders where symptoms may alternate in levels, the symptoms seen in personality disorders tend to be consistent and constant. Treatment is rarely sought because of the person's denial or inability to identify the problem. When treatment is obtained, compliance with the treatment plan is doubtful and less successful.

People with personality disorders tend to share some common characteristics that define them as having inflexible and maladaptive behaviors. Because behavior is the result of the way we perceive and think about the world around us, these characteristic differences tend to permeate their personal and social lives. They tend to view their life in terms of all good or all bad with little understanding that something or someone can have both qualities. They tend to be arrogant and self-indulgent; often they are unable to delay satisfaction of their needs to allow for the wishes of another. Many have unmet needs for dependency that relate back to inconsistent nurturing during the early developmental years.

In addition, there is a **passive-aggressive** tendency in which the person indirectly and subtly acts on hostile feelings. This may be seen as an ambivalent mind-set in which the person displays a passive and pleasant affect whereas actions are based on underlying pessimism and bitterness. The person is torn between feelings of dependence and independence, love and hate, and action and inaction, with resulting moodiness, frustration, and stubborn self-will. This ambivalence is demonstrated in acting out behaviors that allow the person to avoid thinking about the underlying psychologic conflict. These behaviors may take the form of self-destructive acts meant to manipulate others into conforming to their wishes. Faults are projected to others to avoid feelings of inadequacy and incompetence. Deadlines are avoided with procrastination and other delay strategies to sabotage the efforts of others. If the passive manipulation fails, the resulting anxiety can precipitate angry emotional outbursts.

There are a number of personality disorders that have been identified, each having a particular set of behaviors and symptoms. The *DSM-IV-TR* groups the disorders into three categories or clusters according to the range of characteristics exhibited.

Cluster A Personality Disorders

Cluster A personality disorders include paranoid, schizoid, and schizotypal variations. Persons with these disorders tend to demonstrate odd or eccentric behaviors.

Paranoid Personality Disorder

Paranoid personality disorder is defined ʌ persistent pattern of suspicion and mistrust ʌ which the actions or motives of others are seen as intentionally threatening or humiliating. Although there is no obvious reason for the suspicion, the person may become hostile and attack without warning. Often people with this disorder think it is necessary to "attack first" before others have the opportunity to harm them.

Common Signs and Symptoms. People with paranoid personality disorders are often viewed as being cold and aloof. Their suspicious nature leads them to be watchful, resentful, and guarded in their interactions with others. They are unable to believe that others can be good to them. There is a reluctance to share personal information with others for fear that it will be used against them later. Angry or hostile outbursts are perceived as necessary to defend against the disloyalty and deceit of others. The person with this disorder is unable to accept constructive criticism while being critical of others. Grudges are maintained with no hint of forgiveness for a perceived insult or injustice.

There is usually a long history of inability to achieve closeness in interpersonal relationships. Many jealous accusations of infidelity and indiscretion are made toward partners or spouses. They attempt to maintain control of the relationship by confronting the partner with demanding questions concerning places they have gone or their intent for going. Vehicle mileage may be monitored to support the perceived disloyalty. This suspicion is further seen in their projection of blame for their own faults onto others. Their need to counterattack for a perceived injustice often leads to lawsuits against those blamed for the action. Their rigid, inflexible nature prevents any type of mutual agreement to resolve a problem. Although they tend to work better independently, these people are often quite efficient and dedicated to their employment situation. Their interests are often in areas

At a Glan...
and Sympton...
Personality Dis...

- Cold and aloof ma...
- Rigid and inflexible
- Doubts about loyalty and honesty of others
- Watchful and guarded
- Resentful, accusing, and argumentative
- Inability to tolerate criticism
- Mistrustful and unable to confide in others
- Feelings that others are out to deceive them
- Angry or hostile outbursts
- Maintenance of grudges against others
- Controlling relationships
- Extreme jealousy
- Projection of faults to others
- Inability to perceive self as a problem
- Self-sufficiency

Mind Jogger
How would the person with a paranoid personality disorder respond to being given a compliment by a co-worker?

Incidence and Etiology. Paranoid personality disorder is more prevalent in men. Typical behaviors are often seen by early adulthood. A possible genetic link to schizophrenia is seen in the tendency for those with this disor-

...ual ...this to ...nought pro... ...rs.

...sonality Disorder

...with a schizoid personality disorder ...withdrawn and secluded and demonstrate an emotional indifference toward social relationships. The behavior characteristics are seen in most aspects of the person's life by the early adult years.

Common Sign and Symptoms. Because they are usually self-absorbed in their own feelings and thoughts, people with this disorder tend to avoid close relationships and intimacy. They are viewed as being "loners," usually choosing to pursue activities and interests alone. The person with this disorder derives less pleasure from things that are soothing and sensuous such as music, romance, or beauty. Sexual experiences are usually not desired. Facial expression or affect is usually bland and unresponsive to positive emotions in others. Emotions such as elation or anger are seldom felt or displayed. Delusional thinking can be precipitated by stressful events.

At a Glance 10-2 Signs and Symptoms of Schizoid Personality Disorder

- Withdrawal and seclusion
- Emotional indifference
- Self-absorbed attitude
- Avoidance of close relationships and intimacy
- Loners
- Preference for solitary activities
- Decreased pleasure experience
- Decreased interest in sexual experiences
- Bland facial expression
- Daydreaming
- Emotional barrenness
- Social avoidance

These people are often described as daydreaming, fantasizing, and without purposeful goals. Working situations that require social interaction are usually avoided. However, they may do well in an employment setting where interaction is not necessary and they can work alone. Their interests are often in the areas of mechanics or art.

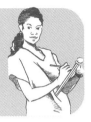

Just the Facts
The schizoid person is usually not concerned with how his or her behavior is perceived by others.

Incidence and Etiology. This disorder is somewhat more common in men than women. There is an increased incidence in those who have a family history of schizophrenia or other personality disorders.

Schizotypal Personality Disorder

In addition to being secluded and withdrawn from social situations, persons with schizotypal personality disorder exhibit strange and unusual patterns of thinking and communicating.

Common Signs and Symptoms. The thinking patterns and opinions of these people are unusual and bizarre, often with paranoid undertones. They often display a sort of **magical thinking** in which they propose to forecast the future or read the minds of others. **Ideas of reference** are seen in which the person believes that everyday occurrences have a special and significant personal meaning. Perceptual distortions and illusions are common. Emotions are rigid and inflexible, and these individuals have little ability to respond to feelings and expressions of others. Dress habits and mannerisms may be eccentric or unusual.

At a Glance 10-3 Signs and Symptoms of Schizotypal Personality Disorder

- Weird and bizarre thinking and beliefs
- Paranoia and suspiciousness
- Magical thinking
- Ideas of reference
- Perceptual distortions, illusions
- Inflexible emotions
- Eccentric dress habits
- Social isolation
- Remorse over lack of social relationships

Increased fear and anxiety are experienced in social situations. This results in a diminished ability to form interpersonal relationships. The person is often unhappy about not having social friends and relationships but is unable to overcome the social ineptness and suspiciousness of others. Psychotic behavior may occur in brief episodes of minutes to hours. It is believed that this disorder is a mild form of schizophrenia but without the continuous thought alterations.

Incidence and Etiology. Schizotypal personality disorder typically is apparent during childhood and adolescence. The odd behavior is often the target of ridicule by other chil-

Case Study: Uneasy Predictions

Margie is a 25-year-old client who was admitted to the psychiatric unit after employees of a clothing store called the police about a lady who was "acting weird" and saying "all this crazy stuff." Her history reveals that as a child she had very few friends and people called her "odd." She has always worn clothes that were unusual and don't match.

She expresses little emotion as she walks around the unit. Margie seems superstitious, because she avoids mirrors and steps over cracks in the tile floor. It is not unusual to see her gazing out the window with nodding and hand gestures, seeming to indicate she is communicating with someone. Today the nurse walks into the day room and finds Margie looking into a flower vase making predictions for the future of several other clients. One of the clients becomes quite disturbed over Margie's comments to him.

How should the nurse approach Margie?

_____

_____

What characteristics of schizotypal personality does Margie demonstrate?

_____

_____

How could the nurse help Margie continue a therapeutic type of interaction with other clients on the unit?

_____

_____

dren, leading to early social isolation. It is more common in men than in women. Prevalence is also seen in first-degree biologic relatives of people with schizophrenia. Treatment is usually sought for symptoms of anxiety or depression rather than for the symptoms of the personality disorder itself.

Cluster B Personality Disorders

Dramatic, emotional, or erratic behavior is characteristic of individuals with a cluster B personality disorder. The category includes the antisocial, borderline, histrionic, and narcissistic personality disorders.

Antisocial Personality Disorder

Those with an antisocial personality disorder exhibit a persistent pattern of disregard and infringement on the rights of others in a society. A false sense of privileged revenge against others is demonstrated by their basic cold indifference to the laws of society and humanity.

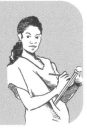

Just the Facts

Also referred to as a sociopath, the person with antisocial personality disorder is selfish and seemingly has no conscience.

Common Signs and Symptoms. The person with this disorder is suspicious and feels betrayed by the world. Thinking that humans are basically evil and out to undermine, the person performs actions impulsively and recklessly to avoid being sabotaged. Vandalism, fighting, explosive anger, and verbal assault are common. School expulsion, truancy, and delinquency are among the problems in

the person's history. Their interactions with others are full of lying and dishonesty. They victimize others for materialistic self-gain and are often described as "con-artists." Their way of thinking is cold, calloused, insensitive, arrogant, and ruthless, with insensitivity to the feelings of others. Their behavior results in continued and frequent encounters with law enforcement officials. Despite the continued conflict with the law, these people do not feel remorse or responsibility for the consequences of their behavior. Rarely do they benefit from incarceration or treatment programs. Projection of blame to others is typical as they try to rationalize and minimize their vengeful actions.

Individuals with antisocial personality disorder may use alias names, relocate, or change jobs in an attempt to avoid recognition. Little regard is given to dependent or financial responsibilities. They often display superficial charm, smooth conversation skills, and excessive self-assurance as they manipulate others

At a Glance 10-4 Signs and Symptoms of Antisocial Personality Disorder

- Suspiciousness of others
- Impulsive and reckless behavior
- Vandalism, fighting
- Explosive anger
- Deceitfulness and dishonesty
- Lying
- Coldness and insensitivity
- Arrogance
- Violation of rights of others
- Lack of remorse or guilt
- Manipulation
- Projection of blame
- Irresponsibility
- Alias names
- Charm and scheming
- Recklessness
- Sexual promiscuity and exploit
- Dysphoria

Mind Jogger

How is the antisocial personality reflected in the mind of the criminal who thinks that getting caught is failure to achieve success?

for their personal gain and pleasure. There is a reckless disregard for the safety of others as seen in careless driving, actions that put others in danger, or destruction of property. Sexual promiscuity and exploitive relationships with a lack of concern for partners is common. Unable to tolerate boredom, the person may become dysphoric and may look for something stimulating such as sex, alcohol, gambling, or other compulsive self-indulgence to compensate for this feeling.

Incidence and Etiology. Most people with antisocial personality disorder have a history of conduct disorder with an onset before the age of 15. Situations of child abuse, unstable parenting, and inconsistent parental discipline may increase the chances of a person developing antisocial personality disorder by the age of 18. The disorder tends to be more prevalent in men and is most often associated with those in low socioeconomic class and crowded living situations. There is a higher incidence among the prison population and those who have a history of substance abuse. There tends to be a familial pattern with it occurring more often in those who have first-degree biologic relatives with antisocial personality disorder. The disorder tends to be chronic but may become less evident as the person ages.

Borderline Personality Disorder

Persons diagnosed with borderline personality disorder have a persistent pattern of unstable interpersonal relationships, insecure self-image, and mood swings. They are impulsive and intense in their outbursts of anger.

Common Signs and Symptoms. There is a chronic sense of emptiness and abandonment accompanied by continued anxiety and efforts to avoid the perceived rejection. The fear often leads to clingy, dependent, and needy behavior with rapid attachment to a nurturing partner. They quickly become overinvolved and attached in the relationship, but soon feel threatened the partner will leave. Without warning, the person may suddenly view the caring partner as evil and cruel, pushing them away to avoid future rejection. While rallying between the labile emotional states of self-admiration and self-dislike, the person with this disorder becomes confused about self-identity. There are intense episodes of dysphoria and irritable moods that may last hours or days. The quick change from clingy and dependent extremes to angry outbursts in a short period of time is typically referred to as a "Jekyll and Hyde" characteristic. This is very frustrating to those who try to befriend them and dampens most of the person's relationships.

Along with the mood change, the person usually demonstrates an extreme view, or **splitting,** of their relationship to the world. Things are seen as all or none, black or white, love or hate, with no neutral ground (e.g., loss of a partner means I am a bad person). When a relationship ends, the person believes it proves his or her feelings of worthlessness. Dissociation may occur to escape the feeling of being alone. At times, there may be brief episodes of paranoia and hallucinations, because the person's ability to maintain a reality state is unstable. This is often the time when repeated threats of suicide or self-mutilation are exhibited. **Self-mutilation** is not meant to be lethal, but it serves to restore the person's sense of realism and value. It may include actions such as burning or cutting the body or overdosing. The person also may engage in impulsive behaviors that have the potential for self-destruction such as substance abuse, gambling, sexual promiscuity, reckless activity, or excessive eating patterns.

People with this disorder may demonstrate caring for others, but with expectation for self-gain. Rarely do they experience any positive emotions of happiness or well-being. If their wishes are ignored, the display of acting-out behaviors demonstrates their inability to delay satisfaction of their needs. These behaviors are usually in the form of temper-tantrums, impulsive anger, and sarcasm directed at others. They are easily enraged if authority figures do not provide instant response to their wishes. This behavior often tends to undermine their successes because they often quit before a goal is achieved. Multiple employment losses, broken relationships, and unfinished education are common.

Just the Facts

Persons with borderline personality disorder tend to engage in self-destruction by repeatedly becoming involved in no-win relationships with others who are emotionally unstable or abusive.

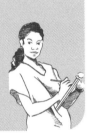

At a Glance 10-5 Signs and Symptoms of Borderline Personality Disorder

- Unstable relationships
- Insecure self-image
- Mood swings
- Dissociation
- Impulsive outbursts of anger
- Chronic sense of abandonment
- Clingy, dependent behavior
- Splitting
- "Jekyll and Hyde" characteristic
- Self-mutilating acts
- Suicide threats and gestures
- Inability to delay gratification of needs

Incidence and Etiology. Borderline personality disorder tends to occur more in women than in men. It is more common in those with

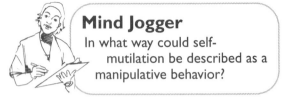

Mind Jogger

In what way could self-mutilation be described as a manipulative behavior?

a family history of the disorder. There seems to be more instability during the early adult years, with some stabilization of moods seen by the 30- to 40-year-old age-group. The incidence of suicide in this group is the highest during young adulthood.

The exact cause of this condition is not known. It is believed that perhaps instances of parental neglect, separation from the primary caregiver, and child abuse may contribute to development of the disorder. An infant who is suddenly removed from the emotional attachment figure learns that a comfortable trusting relationship is followed by anxiety when that person is no longer available. Trust is lost and the separation is viewed as abandonment. Once the security and comfort of the good relationship changes to anxiety in a bad situation, the child learns to see "all good" and "all bad." There is continued difficulty in being able to integrate these two conditions as coexistent in the same person. This leads to splitting, in which the person reacts to people in either a very positive or very negative way.

Narcissistic Personality Disorder

The term *narcissism* is derived from the Greek, meaning "excessive love and attention given to one's own self-image." The person with a narcissistic personality disorder has a continued need for lavish attention and admiration with little regard for the feelings of others. Other people may be used unfairly to satisfy this person's desires.

Common Signs and Symptoms. The narcissistic person has an exaggerated and grandiose sense of importance. This is ex-

Case Study: Hidden Ambivalence

Sherry is a 24-year-old woman who is admitted to the psychiatric unit for self-mutilation: she cut her forearms 28 times with a kitchen knife. She had just discovered that her live-in boyfriend of 2 years had moved out. Her history reveals many broken relationships and four previous suicide attempts, including two overdoses, walking in front of a fast-moving vehicle, and a gunshot wound to her left leg. Before the present incident, she had telephoned her boyfriend, who abruptly hung up on her. Her mother tells the nurse that she doesn't understand why this is so upsetting to Sherry. She says that 2 months ago Sherry told her boyfriend to "get lost." In between episodes of crying, Sherry tells the nurse, "I must have done something bad for him to do this. If I were a good person he would still be there."

How does Sherry's behavior demonstrate her underlying sense of insecurity?

_____

_____

How is "splitting" evident in her behavior?

_____

_____

How should the nurse respond to Sherry's last statement?

_____

_____

_____

hibited as arrogance and claims of **entitlement** that others owe them because of their superiority. When shopping for services or merchandise, the person will ask to see the manager or owner of the establishment, indicating their sense of importance. Any personal achievement is overexaggerated with demands for praise and approval. Fantasies of power, beauty, and success are believed to be superior and only understood by others who are on this level. They may talk at length about themselves not realizing that others are not showing an interest in the conversation.

Although people with this disorder perceive an awesome superior self, there is an underlying feeling of inferiority and envy of others. They may inwardly resent and dislike those who are awarded more respect or attention and are usually overly sensitive to failure, which results in feelings of insecurity. The grandiose overinflation of the self is seen as overcompensation for their low self-esteem. Because of their extreme sensitivity to criticism, they may experience humiliation, intense anxiety, and shame if reprimanded or disappointed. The need for admiration increases to overcome these feelings of being "bad" if they are not receiving attention. They do not have insight into their behavior and unrealistic thinking. Social withdrawal and mood alterations are common during periods of frustration and anxiety.

At a Glance 10-6 Signs and Symptoms of Narcissistic Personality Disorder

- Grandiose sense of self-importance
- Intense need for admiration and approval
- Lack of empathy for others
- Exploitation of others for own needs
- Sense of entitlement
- Demand for the best of everything
- Fantasies of power, beauty, success
- Underlying feelings of inferiority
- Hypersensitivity to criticism
- Anxiety
- Social withdrawal
- Poor insight into behavior

Mind Jogger

How are narcissistic attitudes fed by a culture that places excessive value on physical appearance?

Incidence and Etiology. Although there is a tendency for adolescents to have a narcissistic view of themselves as they search for their identity, this does not mean that a personality disorder exists. It is only when the narcissistic traits become inflexible and maladaptive enough to cause dysfunction in the person's life that a disorder may be diagnosed. People who develop the disorder rarely seek treatment and often blame the negative results of their behavior on society. Narcissistic personality disorder is more common in men than women.

Histrionic Personality Disorder

Typically, the person with histrionic personality disorder displays a pattern of egocentric and excessive emotion in a demanding manner to gain personal attention. They are uncomfortable in situations where center-stage is not afforded them.

Common Signs and Symptoms. People with this disorder are overly dramatic and may seem fake or exaggerated in their behavior. By creating a scene that gets the attention of others, they usually receive sympathy or affectionate gestures in return. As a result, they may develop attachments easily but tend to be superficial and easily dissatisfied with the relationship. They may also demonstrate unexpected sexual advances in their interactions with others. Relationships are often described in detail as involving more intimacy than is actually present. Casual acquaintances may be introduced as a best friend or a wonderful, dear person. Provocative dress and mannerisms are often used to draw attention. Speech tends to be melodramatic with numerous hand gestures but is vague and lacking in content. The behavior is described as a manipulative ploy to satisfy underlying needs of dependency and protection. Individuals with this personality disorder may be easily influenced by others and overly trusting of those perceived as able to solve all their problems.

At a Glance 10-7 Signs and Symptoms of Histrionic Personality Disorder

- Attention-seeking behavior
- Extreme egocentricity
- Overly dramatic and exaggerated behavior
- Shallow, superficial relationships
- Provocative sexual behavior
- Melodramatic but vague speech
- Manipulation
- Unmet dependency needs

Incidence and Etiology. Histrionic personality disorder tends to occur more often in women but is seen also in men. The available statistics are limited. There is a strong association between the disorder and dissociative symptoms. It is also common for these clients to demonstrate several personality features of other disorders. There is speculation that symptoms may stem from the childhood experiences in which recognition was only received if parental expectations were met. Only when the histrionic traits of the person become maladaptive and impair functioning is it considered a disorder.

Cluster C Personality Disorders

Persons with cluster C personality disorders exhibit anxious and fearful types of behavior such as the avoidant, dependent, and obsessive-compulsive personality disorders.

Avoidant Personality Disorder

The person with an avoidant personality disorder is typically shy and very sensitive to negative comments from others. Feelings of inadequacy and intense discomfort are felt in social situations that involve people other than family.

Common Signs and Symptoms. Because of their extreme fear of ridicule or disapproval, people with this disorder tend to avoid events or situations that involve interaction with others. Educational and work-related opportunities may be rejected out of fear that criticism may follow. The person is afraid that others might become aware of the self-doubt and tend to withdraw from relationships if there is a chance these feelings might be exposed. Intense anxiety is experienced when in a group of people. This feeling is related to those of inferiority and incompetence. Any indication of disapproval will prevent these individuals from becoming involved, though they may be encouraged and offered support by others in the group. There is a perception of rejection even when it does not exist. Unless they are certain of being liked, they are usually not willing to trust the environment. Although they

desire to have intimate interpersonal relationships, this guardedness often prevents them from doing so.

At a Glance 10-8 Signs and Symptoms of Avoidant Personality Disorder

- Extreme shyness
- Sensitivity to rejection
- Feelings of social inadequacy
- Social withdrawal/isolation
- Self-doubt
- Fear of criticism or embarrassment
- Intense anxiety in social setting
- Feelings of inferiority
- Low self-esteem
- Lack of trust in others
- Lack of close friends
- Fear of intimate relationship
- Reluctance to take risks or try new things

Just the Facts
Those who dwell on perceived inadequacies and previous mistakes tend to view themselves as inferior in all aspects of their life.

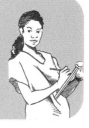

Incidence and Etiology. Avoidant personality disorder is equally frequent in men and women. In persons with this condition, the shyness and fear of new situations exhibited in childhood tends to increase by adolescence. There is some evidence that it decreases with age. People who demonstrate avoidant behaviors often have associated social phobia.

Dependent Personality Disorder

People with a dependent personality disorder demonstrate a consistent and extreme need to be cared for that leads to a reliance on others.

At the same time, they perceive themselves as helpless and incompetent.

Common Signs and Symptoms. People with dependent personality disorder have difficulty making decisions that affect everyday life unless prompted and reassured by others. They relinquish control and priority for their own needs to someone else. Feelings of insecurity and doubt prevent them from making self-care decisions. They may not be able to select items to wear, requiring another to choose their daily attire. Although they may disagree with those caring for them, they do not express these feelings for fear of upsetting the other person. It is not uncommon for these people to demonstrate acting-out behaviors to show their inability to make a decision or know what to do in a given situation. This is illustrated by a woman who shoves a shopping cart into the wall of a grocery store when her husband asks her to select a package of bacon from the shelf. She states she does not know what brand he wants. Afraid of making her husband upset and being left alone, she relinquishes the selection of groceries to him.

People with dependent personality disorder will search at length to find relationships where the hovering support will continue. Because of the extreme anxiety experienced when someone is not present to make decisions for them, a replacement figure is needed if a relationship ends. Independent or self-initiated involvement in activities is not an option for these individuals (e.g., a man needs shampoo to wash his hair, but will not buy it until someone tells him what brand to buy). There is an increased incidence of abuse that is tolerated in these relationships. Because the abused person is so afraid of being alone, the abuse is endured even when help is offered to leave the situation. Their passive nature and fear of abandonment overrides any expression of unmet personal needs. For example, a 28-year-old woman who is in an abusive relationship wants to take college classes, but is afraid her husband will leave her if she has skills for making her own living. She does not pursue her dreams and remains dependent on his support. This person is so afraid of being unable to make decisions for living by herself, she remains in the clutch of a controlling and cruel relationship.

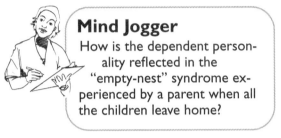

Mind Jogger
How is the dependent personality reflected in the "empty-nest" syndrome experienced by a parent when all the children leave home?

At a Glance 10-9 Signs and Symptoms of Dependent Personality Disorder

- Inability to make decisions
- Extreme reliance on others
- Insecurity and self-doubt
- Extreme fear of being alone
- Excessive anxiety
- Feelings of incompetence
- Constant need for reassurance
- Self-sacrificing behavior
- Relinquishment of control to others
- Submissive behavior

Incidence and Etiology. Dependent personality disorder is diagnosed more often in women than in men. It is one of the most frequently reported personality disorders. Age and cultural factors can contribute to the behavior. In some cultures, women are expected to be subservient to men. The distinction between what is considered respectful and what is excessive must be made. Children and adolescents who experience chronic physical illnesses or separation anxiety disorder have an increased risk of developing this disorder.

Obsessive-Compulsive Personality Disorder

People with obsessive-compulsive personality disorder are conscientious, highly organized, and preoccupied with order and perfection. They are usually dependable but want rigid control and lack the flexibility to allow for compromise.

Common Signs and Symptoms. Excessive attention is paid to details and rules to the point that tasks are left unfinished. For example, a businessman is so concerned that Robert's Rules of Order be maintained during a meeting that nothing is accomplished. Compulsive people tend to insist that their way is the only right way to do things. As a result, they have difficulty delegating to others, preferring to do the task their way so it is done right. If tasks are assigned, lengthy detailed instructions are given. They are highly critical of others and of themselves if mistakes are made or deviations made from the instructions. It is difficult for these people to feel satisfaction for their accomplishments. They experience high anxiety levels if deadlines or prioritizing are expected of them.

Miserly spending and hoarding are part of their stubborn refusal to waste or throw away items that "might be needed" at some future time. It is common for items such as magazines or paper sacks to be saved and arranged precisely in piles with all corners exactly in line to perfection. Their need to keep things is often an annoyance to those around them. These people rarely take time off from work for leisure activities or vacation, believing that to do so is a waste of time. Relationships are often more serious and shallow. The person believes that public display of emotion or affection is foolish and typically exhibits a limited ability to express feelings or intimacy toward another.

At a Glance 10-10 Signs and Symptoms of Obsessive-Compulsive Personality Disorder

- Preoccupation with orderliness
- Rigidness and controlling behavior
- Focus on details
- Unrealistic expectations
- Missed deadlines
- Inability to relax
- Rigid moral and ethical standards
- Hoarding of items
- Inability to delegate
- Stubbornness
- Miserly with material things
- Shallow display of emotions

Incidence and Etiology. Obsessive-compulsive personality disorder is seen twice as often in men than in women. People with this disorder are often employed in situations such as research where precision and detail are required. They rarely seek treatment because to do so would require change. Any diversion from their rigid nature is highly threatening to them. There is usually little insight into the psychologic origin of their discomfort.

Application of the Nursing Process

Nursing Assessment

It is not often that a client is admitted with a personality disorder as a primary cause for treatment. Treatment may be sought by the

Just the Facts

The person who has an unconscious feeling of powerlessness may attempt to achieve self-control by controlling others.

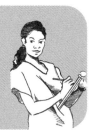

person or family members as the maladaptive traits become problematic and disrupt the person's life. Other disorders such as depression, substance abuse, or suicidal acts may be the trigger that leads to admission. It is important that the nurse first develop a trusting relationship by using an empathetic and nonjudgmental approach.

Some assessment techniques that could be used are:

- Use direct questions to find out what events or behaviors led to the admission.
- Observe nonverbal behaviors and symptoms that indicate appropriate affect.
- Assess thought processes for content and clarity, all or none thinking, magical thinking, or narcissism.
- Look for inconsistencies between what is said and mannerisms or behavior.
- Determine social habits and present or past relationships in which the person is involved.
- Assess the level of anxiety and emotional state during the initial history intake.
- Note any resistance to questioning or indication of impulsive reaction to requested information.
- Ask about usual coping methods used to deal with life stressors.
- Note any scars or cuts that may indicate self-mutilating behaviors.
- Ask if suicidal thoughts have occurred and verify whether a plan has been made.
- Establish what type of situations may have led to the self-destructive behavior.

Because clients with personality disorders tend to be irritating and demanding, it is important for the nurse to recognize and deal with his or her own feelings. The feelings experienced by the nurse are often the same feelings being demonstrated in the client and caregivers. The client with a personality disorder can be manipulative and conniving with nurses and other clients. It is important to view the situation objectively. Therapeutic intervention can only occur if self-awareness allows the nurse to project an appropriate attitude of caring and concern for the well-being of the client.

Nursing Diagnoses

A nursing diagnosis is made after a thorough analysis of the data collected through the nursing assessment process. Any data that can provide new or useful information should be considered when developing the diagnosis statement. Nursing diagnoses may be applicable for more than one personality disorder because many share similar symptoms and problems. These may include:

- Social isolation, related to suspicious view of others
- Anxiety, related to unconscious conflicts
- Impaired communication, related to social withdrawal
- Ineffective individual coping, related to suspiciousness, ambivalence, or projection
- Impaired social interaction, related to indifference toward others
- Personal identity confusion, related to social withdrawal
- Risk for violence: self-directed, related to self-mutilating behaviors
- Risk for violence: directed at others, related to rage and inability to tolerate frustration
- Self-esteem disturbance, related to unmet dependency needs
- Powerlessness, related to extreme feelings of dependency
- Personal identity disturbance, related to splitting and unmet dependency needs
- Decisional conflict, related to ineffective problem-solving ability
- Family coping, ineffective, related to maladaptive relationships
- Hopelessness, related to feelings of inadequacy and incompetence

Expected Outcomes

Expected outcomes provide criteria by which the effectiveness of nursing interventions can be measured. Nurses and clients work together to facilitate change within a reasonable time. If the expected changes have not occurred within the given timeframe, the plan of care is revised at the time of evaluation. Anticipated outcomes may be that the client can:

- Express thoughts and feelings appropriately
- Increase interaction with others
- Exhibit decreased hostility and anger
- Exhibit relaxed posture
- Participate in unit activities
- Conform to unit rules
- Gain control over impulses
- Decrease manipulative behaviors
- Manage anxiety without acting-out behaviors
- Refrain from harming self or others
- Associate anxiety with precipitating factors
- Refrain from using splitting or clinging behaviors
- Claim ownership of own feelings and thoughts
- Verbalize positive qualities about self
- Make independent decisions about self-care

Nursing Interventions

Providing care for people with personality disorders is very challenging for nurses. The nurse must identify personal feelings about the client's behaviors and maintain a continuous awareness to provide appropriate interventions. Nursing actions may include the following:

- Show acceptance of the person at all times by separating the person from the behaviors.
- Provide a safe environment, especially important for clients who exhibit self-mutilating behavior.
- Set and maintain limits with consequences.
- Explain all unit rules and enforce them fairly and consistently.
- Require the client to take responsibility for his or her own behavior.

- Identify inappropriate behavior and discuss possible alternative behavior with the client.
- Do not make exceptions or show favoritism.
- Encourage the client to openly express feelings and thoughts.
- Identify triggers of acting-out behaviors.
- Maintain alertness to manipulative behaviors of clients.
- Communicate problems with manipulative clients to other team members.
- Provide positive feedback to clients who are making efforts to change behavior.
- Approach clients from the front and speak clearly. This is especially true for the client with paranoia.
- Monitor for cheeking of medication.
- Encourage the client to participate in unit activities.
- Assess for suicidal ideation.
- Develop a no-harm contract with the client with self-destructive tendencies.
- Assist and educate the client in the problem-solving process.
- Demonstrate a matter-of-fact attitude when clients act-out or exaggerate events.
- Point out "all or none" behavior to the client when it occurs.
- Encourage the client to keep a private journal of thoughts and feelings.
- Discuss with the client how his or her behavior affects others and assist to explore alternative actions.
- Observe and intervene before escalation of behavior occurs.
- Use time-out for curbing acting-out behavior if client is resistant to redirection.

Other Treatment Modalities. Other members of the mental health care team join the nurse in providing an environment in which the client with a personality disorder can effect behavior change. To do this, the client must gain perspective into the problem underlying his or her maladaptive response to the world. This is often difficult because most people with these disorders lack insight and resist attempts to impose change. If the person is admitted for an associated disorder, he or she may comply with treatment for that problem while avoiding the personality symptoms completely.

- Group therapy helps clients improve interaction skills in addition to gaining an understanding of how they are perceived by others. Clients can learn how to ventilate anxiety and trust others in a safe environment. Problem-solving methods can be practiced within the group to resolve community issues. Individual therapy helps clients gain insight into their thinking and behavior. Ways can be explored for them to modify their behavior to a more functional level.
- Occupational therapy allows clients to increase their level of functioning so that they become more independent. Task completion skills can also be evaluated and enhanced by these activities.
- Recreation therapy can assist clients to ventilate feelings and increase socialization skills.
- Interaction and guidance by the therapist can provide clients with constructive ways to deal with anger and other self-destructive behaviors.

Evaluation

The effectiveness of implemented interventions for clients with personality disorders is difficult to measure. Changes do not occur quickly and are often not recognizable during the brief treatment period. The ability of the nurse to set boundaries and maintain a therapeutic approach to the behaviors is often one indicator of progress. Short-term outcomes that involve interaction with other clients and impulse control can be evaluated within the confined milieu. The client's behavior following discharge will demonstrate whether actual improvement has occurred. Regardless of efforts expended by the mental health team, the potential for improvement is limited by the deeply ingrained patterns of pervasive be-

haviors that have developed over time. Unlike an acute medical problem, the maladaptive personality traits are usually hidden to those who exhibit them. They cannot solve the problem because they are unable to identify the reason for the problem.

Summary

Although everyone has unique traits and characteristic patterns of behavior, those with traits that are deeply embedded, inflexible, and maladaptive are viewed as an abnormal segment of society. The paradox of this picture is that although the feelings that accompany the disorder cause misery, the person does not recognize the problem and sees the behavior as normal. Unfortunately, this failure to see the problem is what contradicts the benefit of treatment programs and interventions. Most of these people endure a lifetime of unsuccessful attempts to secure stability in their personal and social situations.

Personality disorders cover a wide range of behavior manifestations. These are categorized by the *DSM-IV-TR* in cluster groups according to the typical pattern of the behavior. Three clusters have been identified to provide organization. Regardless of the disorder, people with maladaptive personality characteristics tend to have some common tendencies. Viewing the world from an ambivalent perspective, the person conforms to rigid thinking that objects, people, and events are either all good or all bad. This tunnel vision rejects the possibility of these two extremes coexisting in one situation. With this type of mindset, the person often passively and indirectly projects hostility to others in subtle, deceitful ways.

Most clients receive treatment in connection with care received for another disorder. In many instances, the person may have engaged in self-destructive behaviors that bring them to the attention of the health care system. The ability of nurses to participate in the treatment plan is diverted by the manipulative, annoying, and disruptive nature of the behaviors. It is easy to become very frustrated and irritated. Although the maladaptive behavior may be obvious to the nurse and others, people with these disorders are oblivious to the impact their behavior has on others. When confronted with the irrational nature of their actions, they often become angry and belligerent. It is important that boundaries and limits be set and strictly enforced for behaviors. Nurses must have an awareness of their own feelings and be alert for the manipulative efforts of the client. Many times the feelings of the nurse are the same as those the client may be experiencing. A therapeutic climate mandates that the nurse be accepting and nonjudgmental as attempts are made to evoke change in the client who is so resistant to it.

Bibliography

American Psychiatric Association (2000). *Diagnostic and statistical manual of mental disorders text revision* (4th ed). Washington, DC: American Psychiatric Association.

Berkow, R., & Fletcher, A. J. (2002). Personality disorders. *The Merck manual* (18th ed., Section 15, Chapter 191). Rahway, NJ: Merck & Co.

National Mental Health Association. "Personality disorders," Fact Sheets. Available at http://www.nmha.org/infoctr/factsheets/al.cfm. Accessed July 7, 2004.

Sternberg, R. J. (1994). *In search of the human mind* (pp. 668–670). Philadelphia, PA: Harcourt Brace.

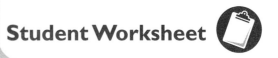

Student Worksheet

FILL IN THE BLANK

Fill in the blank with the correct answer.

1. The symptoms in personality disorders tend to be _____ and _____.

2. People with personality disorders tend to have a(n) _____ mind-set in which underlying hostility is indirectly exhibited in subtle behaviors.

3. _____, secluded, and indifferent behavior is typical of the schizoid personality.

4. The person who proposes to forecast the future or read the minds of others is displaying _____.

5. When everyday occurrences are seen as having a special and significant personal meaning, the thinking is referred to in terms of _____ of _____.

6. A persistent pattern of disregard and infringement on the rights of others in a society is characteristic of the _____ personality.

7. _____ acts are a distorted way in which the person restores a sense of realism and value to neutralize intense feelings of self-dislike.

8. A type of self-destruction is involvement in _____ relationships with people who are emotionally unstable and abusive.

9. Those who exhibit a sense of _____ feel that others owe them because of their superior and powerful status.

10. Creating an overly dramatic scene of emotional behavior to attract the attention of others is typical in the _____ personality.

MATCHING

Match the following terms to the most appropriate phrase.

a. Defense mechanism in which faults are attributed to others.

b. Person who disregards the rights of others without remorse.

c. Withdrawal related to extreme self-doubt and fear of disapproval.

d. Aggressive response to underlying negative feelings.

e. Extreme view of all good or all bad.

f. Persistent ways of viewing and relating to the world.

g. Perceived state of helplessness leading to extreme reliance on others.

h. Extreme mood shift from clingy dependent behavior to angry outbursts.

i. Grandiose sense of self-importance.

1. _____ Personality traits

2. _____ Splitting

3. _____ Narcissism

4. _____ Dependency

5. _____ Projection

6. _____ Acting-out behavior

7. _____ "Jekyll and Hyde" characteristic

8. _____ Sociopath

9. _____ Avoidance

MULTIPLE CHOICE

Select the best answer from the multiple-choice items.

1. The nurse is caring for a client admitted with self-inflicted burns to her abdomen. While the nurse is doing an assessment of the wounds, the client says, "I deserve to be in pain." Which of the following best describes the underlying feelings in this statement?

    a. Arrogance

    b. Worthlessness

    c. Suspicion

    d. Egocentricity

2. The nurse notes that a client is monopolizing most of the conversation during breakfast. He is loud and criticizing other clients. Which of the following is the most appropriate intervention for the nurse to make at this time?

    a. Reprimand him for his inappropriate behavior.

    b. Provide him with medication to calm him down.

    c. Put him in seclusion until he can control his actions.

    d. Redirect and reinforce limits on his behavior.

3. Which of the following statements is true regarding clients with personality disorders?

    a. They are aware that they have a behavior problem.

    b. Manipulative patterns often render treatment ineffective.

    c. Most have a sincere motivation to change behaviors.

    d. Most recognize how their behavior affects others.

4. By cluster grouping, the person with avoidant personality disorder will have predominant behavior characteristics described as:

    a. Anxious and fearful

    b. Odd and eccentric

    c. Magical and unusual

    d. Dramatic, emotional, and erratic

5. A client diagnosed with schizotypal personality disorder would most likely exhibit which of the following behavior patterns?

    a. Aggressive, hostile, impulsive

    b. Trouble seeking without remorse for acts

    c. Magical thinking with ideas of reference

    d. Hostile aloofness, splitting, and attention seeking

6. Which of the following would be most typical of the person with an obsessive-compulsive disorder?

    a. Harsh and inconsistent parental boundaries

    b. An overprotective and clingy mother figure

    c. Reluctance to take risks or try new things

    d. Rigid preoccupation with details and orderliness

7. A client receives a paper cut on her right forefinger. She suddenly cries out loudly, "Someone needs to help me—I nearly cut off my finger!" The nurse assesses that a small amount of bleeding is present and reassures other clients that nothing major has occurred. This client is demonstrating behavior typical of which disorder?

   a. Histrionic personality

   b. Schizotypal personality

   c. Dependent personality

   d. Borderline personality

SEEK AND FIND

Find the incorrect information in the following statements.

1. The person who has an unconscious feeling of excessive power may attempt to achieve self-control by exerting control over others.

2. Those who dwell on their perceived inadequacies and previous mistakes tend to view themselves as able to excel in all aspects of their life.

3. The person with antisocial personality often views getting caught as a personal gain toward success.

4. The schizoid person is usually very concerned with the perception others have of his or her behavior.

SCENARIO: SMOOTH CHARACTER

Ed is a 28-year-old man who was admitted to the psychiatric unit yesterday under a court order. He was diagnosed with conduct disorder at age 10 and has been in conflict with law officials many times during his adolescent years. He has been in custody for driving under the influence of drugs. Because this is not his first substance-related offense, he is court-ordered to receive treatment for substance abuse and anger management.

Ed is very charming and good looking. His manner is very convincing as he freely gives polite compliments and makes friendly gestures. Today Ed tells a female nurse that he is really attracted to her and has never felt this way before. He asks for her phone number so he can call her when he is discharged.

How should the nurse respond to Ed's request?

_____

_____

In addition to substance abuse, what personality disorder is demonstrated by Ed's behavior?

_____

Why is limit-setting so important in dealing with Ed's behavior?

_____

_____

When confronted with his manipulative behavior, Ed becomes enraged and tells the nurse, "You wouldn't recognize a good thing if you saw it. You're nothing but a slut anyway." How would the nurse describe Ed's actions at this point?

_____

_____

What are the chances that Ed will benefit from the treatment process?

_____

_____

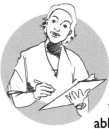

LEARNING OBJECTIVES

After learning the content in this chapter, the student will be able to:

1. Define psychosis.
2. Describe common characteristics of schizophrenia.
3. Perform a nursing assessment of the client with schizophrenic disorder.
4. Formulate appropriate nursing diagnoses for the client with schizophrenia.
5. List expected outcomes for problems seen in the client with psychosis.
6. Identify appropriate nursing interventions for people with schizophrenia.
7. Evaluate effectiveness of nursing care delivered to those with schizophrenia.

Schizophrenia

KEY TERMS

Avolition
Catatonic
Delusion of reference
Delusions
Derailment
Grandiose
Hallucinations
Illusions
Loose associations
Neologisms
Persecution
Poverty of speech
Prodromal phase
Psychosis
Thought broadcasting
Thought insertion
Thought withdrawal
Water intoxication
Waxy flexibility
Word salad

Psychosis

The term **psychosis** is linked with a variety of meanings. Most often it makes reference to a set of symptoms that demonstrate disorganization in the mental processes. These symptoms reflect the behavior, emotional response, and thought processes of the person who has lost contact with reality. Most people associate the disturbances of "hearing voices" or other strange behaviors with this psychosis. Those who experience these symptoms also tend to withdraw from society and retreat into their own unreal world. For us to understand the peculiar and abnormal state of psychosis, we must first look at the characteristic symptoms that define this disturbance.

Perceptual Disturbances

Hallucinations are false sensory perceptions that have no relation to reality and are not supported by actual environmental stimuli. When a hallucination occurs, the person has the perception of seeing (visual), hearing (auditory), smelling (olfactory), feeling (tactile), or tasting (gustatory), although there is no stimulus present. Although all of these may occur, auditory hallucinations are the most common. Most of these are in the form of voices or sounds that can only be heard by the person experiencing them. The voices may originate inside or outside the person's head and may be talking to the person or commenting on his or her behavior. Many of the voices are commanding, telling the person to harm himself or others and are very frightening to the person.

> ### Mind Jogger
> Considering that the client hearing commanding voices is not in touch with reality, what is the best approach to this person?

Visual hallucinations are less common but may involve seeing people or images that are not actually present. Feeling that something is crawling on the skin or moving inside the body parts are typical of tactile hallucinations. Olfactory (smell) and gustatory (taste) misperceptions account for a small percentage of perceptual disturbances.

Illusions are experienced when sensory stimuli actually exist but are misinterpreted by the person. For example, the person may refer to spots on the floor as insects or to an electric cord as a snake.

Disorganized Thinking

In psychosis, the thought processes become confused and disrupted, leaving the person with an inability to carry on a logical conversation. **Delusions** consist of false constant ideas that cannot be changed by reasoning. These thoughts usually involve a theme that is dominant in the mind. For example, the client who thinks someone is trying to kill him will demonstrate this both verbally and behaviorally. The client might say, "I'm not taking this medication because you are trying to poison me," or "I'm not eating my supper because the FBI put poison in my food." The content or theme of the delusions can include depressive (they have committed terrible deeds), somatic (their body is disintegrating into another substance or infested with insects), **grandiose** (they are very important and powerful), and **persecution** (others are out to get them). Others may be **delusions of reference** in which something such as a newspaper article or television commercial is believed to be sending a special message to the person. Content can also include a belief that **thought broadcasting** occurs in which the person's thoughts can be heard by others. This person might say, "I have a direct wire attached to the commander of intelligence to rule the underground." **Thought insertion** may also be claimed in which the person believes the thoughts of others can be inserted into his or her mind (e.g., "Men from Mars are implanting seeds of destruction into the layers of my mental dirt."). **Thought withdrawal** indicates a belief that others are robbing thoughts from one's brain (e.g., "Those who steal the knots of my wisdom are employed in drawers of the intelligence bureau.").

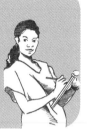

Just the Facts:

The most common delusional themes in the person with schizophrenia tend to be related to themes of persecution, religious ideas, or somatic reference.

As the normal brain organizes and directs thought processes into spoken words, there are associations or connections that give meaning or logic to the content. *Content* refers to the meaning of the words or conversation that is spoken. People with disorganized thinking convey the fragmented content in the way they speak. They may be talking and suddenly change the course of the conversation to something with no logical connection to the original topic. The inability to organize and connect one concept to another related thought is referred to as **loose associations** or **derailment,** meaning that the content is off track (e.g., "This meat is tough, but I saw meat in the store and nails are keeping it together until the cows get home."). **Poverty of speech,** or a decrease in the amount or speed of speech, may occur, in which the person may not answer questions or may stop in the middle of a thought.

Word salad refers to a jumble of unconnected and disorganized thoughts that indicate severe impairment (e.g., "You see I am living in the sky where it snowed yesterday with thunderous wires darting in and out of the highway . . . brilliant colors keep the orchestra moving the ball down the railroad track toward the divine intellect of my intes-

tines."). The person may make up new words that have special personal meaning such as, "The *malitars* are coming to get me." These new words or **neologisms** are indicative of disconnected thought processes. Clang associations may also be demonstrated with insignificant rhyming of words (e.g., "The sky is blue, so are you . . . two plus two, much to do so to fear, far and near, let's have a beer . . .").

Behavior Alterations

Psychotic behavior may be described as agitated, aggressive, childlike, inappropriate, silly, and unpredictable. Wild, purposeless, agitated movements are described as frenzied motor activity. Disorganized behavior can lead to an inability to perform activities of daily living (ADLs) or carry out goal-directed activity. The person may appear very unkempt and dress inappropriately for the situation. Many times the person will wear multiple layers of clothing regardless of the environmental temperature. Because the person with psychosis has poor impulse control, behavior may also be sexually inappropriate, unpredictable, and include sudden explosive outbursts. The person is unable to recognize what is considered by most as a norm of society. For example, most people refrain from going without clothes or masturbating in public because this is not acceptable. In psychosis, however, the person displays behavior that reflects his or her own personal thought process and is oblivious to moral boundaries.

Catatonic behaviors involve a decreased reaction to environmental surroundings. Movements may be severely decreased or absent and accompanied by a lack of awareness and orientation. The person with catatonia may assume a rigid posture and resist efforts to be moved. Inappropriate and bizarre postures can also be observed. During an excitement phase, the person may have purposeless movements. This behavior involves excessive motor activity that is not triggered by any stimulus. **Waxy flexibility** occurs when the person remains in one position until someone changes it. An arm, leg, or other body part can be moved by another person and it will remain in that position until moved again.

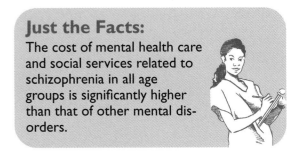

Mind Jogger

Homeless people without shelter or housing have a sense of isolation and rejection. What might contribute to the fact that many people with psychotic disorders become part of this population?

Psychotic Disorders

There are a number of different situations in which the symptoms of psychosis are manifested. They may be evidenced in some medical conditions, delirium, drug toxicity, dementia, mood disorders, and other delusional disorders. In most situations, the symptoms are not present at all times. The major symptom of these disorders is the occurrence of delusions and hallucinations. Some individuals may experience this as a single psychotic event, such as that seen after an extremely stressful event or trauma. The episode may last a few days but usually resolves within several weeks. In other situations, such as in schizoaffective disorder, there is a combined

At a Glance 11-1 Associated Causes of Psychosis

- Depression
- Bipolar disorder
- Epilepsy
- Brain tumor
- Dementia
- Stroke
- Alcohol or other drug use

presence of schizophrenic symptoms and those of a mood disorder. The most common and severe form of psychosis is seen in those with schizophrenia. Because this disorder is most associated with a psychotic disorder, our discussion centers on this illness.

Just the Facts:

The cost of mental health care and social services related to schizophrenia in all age groups is significantly higher than that of other mental disorders.

Schizophrenia

Schizophrenia is a form of psychosis in which there are disorganized thoughts, perceptual alterations, inappropriate affect, and decreased emotional response as the links to reality are lost. It is a chronic and disabling mental illness that causes the person to withdraw into a world of delusional thoughts and misperceptions. The word *schizophrenia* derives from the Greek, meaning "split mind." The person's ability to distinguish real from unreal becomes painfully disordered. This does not mean, however, that the personality is disintegrated as in multiple personality disorder. Although not all people suffering from schizophrenia experience all the symptoms, the impact to their personal, family, and social life is severe.

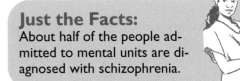

Just the Facts:

About half of the people admitted to mental units are diagnosed with schizophrenia.

Common Signs and Symptoms. In most cases, the onset of symptoms is insidious, with the person experiencing them for some time before the first full-blown psychotic episode occurs. This period is often referred to as the **prodromal phase** and actually indicates the beginning of the illness. The person may have increasing anxiety with inability to concentrate or complete goal-oriented tasks. In the case of the student, there is a loss of connections, which destroys the ability to think and learn. There may be an alternation between hyperactivity and inactivity. As the deterioration continues, the person becomes more distracted and feels that something is happening or expresses fear of "losing my mind." The person may misread things that are happening in the environment, often becoming paranoid about being followed or poisoned. Delusions may center on imaginary people who appear and harass or ridicule the person. Gradually the delusions and hallucinations become a part of each day with jumbled speech patterns and bizarre behaviors. Social relationships deteriorate to the point that the person is unable to function in a romantic, peer, or work relationship. Interest is lost in any type of competition or planning for the future. This tends to be the point at which many individuals turn to drug use to compensate for a loss of self-confidence and self-esteem.

Associated with psychotic disorders such as schizophrenia is the potential for clients to overhydrate by drinking excessive liquids, sometimes as much as 10 to 15 liters a day. The client is seen constantly carrying a cup or container with frequent trips to the water fountain or requests for something to drink. Some have been observed drinking from the toilet bowl or sink. The continued intake of fluid can lead to **water intoxication** or a psychosis-induced metabolic state of fluid overload. This can lead to cerebral edema and other potentially lethal situations. It is thought that a possible cause of this overload is related to the effects of antipsychotic drugs on the pituitary gland, which produces antidiuretic hormone (ADH) and thus inhibits the excretion of water.

The symptoms of schizophrenia are primarily categorized as positive and negative.

Positive Symptoms. Positive symptoms are evidenced early in the progress of the disorder. These are usually demonstrated in the initial contact that the person has with the health care system. This is usually a hospitalization for what is called *acute schizophrenia.* These symptoms include alterations in thinking, perception, and behavior.

The delusional patterns seen in schizophrenia are distorted and often bizarre with no logical connections. In the case of psychosis, the behavior that occurs while thoughts are processed and spoken actually provides more information than the content of what is said. The fragmented and disorganized thought processes are demonstrated in speech patterns of word salad and derailed loose associations. These jumbled words can reflect the theme of what the person is experiencing within his or her head. However, the theme reference and feelings can also be reflected in behavior. For example, the person who has recurring delusions of persecution may demonstrate fear by constantly looking to the side or over a shoulder as if someone is lurking behind or following him or her. Themes of persecution are the most commonly experienced delusions in the schizophrenic client. This type involves a false belief that someone is plotting to harm him or her. Often the person believes this is being devised by very important people or alien powers (e.g., a client believes the CIA is sending signals through telephone wires that will electrocute her). Beliefs such as these may hold some resemblance to life experiences such as a young man who was abused as a child and believes his father will electrocute him using the light switches. Others are more bizarre and have no realistic theme. For example, a client thinks there is a machine in her stomach that is timed to explode on New Year's Eve. The delusional thinking persists regardless of evidence that proves it inaccurate. Delusions of grandeur centralize on false beliefs that one is a very powerful and important person. These delusions often tend to have religious or governmental themes. For example, a client may believe that he is a disciple sent by God to lead the world through the Internet.

Perceptual alterations may include all sensory types of hallucinations. Auditory and visual hallucinations are perhaps the most common in people with schizophrenia. Hearing voices or sounds, both within the confines of the mind or externally, is perhaps the most familiar of these alterations. These individuals may respond to the voices, which often talk directly to them or make remarks about their actions. This is illustrated by the young man who thought his girlfriend was talking to him from his shirt pocket. He would face the wall as if wanting privacy, open the flap of the pocket, and answer the voice.

Misperceptions of personal identity are also seen, with the inability to distinguish oneself from the realness of another. They are often confused about their sexual identity, feeling that parts of others are meshing with their own body parts. They may feel disconnected to their own body or depersonalize themselves. For example, a woman views her blood vessels as worms floating through the air.

Patterns of strange, bizarre, and unusual behavior can occur in many forms. The person may dress oddly, assume strange positions, or demonstrate restless physical movements. The person may have stereotyped behavior without purpose such as picking up

Case Study: Antonia's Internal Threat

Antonia is a client in the psychiatric unit with a diagnosis of undifferentiated schizophrenia. She has a history of noncompliance with medications. She approaches the nurse and states, "The president told me to tell you meteors are descending toward the earth. They are going to get into the brains of all women to prevent the overpopulation of the outer planets." Antonia runs frantically and finally crawls under the coffee table in the day room.

What type of theme does Antonia's delusional thought process indicate?

_____

_____

Describe the speech pattern of this client:

_____

_____

How should the nurse approach Antonia regarding her behavior?

_____

_____

_____

trash items but not depositing them in a trashcan. Many clients with schizophrenia demonstrate a negative response to directions or instructions by doing the opposite of what is asked of them. The person who is told to sit down and eat may get up and start pacing in the hall. Agitation is often relieved by pacing, with some clients walking great distances without realizing how far they have gone.

Negative Symptoms. Negative symptoms develop slowly over time. They are reflected in the person's inability to deal with the way their illness affects their life. The devastating effects result in isolation and withdrawal from the uncomfortable inability to interact with others in a meaningful way.

Affect is perhaps the most noticeable of these symptoms. The person with schizophrenia typically has a blunted or flat affect that is expressionless and blank. The affect can also be inappropriate, such as smiling when the situation is sad. Other times, the person may exhibit bizarre expressions such as giggling while mumbling to a water faucet in the bathroom. The behavior is often described as autistic, referring to a focus on an inner fantasy world while excluding the external environment.

As the disorder takes over the person's life, interrelating with others and maintaining relationships becomes impossible. The person experiences **avolition,** lacking motivation to make decisions or initiate self-care such as hygiene and grooming. Dress becomes unkempt and inappropriate. Anergia or decreased energy and a passive lack of ambition are evident. Anhedonia is seen as little interest is shown in activities that were previously enjoyed. Speech may regress to brief phrases, a one-word response, or mutism.

Substance abuse, suicide, and violence are common associated symptoms that accompany the devastating effects of schizophrenia. Depression with a suicidal end to the helpless and isolated pattern of living is not uncommon. Both psychoactive drugs and illegal substances are abused by people with schizophrenia. Use of alcohol, marijuana, cocaine, and others are used to offset the haunting symptoms of the illness. Often the use of these drugs contributes to violence and severe acts of cruelty toward others.

Mind Jogger

It is said that most people with schizophrenia who attempt suicide are also in major depression. What factors might be contributing to this state?

At a Glance 11-2 Signs and Symptoms of Schizophrenia

Positive Symptoms

- Delusions
- Word salad
- Clang associations
- Thought broadcasting
- Thought insertion
- Loose associations
- Neologism
- Hallucinations
- Illusions
- Depersonalization
- Bizarre behavior
- Agitation
- Catatonia
- Autism

Negative Symptoms

- Blunt or flat affect
- Lack of energy
- Failure to find pleasure in activities
- Lack of motivation
- Inability to initiate self-care skills
- Inability to interact with others
- Impoverished speech
- Substance use
- Depression and suicidal acts
- Violent behavior

Incidence and Etiology. Schizophrenia affects approximately 1% of the world's population. The onset typically occurs between late adolescence and mid-30s. There are instances where schizophrenia begins in childhood, and there is a late-onset type that occurs after age 45. There is evidence that indicates that this disorder manifests differently in men than in women. For men, the average age of onset is between 18 and 25 years, and that of women occurring between 25 and 30 years. Late onset is more common in women than in men. Women tend to experience less severe symptoms with fewer hospitalizations than men. This disorder is prevalent in all populations without bias as to race, gender, culture, or socioeconomic groups. There is a higher risk in those who have first-degree biologic relatives with the disorder. Most people who develop schizophrenia have the symptoms for the remainder of their lives.

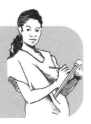

Just the Facts:
Approximately 10% of persons with schizophrenia attempt or commit suicide.

There is no particular single cause of schizophrenia. It has long been known that a genetic factor exists, but the hereditary mechanism is not clear. Research regarding a connection to brain chemistry is providing possible links to an imbalance in the neurotransmitters dopamine and glutamate. Other studies show abnormalities in the brain structure of those with schizophrenia. All research efforts are being made to identify the genes and contributing factors for the development of this debilitating illness.

Subtypes of Schizophrenia

Along with the diagnosis of schizophrenia, a further distinction is usually made based on the symptoms that are exhibited.

Paranoid Type. People with paranoid type of schizophrenia experience prominent hallucinations and delusions. The hallucinations are often auditory in nature with delusions of being persecuted or followed. The delusions are usually very organized and focus on the theme. For example, one person may think that everyone who wears black is sent by the devil to harm him. Everything the person does is centered on this theme. Because this is threatening to the person, he or she assumes a defensive behavior toward anyone who is wearing black. This can endanger others if the delusion is severe.

Disorganized Type. Those with disorganized type of schizophrenia exhibit disorganized and unintelligible speech, bizarre behavior, and a flat affect. Delusions do not center on any particular theme but tend to be fragmented and varied in focus. Unusual mannerisms and posturing may prevent these individuals from eating, toileting, or attending to personal hygiene. They may demonstrate inappropriate laughter or be strangely silly. It is not unusual to see these individuals sitting in an empty room laughing and acting theatrical.

Catatonic Type. The catatonic type of schizophrenia is characterized by a severe decrease in motor activity and responsiveness to the environment. The person may be mute and suddenly start repeating words heard at an earlier time. These individuals may make strange motions with their arms while walking with rigid posture or make stereotyped movements that mimic the actions of others. When assuming a rigid, fixed posture for extended periods, these individuals usually have waxy flexibility and can be repositioned without a return to the previous pose. This type is rarely seen as a single diagnosed condition.

Undifferentiated Type. The person with schizophrenia of the undifferentiated type exhibits a number of classic symptoms such as delusions, hallucinations, disorganized speech, strange behavior, and blunted affect. The symptoms are not defined to meet the criteria for any other subtype. The person may exhibit the prominent symptoms but none that are specific to any one type of the disorder.

Residual Type. The person with residual type of schizophrenia has experienced prominent psychotic symptoms with a previous diagnosis of schizophrenia but no longer has them. There is lingering evidence of unusual behavior, a blunted affect, some unrealistic thinking, or social withdrawal.

Mind Jogger

Many people with schizophrenia are caught in a cycle that takes them from acute care management, to a supervised milieu, and back to the community only to be readmitted with an acute exacerbation of the illness. Why do you think this pattern exists?

Application of the Nursing Process

Nursing Assessment

A nursing assessment will include information regarding any previous incidence of mental illness or psychotic episodes. Because the person may not always be a reliable source of information, family members or other people familiar with the client should be consulted.

Data are most often compiled according to the nature of the symptoms, including perceptual alterations such as hallucinations or illusions.

- Identify the type of disturbance the client is experiencing.
- Ask the client about feelings while thought alterations are evident.
- Determine the theme and content of delusional thinking. If the delusion is persecu-

tion oriented, assess the nature of the threat and whether there is a risk for violence as a result.

- Assess speech patterns associated with the delusions. Delusional thinking is characterized by speech in which the person jumps from one unrelated subject to another. Remember that the manner in which speech is manifested and the accompanying behavior usually provide more information about the delusion than the content.
- Note the affect and emotional tone of the client and whether they are appropriate in relation to the present situation. Apathy or a lack of interest in the environment and flatness of affect are characteristic signs of schizophrenia.
- Observe behavior patterns, activity, sleep habits, and interactions with other clients.
- Observe for posturing or other psychomotor disturbances.
- Assess the person's appearance, hygiene, and ability to perform self-care activities.
- Determine any suicidal intent or recent attempts that may have been made.

Nursing Diagnosis

After careful review of the data, nursing diagnoses can be formulated. Approaches to treatment are usually selected on their ability to reduce and control the symptoms. Nursing care should be planned to focus on symptomatic relief as well, with careful attention to the physical, emotional, and social needs imposed by impaired mental functioning. Nursing diagnoses for the client with schizophrenia may include:

- Verbal communication impaired, related to fragmented delusional thinking
- Violence, high risk for: self-directed or directed at others, related to suspiciousness or command hallucinations
- Family process alteration, related to chronic illness
- Individual coping ineffective, related to chronic illness, substance use

- Self-care deficit, related to withdrawal and apathy
- Altered thought processes, related to delusional thinking
- Social isolation, related to lack of trust
- Role performance alteration, related to decreased functional ability
- Sensory/perceptual alterations, related to stress and withdrawal
- Low self-esteem, related to chronic illness
- Noncompliance, related to denial of illness
- Knowledge deficit, related to drug therapy
- Hopelessness, related to chronic low self-worth

Expected Outcomes

The anticipated outcomes will depend on the level of functioning demonstrated by the client. This will depend on the severity of symptoms and the effectiveness of antipsychotic drug therapy or other therapeutic approaches. It is important that the goals and timeframe for improvement be realistic. Expected outcomes for the schizophrenic person may include that he or she:

- Develops reality-based ways to communicate and meet self-needs
- Remains oriented to self and the environment
- Interacts appropriately with others
- Has not injured self or others
- Family members express realistic expectations of individual member
- Performs self-care and hygiene with minimal prompting
- Demonstrates increased trust of others
- Exhibits increased ability to associate behavior with misperceived environmental stimuli
- Participates in unit activities with appropriate behavior
- Identifies realistic self-expectations and perceptions
- Has reduced incidence of hallucinations
- Cooperates with staff in taking medications

Nursing Interventions

Selecting appropriate interventions that the client can tolerate requires careful planning. It is important to avoid expecting too much, but at the same time it is important to encourage clients to maximize their ability to function. Understanding the client's ability to focus, process, and follow instructions provides direction for the selection of nursing interventions. It is important to consider the holistic picture of the client, including physiologic, emotional, cultural, and spiritual needs. Interventions for the client with schizophrenia may include:

- Show acceptance of the client, separating the person from the behavior.
- Provide a safe environment by removing unsafe objects and diffusing potentially violent situations before they escalate.
- Maintain a reality-based approach to communication with the client.
- Provide a nonstimulating environment that reduces external stimuli.
- Monitor for behavioral clues that indicate hallucinations or delusions (e.g., staring at an inanimate object, whispering, inappropriate giggling, facial, or hand gestures).
- Acknowledge the perceptual or thinking alteration as being real to the client while reinforcing reality (e.g., "I understand that the voices must be frightening to you, but I do not hear them."), which helps the client to recognize symptoms as part of the illness.
- Set and maintain limits on unsafe or inappropriate behavior.
- Reinforce the importance of consistent compliance with medication therapy.
- Provide positive feedback for appropriate behaviors.
- Encourage the client to ventilate feelings associated with altered thoughts and behaviors.
- Avoid abrupt touching of the client, which can be perceived as threatening.
- Provide prepackaged foods for clients who are paranoid. (Clients are more likely to eat foods they can open themselves than foods

already prepared. Food such as casseroles, mashed potatoes, meats, and gravy should be avoided during time of increased paranoia. Instead, items such as cheese slices, potato chips, crackers, milk, and complete nutrition prepackaged drinks can be offered as supplemental foods.)

- Monitor number of hours client sleeps each 24-hour period.
- Encourage participation in social interaction with others and recognize that a group activity may be threatening to the client with paranoia.
- Promote independence in self-responsibility for hygiene and self-care needs.
- Promote client and family understanding of the illness and treatment regimen.
- Monitor for extrapyrimidal side effects of antipsychotic drug therapy.
- Monitor client's fluid intake, especially when in agitated or frenzied state.

Medications for Psychosis. Medications can provide relief for people who are experiencing positive symptoms of psychosis. These medications and their side effects are discussed in Chapter 20. It is of particular importance in the case of antipsychotic drugs to monitor for the extrapyramidal side effects. These are often monitored using the AIMS assessment tool (see Chapter 20). The effects of tardive dyskinesia are potentially irreversible and affect the functional ability of the client. The masklike facial appearance, tremors, shuffling gait, cogwheel rigidity, pill-rolling, and stooped posture are common indications that long-term use of these drugs has occurred. The physician can make dosage adjustments or prescribe medications to counteract these effects if they occur and are recognized early.

Use of Seclusion. It is important to assess the client for escalating behavior and intervene before an "out of control" situation occurs. In some instances, when other interventions do not work and the client is at risk of harming self or others, the client may be tem-

porarily restrained with a time-out in seclusion imposed to allow the client to regain self-control. When this situation occurs, nurses must use every measure to show respect for the client. Limits for behavior are reinforced and explained, reassuring the client of the temporary nature of these restrictions. Nutritional, hygiene, and toileting needs should be met in accordance with unit policies.

Evaluation

When evaluating the effectiveness of planned interventions, the nurse should look for signs that indicate improved functioning of the client. It is anticipated that compliance with drug therapy will diminish the positive symptoms of psychosis the client experiences. Hopefully, this is accompanied by an increase in the client's understanding of actual and real events that precipitate the perceptual and delusional alterations. This is demonstrated as the client is able to identify these factors and practice diversional techniques to avoid the anxiety that encourages the psychotic behavior.

Communication with staff and other clients in an appropriate and reality-based conversation is evidence of improved thinking processes. A decrease in bizarre and inappropriate behavior will occur as thoughts and perceptions decrease the need for their use. Reduced suspiciousness is evidenced by increased willingness to trust staff and other clients. This is a slow process for a client who has lived with a world of perceived threats and injustice. Any small gain should be viewed as progress. Compliance with taking medications and increased food intake are also evidence that the client has decreased fear of poisoning by ingested substances.

Living with a life of losses in personal and social acceptance is difficult for clients with schizophrenia. Their feelings of hopelessness and worthlessness are ongoing. Expression of these feelings is a positive step as they move toward identification of peer and social support systems. Involvement in unit activities is a demonstration of their willingness to engage in the company of others. This also may be seen in the client who follows a task to completion such as in occupational therapy, clearing tables in the dining area, or taking a shower and dressing without assistance.

Summary

Psychosis is severe disarray in the mental processes of thinking, perceiving, and behaving. Because behavior is directly linked to our perceptions and thoughts about environmental stimuli, it seems logical that behavior changes occur when these processes are distorted and disorganized. This is what happens in psychosis. The characteristic symptoms reveal a loss of touch with reality and those things that give life meaning. Loss of the ability to communicate meaningfully with others leads to a deterioration of relationships and contact with society.

Schizophrenia is the most common form of psychotic disorder. It inflicts a devastating downward spiral of losses in the person's ability to interact with the world. A prodromal period often precedes the actual first psychotic event. During this period the person may begin experiencing inability to concentrate and finish things. Thoughts may become distorted and speech patterns reflect a jumble of misplaced words. The person may struggle with feelings of inadequacy and resist any sort of competition with others. This usually leads to withdrawal from personal, work, and social relationships. The losses result in an overwhelming feeling of loneliness, worthlessness, and apathy. As the illness progresses, the disorganization becomes the central theme of each day.

Treatment and nursing care of the client with schizophrenia centers on reduction of the debilitating symptoms. Most of the positive symptoms can be managed by consistent compliance with antipsychotic drug therapy. The effectiveness of these drugs is often limited by the incidence of side effects and noncompliance. This is compounded by the indigent existence that is led by many people with schizophrenia. Rejected by society, many turn to illicit drugs to drown their feelings of worthlessness and emptiness. Unless appropriate interventions and treatment is afforded them, they may become suicidal, and many succeed in their attempts.

Bibliography

Pawar, A. V., & Spence, S. A. (2003). Defining thought broadcast: semi-structured literature review, *British Journal of Psychiatry, 183* (October), 287–291.

American Psychiatric Association (2000). *Diagnostic and statistical manual of mental disorders text revision* (4th ed.). Washington, DC: American Psychiatric Association.

Modestin, J., Huber, A., Satirli, E., Malti, T., Hell, D. (2003). Long-term course of schizophrenic illness: Bleuler's study reconsidered. *American Journal of Psychiatry, 160,* 2202–2208.

National Institute of Mental Health. Schizophrenia. Available at http://www.nih.gov/ healthinformation/schizophreniamenu.cfm. Accessed on July 7, 2004.

Pallanti, S., Quercioli, L., & Hollander, E. (2004). Social anxiety in outpatients with schizophrenia: a relevant cause of disability. *American Journal of Psychiatry, 161,* 53–58.

Howard, R., Rabins, P. V., Seeman, M. V., et al. (2000). Late onset schizophrenia and late-onset schizophrenia-like psychosis: an international consensus. *American Journal of Psychiatry, 152(2),* 172–178. Available at http://ajp. psychiatryonline.org/cgi/search. Accessed July 7, 2004.

Student Worksheet

FILL IN THE BLANK

Fill in the blank with the correct answer.

1. Symptoms of psychosis most often make reference to a(n) _____ in the mental processes.

2. _____ are perceptual disturbances in which the person misinterprets sensory stimuli that actually exist.

3. About _____ of the people admitted to mental units are diagnosed with schizophrenia.

4. A psychosis-induced metabolic state of overhydration in the schizophrenic client is referred to as _____ _____.

5. Auditory hallucinations may involve _____ voices that tell the person to harm himself or others.

6. Delusions of _____ centralize on false beliefs that the person is very powerful and important.

7. The person with schizophrenia typically has a(n) _____ affect that is expressionless and blank.

8. A(n) _____ period of symptoms often occurs prior to the first actual psychotic episode in those diagnosed with schizophrenia.

9. _____ type of schizophrenia includes those situations where the classic symptoms are demonstrated but do not meet criteria of any one subtype.

10. It is of particular importance to monitor the client taking antipsychotic drug agents for the incidence of _____ side effects.

MATCHING

Match the following terms to the most appropriate phrase.

a. Person remains in one position until changed by another person.

b. "I know all the judges can hear what I am thinking."

c. Lack of motivation to make decisions or do self-care.

d. "Our bowl is loud star to a wet red noodle carried by the military in excess of the earth."

e. "Take the pill up the hill winter kill . . ."

f. "Tom Brokaw is telling me I hold the key to security in outer space."

g. Loose associations that are off track or not connected to each other.

1. _____ Avolition

2. _____ Derailment

3. _____ Clang associations

4. _____ Thought broadcasting

5. _____ Word salad

6. _____ Waxy flexibility

7. _____ Delusion of reference

MULTIPLE CHOICE

Select the best answer from the multiple-choice items.

1. The nurse is assessing a client who states, "The radio is sending signals to my intellectual processes to inflict damage on myself." Which of the following would the nurse include in documenting the delusional pattern of this client?
   a. Experiencing auditory hallucinations
   b. Having delusions of persecution
   c. Demonstrating thought insertion
   d. Speaking in loose associations

2. Which of the following statements best describes poverty of speech?
   a. A jumble of unconnected and disorganized thoughts
   b. Insignificant rhyming of words
   c. Thoughts of others can be inserted in one's mind
   d. Decrease in amount or speed with which a person talks

3. A client approaches the nurse and states, "This little elf keeps following me with a leash, and it really is getting on my nerves." Which of the following would be the most appropriate response for the nurse to make at this time?
   a. "I know seeing the elf is frustrating to you, but no one else sees it."
   b. "Why don't you just tell the elf to sit down and leave you alone."
   c. "That is silly. There is no one following you."
   d. "You are only making that up in your mind."

4. The nurse is serving lunch to a client with paranoid delusional thoughts of being poisoned by insecticides. Which of the following foods will this client most likely eat?
   a. Beef stew
   b. Squash casserole
   c. Sealed container of pudding
   d. Apple slices with packages of peanut butter

5. Which of the following nursing diagnoses is best supported by data that describe a client as "wiping the water fountain vigorously with his hands and making loud comments telling it to shut up?"
   a. Individual coping ineffective
   b. Hopelessness
   c. Altered thought processes
   d. Sensory/perceptual alteration

SEEK AND FIND

Find the incorrect information in the following statements.

1. The person with schizophrenia typically has a blunted affect that is responsive and receptive to the environment.

2. The negative symptoms of schizophrenia are what usually brings those with this disorder to treatment.

3. Thought insertion indicates a belief that others are robbing thoughts from one's brain.

SCENARIO: DELUSIONAL EROSION

Elaine is admitted to the psychiatric unit with a history of psychosis and noncompliance with medication therapy. During an interaction with the nurse, Elaine states, "I have a scientific machine in my colon that clips off pieces of my internal organs to ship to the FBI. They are trying to kill me."
How should the nurse respond to Elaine's statement?

_____

_____

What type of delusion is Elaine experiencing?

_____

Later that day, Elaine refuses to eat. She states, "I can't eat because food makes the machine interrogate faster." What are the appropriate nursing interventions at this point?

_____

_____

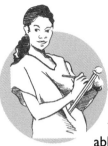

LEARNING OBJECTIVES

After learning the content in this chapter, the student will be able to:

1. Define the psychophysiologic dynamics of a somatoform disorder.
2. Identify the signs and symptoms of the somatoform disorders.
3. Identify etiologic factors in the development of a psychophysiologic disorder.
4. Perform a skilled data collection in assessing the client with a somatoform disorder.
5. Formulate nursing diagnoses and outcomes to address problems common to clients with psychophysiologic symptoms.
6. Plan appropriate nursing interventions for psychophysiologic behaviors.
7. Describe evaluation methods for determining the effectiveness of planned interventions.

Somatoform Disorders

KEY TERMS

Hypochondriasis
Hysteria
La belle indifference
Primary gain
Pseudoneurologic
Psychophysiologic
Secondary gain
Soma
Somatization
Somatoform

Defining a Somatoform Disorder

The term **soma** is derived from the Greek language and refers to the body. Historically, the connection between stress, anxiety, and physiologic symptoms has been delegated to **hysteria** or a nervous disorder marked by ineffective emotional control. The predictable syndrome of physical complaints and symptoms that are expressed as a result of psychologic stress are defined as **somatization.** In all of the situations, the physical symptoms suggest that a medical condition exists. However, because they cannot be explained by diagnostic findings, the symptoms cannot be attributed to a medical condition and are considered **psychophysiologic** or **somatoform.** Unlike the client who intentionally creates symptoms to remain in the role of patient, the person with somatization is not consciously aware of the psychologic factors underlying the disorder and does not intentionally continue the complaints. The person is not in control of the symptoms, which are an involuntary expression of psychologic conflicts. Somatization is considered a defense mechanism. The somatic symptoms provide a psychologic or **primary gain** as the anxiety is relieved and focus is diverted to the physical problem. **Secondary gain** comes from the subsequent attention the person receives from a physician or family member. Other mechanisms that are used by people with this disorder include repression of trauma or conflict, denial that psychologic factors exist, and displacement of anxiety and conflict to body symptoms.

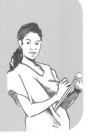

Just the Facts

Somatoform disorders are characterized by disturbances in sensory or motor functioning, while dissociative disorders affect the sense of identity or memory.

Categories of Somatoform Disorders

The somatoform disorders share the common feature of physical symptoms that seem to suggest that a medical condition is their cause, but the clinical findings do not support the existence of a medical problem or other mental disorder. The symptoms are severe enough to cause significant distress and dysfunction for the person in social and work-related settings. The autonomic nervous system response to stress may be associated with an increased awareness of physiologic symptoms such as acceleration of the heart rate, muscle tension, and increased gastrointestinal motility. These symptoms may initially seem to indicate a medical problem for which the person seeks treatment.

Clients with a somatoform disorder often have long histories of medical or exploratory and unnecessary surgical treatments by several different doctors. This fact, in addition to the automatic nature of the symptoms over which the person has no control, tends to complicate the process of distinguishing the symptoms from actual medical problems. The client tends to perceive the presence of an illness or injury despite reassurance to the contrary by the physician.

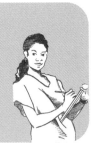

Just the Facts

Somatoform disorders are a significant problem for the health care system because clients with these symptoms overuse physician services and resources.

Somatization Disorder

Somatization disorder, also referred to as Briquet's syndrome, is characterized by multiple symptoms that begin before age 30 and extend over a period of years. This disorder tends to involve several body systems and is the most common somatoform disorder. The client often goes from one physician to another seeking a diagnosis. This in turn leads to a series of repeated diagnostic tests and x-ray studies in an attempt to support a medical problem. The potential hazard of concurrent medical treatments, such as drug interactions or potentiation, is also a definite consideration.

Common Signs and Symptoms. A somatic complaint is considered to be valid if it requires medical treatment such as medication. In this disorder, there are multiple somatic complaints that cannot be completely explained by medical findings. When describing the problem, the client often exaggerates the symptoms with little supportive factual information. Symptoms of moderate to severe anxiety and depression are commonly seen in addition to the somatic complaints. The intensity and persistence of symptoms indicate the person's desperate need to be cared for in all aspects of living. This, in some instances, is suggestive that the person has underlying feelings of unworthiness and guilt.

The somatic complaints include pain in at least four different locations, such as the head, joints, chest, or back. There must be at least two gastrointestinal symptoms present. Nausea and abdominal bloating are frequently seen, whereas diarrhea and vomiting are less common. A complaint of a sexual or reproductive problem other than pain is also a feature of the disorder. Often women complain of menstrual irregularities and men of erectile dysfunction. Finally, at least one complaint must involve a neurologic symptom such as a loss of sensation or coordination in a limb, weakness, or visual problems. The subjective symptoms cannot be controlled by the person and are perceived as real by the person experiencing them. The common threads of the complaints are the primary gain obtained as the anxiety is relieved and the secondary gain, or attention the person receives in response to the symptoms. These factors are usually not apparent to the client demonstrating the behavioral pattern.

The person becomes extremely dependent both in doctor–patient and personal relationships with an increasing demand for attention and emotional support, often getting enraged when they feel their needs are not being met. In an attempt to manipulate others, the demand for attention may in some instances result in threats or attempts to commit suicide.

At a Glance 12-1 Common Signs and Symptoms of Somatization Disorder

- Multiple somatic complaints unexplained by medical findings
- Exaggeration of symptoms without factual information
- Complaints of pain in at least four different locations
- Two gastrointestinal symptoms
- One sexual or reproductive symptom
- One neurologic symptom
- Moderate to severe anxiety
- Depression
- Inability to voluntarily control the symptoms
- Dependency with demanding, attention-getting behaviors
- Secondary gain
- Significant distress or impairment in social or occupational areas

---

Incidence and Etiology. Only a small percentage of the U.S. population is affected by this disorder, and it is seen much more prominently in women than men. Somatization disorder is considered to be a chronic condition that tends to recur throughout the person's life. Initial symptoms may appear as early as adolescence. Menstrual complaints may be the initial symptom in women. The disorder tends to run in families, with a likely occurrence of other mental disturbances as well. Familial patterns of behavior are often replicated by children and adolescents, especially when those behaviors receive the attention of others. This imitation as well as differences in the perception of pain may be factors in the generational tendency. These disorders also tend to be more prevalent in Greek and Puerto Rican cultures. Personality disorders such as narcissistic, borderline, and antisocial disorders are often seen in association with somatization disorder.

Mind Jogger
How might the secondary gain received by the parent with a somatic disorder encourage a child to copy the behavior?

Conversion Disorder

The person with a conversion disorder exhibits symptoms that indicate a sensory or neurologic impairment that is not supported by results of diagnostic testing. Usually there are related stress or trauma factors that have occurred concurrent with the onset of the symptoms. Because the symptoms essentially involve voluntary motor or sensory functioning, they are considered **pseudoneurologic,** or false neurologic, disturbances. The actual conversion aspect of this disorder refers to the transfer of psychologic conflict or stressors into a perceived paralysis of body parts or sensory functioning. For example, a person loses functional use of her dominant arm and hand before a piano recital she does not want to perform.

Common Signs and Symptoms. The conversion symptoms contain the factor of anxiety, which serves to divert attention away from the underlying stress situation. The transfer of this anxiety to a loss of physical functioning serves as a primary gain for the client. The changes in social, work-related, or family circumstances that result from the temporary disability may provide the secondary gain of avoiding unpleasant tasks or responsibilities along with the accompanying attention the person receives. People with conversion disorder may exhibit an attitude of **la belle indifference;** that is, they demonstrate little anxiety or concern over the implications of the symptoms.

Motor symptoms may include impaired coordination or balance, paralysis of a limb, the inability to speak, difficulty swallowing, or urinary retention. Sensory deficits may relate to a loss of pain sensation, visual or hearing malfunction, and hallucinations. Occasionally seizures or convulsions may be seen. The symptoms tend to differ from actual neurologic deficits in that the person's description of the problem does not exhibit a dysfunction of the typical nerve pathway. Typically, the symptoms do not lead to any physical changes or disabilities, as are seen in neurologic disorders. There may be an inability to perform a particular movement, but other functions of the body part may be intact. Sometimes the extremity described as dysfunctional will inadvertently be moved when attention is temporarily directed away. Although a limb is described as nonfunctional, the neurologic reflexes are intact. A conversion seizure will vary from one incident to the other without a distinct pattern of activity and may resemble a seizure that has been described to the individual.

Just the Facts
Family stress and physical or sexual abuse are thought to be the most common cause of conversion disorders in children and adolescents.

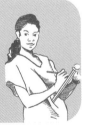

Mind Jogger
What symptoms usually seen in a pathologic seizure might be missing in a conversion seizure?

At a Glance 12-2 Common Signs and Symptoms of Conversion Disorder

- Sensory or neurologic impairment that is not supported by diagnostic testing
- Lack of conscious control over the symptoms
- Loss of balance or paralysis of limb
- Loss of swallowing, speaking, seeing, or hearing
- Loss of pain or touch sensation
- Impaired functioning in social or work-related areas caused by symptoms
- A la belle indifference
- Seizures or convulsion-type behavior inconsistent with usual symptom pattern
- Lack of physical change or disability
- Functional ability and symptoms inconsistent with usual neurologic disorders

Incidence and Etiology. Conversion disorder may begin at any age and does not seem to run in families. Studies show that approximately one third of the population experiences these symptoms over a lifetime, with incidence in women twice as high as that in men. The disorder is more common in people of lower socioeconomic status and those living in rural locations. It is also more prevalent in those who are less educated about medical and psychologic issues. Adolescents with this disorder often have overprotective parents with a subdued need to see their child as "ill." The symptoms then become the focus of the family's attention and lifestyle. Conversion disorder tends to be of short-term duration, with most clients recovering in 2 to 4

weeks without reoccurrence. Those with symptoms of paralysis or loss of speech or vision tend to have a better outcome than those experiencing tremors or seizures.

Pain Disorder

The characteristic feature of pain disorder is severe pain that covers a variety of different complaints. The pain impairs the person's ability to function in social and work settings. Pain disorder may have associated psychologic factors or be associated with both psychologic factors and a medical condition. Psychologic issues are primary in the onset, severity, and continuance of the pain symptoms.

Common Signs and Symptoms. The pain seen in this disorder may severely interfere with activities of daily living. In most instances, the pain is largely due to psychologic factors, although in some cases some of the discomfort may be related to a medical condition. The location or description of the pain does not change. Symptoms may include migraine headaches, back ailments, arthritis, muscle cramping, or pelvic pain. The person may use excessive amounts of analgesics to relieve the pain without ever experiencing relief. Chronic pain may lead to substance dependence, which can complicate the situation. Those with recurrent pain are also at risk for symptoms of depression and contemplated suicide. Social isolation and inactivity may further contribute to the depressive mood. Sleep disturbances are also common in people with chronic pain.

Just the Facts

Male clients are likely to develop conversion disorders in work-related or military-type situations.

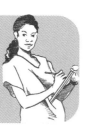

Mind Jogger

In what way might the client's perception of pain contribute to the development of this disorder?

At a Glance 12-3 Common Signs and Symptoms of Pain Disorder

- Severe pain with a variety of different complaints
- Associated psychologic factors
- Unchanging location or description of pain
- Use of excessive analgesia without ever achieving pain relief
- Depression
- Social isolation
- Impaired functioning in social or occupational setting
- Sleep disorders

Incidence and Etiology. Pain that interferes with day-to-day functioning is widespread. The most common form of work disability in the United States is related to back pain. The number of those with severe pain who have a pain disorder is not known. Those with an actual medical condition associated with a pain disorder are more common than those who have the disorder associated with psychologic factors alone. Pain disorder can occur at any age. Chronic pain is more common in older adults, with the female to male ratio nearly equal. Prognosis is highly dependent on the ability of the person to avoid the pain from becoming the dominant factor in his or her lives.

Case Study: Jerry's Displaced Fear

Jerry is a 47-year-old heavy equipment operator. His wife, Angela, has been a homemaker and mother to their three children for the past 12 years. Now that the children are all in school, Angela has decided to fulfill a lifelong dream and enroll in college classes to become a nurse. She has asked Jerry to help her with the children so she can have more time to study. She reminds him that once she is a nurse, she can supplement the family income. Three months after Angela begins her classes, Jerry develops severe back pain that requires him to take a leave of absence from work. He undergoes extensive imaging studies, but no medical reason is found for the pain. He states that the analgesics and muscle relaxants just don't seem to help. He tells Angela that he wants to go to a large medical clinic 400 miles from their home because the local doctors don't know what they are doing. He states that he cannot help with the children or household chores because of the pain. Two months later, Jerry quits his job and Angela must become the family support. She drops her classes and finds a job as a receptionist for a local insurance agency.

What underlying psychologic conflict may be causing Jerry's symptoms?

_____

_____

What are his primary and secondary gains?

_____

_____

_____

Hypochondriasis

Hypochondriasis is characterized by an excessive fear or preoccupation with having a serious illness that is based on a misinterpretation of somatic signs and symptoms. The concerns continue despite medical testing and reassurance that a disease does not exist. The person is not delusional and is able to acknowledge that a disease may not exist. However, the fear continues and creates enough distress to cause difficulty in social or work-related functioning over a period of 6 months or more.

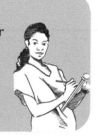

Just the Facts

Hypochondriasis persists over time but tends to occur in sporadic episodes or flare-ups usually associated with stressful events in the person's life.

Common Signs and Symptoms. The unwarranted fear or preoccupation often is related to a minor problem with body functioning that is misinterpreted as being a major illness. The person accesses the health care system repeatedly looking for verification of their fears. The symptoms are usually reported in specific detail as to occurrence, location, and duration. However, these do not tend to follow a recognizable pattern of typical symptoms for the pathologic condition. One or several body systems may be involved in the complaints. The person may become disturbed by reading or hearing information about the illness. Preoccupation and concern with the feared illness become a central focus in the person's life, conversations, and social networking. "Physician-shopping" is common as the person seeks out a practitioner who will substantiate the illness. Medical examinations and verbal reassurance do not convince the person that no disease exists. It is often believed that incompetent medical attention is being rendered. Referrals to mental health professionals are resented and rejected. Because the repeated false symptoms tend to build strained doctor–patient relationships, the presence of a real medical condition may be overlooked. Social and family relationships also become disturbed as the focus is constantly drawn to the person's physical well-being.

At a Glance 12-4 Common Signs and Symptoms of Hypochondriasis

Unwarranted fear or preoccupation with body functioning misperceived as a major illness
- Repeated health care visits seeking verification of fears
- Symptoms reported in specific detail
- Involvement of one or more body systems
- Symptoms that do not follow those typical of pathologic condition
- Perceived illness focal point of existence
- Unconvinced by repeated examinations and reassurance that disease does not exist
- Doctor shopping
- Perception of incompetent medical care
- Rejected referrals to mental health professional
- Impaired social and family relationships

Incidence and Etiology. The actual etiology of this disorder is not known. It is suggested that, like other somatization disorders, it is related to an overindulgence in self-concern with a need to satisfy strong dependency needs. The peak incidence for onset tends to be in the late 30s for men, and late 40s for women. The disorder tends to be chronic in nature, with a pattern that reflects a heightened awareness of body functions with an obsessive preoccupation that a problem exists. Because of the underlying psychologic need for dependency, only a few people are able to associate the somatic symptoms with their mental state. Depression is common as they continue to believe their fears and refuse to accept reassurance to the contrary.

Body Dysmorphic Disorder

Body dysmorphic disorder is characterized by preoccupation with an imagined defect in appearance or overconcern with an existing slight physical defect. The person experiences distress over the defect to the point of impaired functioning in social, school, or work-related settings.

Common Signs and Symptoms. Most people with this disorder focus on facial or head features, but they may involve other body parts—especially those involving sexual attractiveness. Areas of concern may be baldness, complexion flaws, wrinkles or scars, birthmarks, or the shape of the facial lines. Other focal areas include the breasts, buttocks, abdomen, chest, and overall body shape or size. The slight flaw may be seen as a major defect and described as "terrible" or "devastating." The person may alternate between constant viewing of the flaw in lighted magnifying mirrors and avoidance of mirrors entirely. Periods of checking and attempting to alter the defect have an intent of decreasing the anxiety associated with the situation. Excessive exercise, dieting, or clothing changes may be used to alter or hide body shape or size irregularities. Comparisons may be made to others who have "better" or "bigger" breasts, penis, or other body parts. The inability to control their preoccupation with the pain experienced related to their defect may cause discomfort to the point of functional impairment. Feelings of inadequacy and self-consciousness may lead to social isolation. Insight into the psychologic connection to these feelings is usually poor. Reassurance of normalcy is usually not convincing. The person may avoid social activities, drop out of school, or seek employment in positions where job interviews are not required. Some people seek reconstructive plastic surgery or implants to allay the consuming anxiety associated with the defect.

Mind Jogger
The anxiety felt with body dysmorphic disorder is attributed to external flaws. Could a focus on inner self-worth help the person to change his or her thinking?

At a Glance 12-5 Common Signs and Symptoms of Body Dysmorphic Disorder

- Preoccupation with imagined defect in appearance
- Overconcern with minor physical defect
- View of defect as "awful" or "devastating"
- Constant viewing of flaw in magnified mirrors
- Use of excessive means to hide the flaw
- Comparisons to others who have better physique
- Feelings of inadequacy and self-consciousness
- Social isolation
- Poor insight into psychologic connection to discomfort
- Reassurance of normalcy not convincing
- Reconstructive or plastic surgery to remove flaw associated with anxiety

Incidence and Etiology. Body dysmorphic disorder is considered to be a chronic condition with an onset in the late teens and intermittent reoccurrence over a lifetime. The disorder tends to occur in men and women with equal prevalence. An increase in the number of adolescents with this disorder is thought to reflect the preoccupation of society and media with physical attractiveness and appearance.

Application of the Nursing Process

Because the somatoform disorders are associated with physical symptoms, the person is often seen by a physician for the subjective complaints. Before a somatoform determination, a physical examination and diagnostic testing are necessary to rule out any underlying pathology. It is of major importance that nursing observations and data collection contain information that will be of help in this process. Considering that the client is unaware that there may be underlying psychologic issues and is unable to consciously control the symptoms, health care professionals are challenged by clients with this disorder. Most of them are repeat users of health care system services, both outpatient and inpatient.

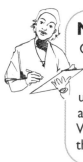

Mind Jogger

Clients who repeatedly access the health care system searching for answers often undergo many diagnostic tests and exploratory surgeries. What risks could this pose for the client?

Nursing Assessment

It is first important for the nurse to create an accepting, safe, and supportive atmosphere that allows open communication with the client and his or her family. This nurturing environment encourages the client to express feelings and needs more honestly. The nurse should focus on the whole person, including psychologic, social, and family factors in addition to the physical symptoms.

A careful assessment of physical complaints should be made, taking into consideration any statements made by the client and the manner in which they are expressed. Note any preoccupation with the symptoms and any inconsistency between what is being described and what is observed in the client. Elicit any pattern of repeated complaints by taking a history of current and past health status. It is important to note the client's attitude toward the symptoms and how he or she may view any limitations caused by them. It should also be noted whether the client is aware of events surrounding the onset of symptoms. In addition, the client's level of stress or anxiety and previous coping skills should be assessed. Questions should be asked to determine whether the symptoms have imposed any limitations related to the person's lifestyle and whether the client's role has changed within the family system. Any behavior that indicates an increased dependency need, such as repeatedly turning on a call light for assistance, should also be noted and documented.

Nursing Diagnosis

Planning care for the client with a somatoform disorder must consider that the client is often frustrated and angered by the implication that the symptoms are psychologic. Nursing diagnoses to address the problems related to these disorders may include:

- Anxiety, severe, related to repressed trauma or unmet dependency needs
- Denial, ineffective, related to avoidance of possible psychologic causes for symptoms
- Chronic pain, related to severe anxiety or unmet dependency needs
- Ineffective coping, related to anxiety, repression, or unrealistic perceptions
- Body image disturbance, related to severe anxiety or low self-esteem
- Self-care deficit, related to perceived loss of function or paralysis of body part
- Sensory/perceptual alteration, related to psychologic stress or chronic pain

- Sleep pattern disturbance, related to anxiety, depression, or chronic pain
- Social isolation, related to preoccupation with self and chronic state of perceived illness
- Knowledge deficit, related to psychophysiologic nature of illness
- Sexual dysfunction, related to perceived loss of body function or fear of contracting major disease
- Self-esteem disturbance, related to repressed unmet dependency needs and unsatisfactory interpersonal relationships

Expected Outcomes

Once problems have been identified for the individual client situation, planning will include realistic outcomes in the course of treatment. These outcomes may include:

- Expresses feelings of anxiety and effective means of dealing with the illness
- Acknowledges understanding and perception of present health problem
- Discusses present health problem with health care provider and family
- Acknowledges that physical pain may be associated with psychologic stress
- Participates in development of a plan for effective pain control
- Demonstrates reduced use of manipulative behavior to secure attention
- Expresses positive feelings about self
- Verbalizes realistic perception of minor body defect and related positive feelings
- Performs self-care needs independently and willingly
- Verbalizes understanding of psychologic factors associated with alteration in physical functioning
- Reports a decrease in sleep-related problems
- Participates in social activities and interaction without discomfort
- Reduces statements that demand a focus on self and physical symptoms
- Identifies realistic illness-related goals and self-perceptions

Nursing Interventions

Establishing a trusting relationship with clients experiencing a somatoform disorder is the first step in helping them overcome a low self-concept. A safe and supportive environment will also help lower their anxiety to a level that allows expression of underlying feelings. The nurse should identify and come to terms with any anger or negative feelings that he or she may have related to clients with this disorder. It must be remembered that they are not consciously trying to be sick or avoid responsibilities. Other interventions may include:

- Recognize that the physical complaints are real to the client even though supportive medical evidence is lacking.
- Avoid any confrontation concerning the psychologic defense nature of the symptoms.
- Respond to client with understanding and patience.
- Encourage discussion of person's life history, recent emotional events, and fears.
- Document observations and behaviors related to physical complaints.
- Continue to monitor physical complaints to assist in ruling out any actual cause for the symptoms.
- Identify unfulfilled dependency needs of the client.
- Identify types of primary and secondary gain achieved by symptoms.
- Minimize time and attention given to physical symptoms.
- Help the client to use words rather than physical means to express feelings.
- Encourage client to keep a diary of daily happenings and feelings, along with physical symptoms.
- Listen actively to determine what the client may be omitting when describing the symptoms.
- Encourage the client to make decisions and take responsibility for situations related to them.
- Help the client to identify more effective coping mechanisms rather than the somatic symptoms.

Evaluation

Evaluation of implemented nursing actions focuses on the client's ability to recognize the underlying psychologic stress and anxiety that are contributing to the physical symptoms. It should be determined if the client has developed an awareness of increased anxiety and initiated more effective coping mechanisms to deal with the stress level. Once the client can look realistically at the connection between repressed emotional turmoil and the somatic symptoms, a decrease in complaints or full recovery from the previous level of altered physical functioning, pain, or preoccupation with body appearance is anticipated. As the need to use somatic symptoms to fill unmet dependency needs is reduced, the client should return to a functional state in self-care activities, social interaction, and family responsibilities. Because these disorders tend to reoccur, it is important to recognize that the symptoms can reappear if psychologic defenses and coping strategies fail.

Summary

Somatoform disorders are characterized by the transfer of anxiety and repressed emotional conflict into somatic or physical symptoms that are unsupported by medical testing or exploratory surgical intervention. Despite reassurance that a disease does not exist, the person remains unconvinced and continues to access other health care options to substantiate their complaints. The person is not consciously aware of the psychologic implications of their disorder. The symptoms are involuntary and cannot be controlled by the person experiencing them.

Two distinguishing factors in the psychologic implications of these disorders are the history of emotional conflict or trauma about the time the symptoms originated and the unmet dependency needs that are objectively evident in the person's behavior. The person experiencing the symptoms is not aware of the underlying feelings and believes the symptoms to be real. The complaint is considered to be somatic if it requires medical intervention to rule out an actual pathologic condition or illness. Once it has been determined that no disease state exists, the person is not content with the outcome. Refusing to believe that the symptoms are not indicative of something serious, the person continues to dwell on the complaints to the point of dysfunctional living. As the symptoms become a focal point within their living environment, a secondary gain is achieved as attention is received from medical personnel and family members. This serves as a reward generated by the behavior.

The goal of treatment is to develop a trusting relationship with the client and family that will foster an understanding of the psychophysiologic symptoms. Interventions are planned to help the person acknowledge the anxiety issues and their connection to the somatic complaints. Once this occurs, the resolution of the symptoms will hopefully follow as more effective coping strategies are employed. Integral to the understanding of the disorder must be the recognition that somatoform disorders tend to reoccur. If the underlying emotional conflict is confronted and resolved, the need for the somatic retreat will be unnecessary.

Bibliography

Adams, D. B. (2004). Somatoform disorders, *Atlanta Medical Psychology.* Available at http://www.psychological.com/somatoform_disorders.htm. Accessed on July 11, 2004

American Psychiatric Association (2000). *Diagnostic and statistical manual of mental disorders text revision* (4th ed.). Washington, DC: American Psychiatric Association.

Berkow, R., & Beers, M. H. (1999). *The Merck manual of diagnosis & therapy* (17th ed.). Rahway, NJ: Merck & Co.

Frey, R. J. (1999). Somatoform disorders, *Gale encyclopedia of medicine.* Gale Research, 1999.

Yates, N. R. (2003). Somatoform disorders. Available at http://www.emedicine.com/med/topic3527.htm. Accessed on July 11, 2004.

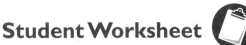

FILL IN THE BLANK

Fill in the blank with the correct answer.

1. A predictable syndrome of physical complaints and symptoms that are expressed as a result of psychologic stress are defined as _____.

2. The attention the person with a somatoform disorder receives from physicians and family in response to the symptoms is referred to as _____.

3. In a conversion disorder, the transfer of anxiety into a loss of physical functioning serves as a(n) _____ as the emotional conflict is avoided and relieved.

4. The lack of concern or anxiety over the implications of functional loss in the person with a conversion disorder is known as _____ indifference.

5. _____ is the term given to the search by the person with hypochondriasis for a physician to substantiate their feared illness.

MATCHING

Match the following terms to the most appropriate phrase.

a. Preoccupation with imagined or slight physical defect

b. Fear of having a serious illness based on a misinterpretation of somatic symptoms

c. Severe discomfort largely due to psychologic factors that is unrelieved by analgesia

d. Exaggerated multiple symptoms that lack a medical reason and occur in at least four different locations

e. Sensory or neurologic impairment not supported by medical testing

1. _____ Somatization disorder

2. _____ Conversion disorder

3. _____ Body dysmorphic disorder

4. _____ Hypochondriasis

5. _____ Pain disorder

MULTIPLE CHOICE

Select the best answer from the multiple-choice items.

1. The nurse is doing an assessment of a client with a known diagnosis of hypochondriasis. Which of the following statements made by the client would the nurse recognize as most typical of a client with this disorder?

    a. "I don't eat much because I will have diarrhea if I do."

    b. "I can't understand why no one can find out what is wrong with me."

    c. "I know I have colon cancer just like my dad."

    d. "I just don't have the energy I used to."

2. Cary has a 5-year history of numerous medical visits for severe migraine headaches. Diagnostic testing reveals no pathologic basis for the symptoms. He tells the nurse he is staying home more often, disabled by the headaches. Cary's symptoms are most characteristic of which of the following somatoform disorders?

   a. Hypochondriasis

   b. Conversion disorder

   c. Pain disorder

   d. Somatization disorder

3. The nurse is caring for a client who was functioning without difficulty until today when she suddenly developed numbness in her right arm. No apparent reason is found for the paralysis. Which of the following is most important for the nurse to remember concerning the client's symptoms?

   a. The cause is related to actual neurologic dysfunction.

   b. The symptoms represent a primary gain for the client.

   c. The client is probably aware that emotions may be the cause.

   d. The inability to use her arm will be of major concern to the client.

4. Which of the following best explains the connection between emotional conflict and the symptoms of a conversion disorder?

   a. The presenting symptom is a transferred sublimation of anxiety and fears.

   b. Feelings that have been suppressed are converted into the presenting symptom.

   c. The temporary disability is a purposeful display of internal anger and resentment.

   d. Repressed feelings are converted into a symptom with special meaning.

5. When interacting with the client with a somatoform disorder, it is most important for the nurse to use which of the following interventions?

   a. Diversion from the sick role to other more productive activities

   b. Supportive interventions to increase feelings of acceptance

   c. Confrontation with the client over the underlying feelings of anxiety

   d. Avoidance of conversation related to fears and recent traumatic events

SEEK AND FIND

Find the incorrect information in the following statements.

1. The person with somatization is consciously aware that the physical symptoms are related to underlying psychologic issues.

2. A temporary disability in the client with a conversion disorder may provide a primary gain—the avoidance of unpleasant tasks or responsibilities that accompany the attention the person receives.

3. The symptoms in a conversion disorder usually show a dysfunctional pattern that is typical of an actual neurologic pathway disorder.

4. In most instances, the pain described by people with pain disorder tends to migrate from one body location to another.

SCENARIO: NATHAN'S SEARCH FOR A CURE

Nathan is a 36-year-old who has been to four different physicians attempting to find an answer to his repeated bouts of chest pain that radiates to his arms and back. Despite an extensive diagnostic work-up by a cardiologist that reveals no cardiovascular abnormalities or problems, Nathan is convinced that he has angina. He believes it is only a matter of time before he has a major heart attack. Last week, his employer told him his sick time had run out. Rather than face having to work everyday, Nathan quits his job. He tells his wife that he is afraid to overwork his heart by going to work every day. He refuses to go with her to family gatherings or outings with their friends, stating he will get too tired and start having chest pain.

Today, Nathan comes into the emergency room stating, "I know I am having a heart attack. The pain is in my chest, then goes down my arms and back. What do I have to do to get someone to listen to me?"

What assessment data should the nurse gather related to the symptoms Nathan is experiencing?

_____

_____

Nathan tells the nurse that there have recently been a lot of layoffs where he worked and that his department was in the process of reorganization before he quit because of his illness. What underlying feelings may be contributing to Nathan's anxiety and somatic symptoms?

_____

_____

What secondary gain does Nathan receive from the physical symptoms?

_____

_____

Identify two nursing diagnoses that would apply to Nathan's situation.

_____

_____

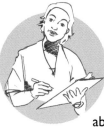

LEARNING OBJECTIVES

After learning the content in this chapter, the student will be able to:

1. Identify the essential feature of the dissociative disorders.
2. Describe characteristics of the four main categories of dissociative disorders.
3. Assess the primary signs and symptoms of mental disorders of dissociation.
4. Identify appropriate nursing diagnoses for the client with a dissociative disorder.
5. Develop expected outcomes for persons with dissociative states.
6. Plan appropriate nursing interventions for the dissociative mental disorders.
7. Evaluate the effectiveness of planned nursing care and make needed revisions.

Dissociative Disorders

KEY TERMS

Continuous amnesia

Depersonalization disorder

Derealization

Dissociation

Dissociative amnesia

Dissociative fugue

Dissociative identity disorder

Generalized amnesia

Localized amnesia

Malingered fugue

Selective amnesia

Switching process

Defining Dissociation

Dissociation is the mechanism that allows our mind to separate certain memories from conscious awareness. These separated parts are kept in the unconscious, or are repressed, and may re-emerge at any time. Painful thoughts and memories often resurface when we encounter a situation similar to the original trauma. We cannot prevent or control the reoccurrence of these thoughts. However, because the unconscious mind also contains learned behaviors, we can go on "automatic pilot" to carry on with routine activities of daily living such as driving the car, parenting, reading, writing, and cooking without really concentrating on these functions.

Just the Facts

Repression, the most basic and widely used defense mechanism, keeps distressing thoughts and feelings buried in the unconscious.

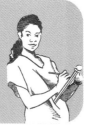

Mind Jogger

In reality, don't we all have periods of "dissociation"? For example, while driving the car, you suddenly realize that you don't remember what has happened during the trip. Or, while listening to someone talk, you suddenly realize that you did not hear part or all of what the person said. Why do you think this happens? Can this be a situation of divided consciousness in which the action and the person's thought go in two different directions at the same time?

Just the Facts

Dissociation, or the "not me," is a systematic process used unconsciously to minimize or avoid certain events or experiences to decrease the anxiety that accompanies them.

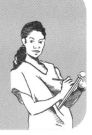

The Dissociative Disorders

The dissociative disorders are described as a disturbance in the ordinarily organized functions of the conscious awareness, memory, identity, and view of oneself in relation to the environment. The disturbance may be sudden or gradual, intermittent or chronic. This disorganization causes significant interference of the person's general functioning, social relationships, and work environment. The disruption of functioning is characterized by a dissociation or interruption in the ability to recognize personal information such as identity, background, and family history. These mental disorders tend to occur in response to severe trauma or abuse. The brain is believed to process and store traumatic events in a different, more distant way than it handles and maintains normal or pleasant memories.

At a Glance 13-1 Categories of Dissociative Disorders

Dissociative amnesia
Dissociative fugue
Dissociative identity disorder
Depersonalization disorder

Dissociative Amnesia

Dissociative amnesia is characterized by an inability to remember important personal information, usually of a traumatic or stressful nature. This lack of recall includes a loss of information beyond ordinary forgetfulness. The void may cover the entire scope of the person's life or may be confined to certain details related to the traumatic event itself.

Common Signs and Symptoms. Localized amnesia usually occurs within a few hours following the event or traumatic incident. This acute form is more common in response to war combat, natural disasters, or severe trauma. For example, a mother who experiences the activity of a tornado may not remember the hours immediately following the storm that has destroyed her home and taken the life of her child. The mother retains an overall understanding of who she is but forgets fragments of her identity. In **selective amnesia,** a person retains memory of some portions of the event, but not all details are remembered. The woman whose home was destroyed by the tornado may remember the storm but not that her child was killed by flying debris. A person with **generalized amnesia** is unable to recall any aspect of his or her life. **Continuous amne-**

sia encompasses a period up to and including the present that is lost from conscious recollection.

At a Glance 13-3 Associated **Signs and Symptoms of Dissociative Amnesia**

- Inability to recall portions or all of memory or identity
- Depression
- Anxiety
- Depersonalization
- Trance state
- Loss of sensation
- Regression
- Sexual dysfunction
- Impaired social and occupational relationships
- Self-mutilation
- Aggressive acts
- Suicidal gestures or acts

Incidence and Etiology. Dissociative amnesia can occur in any age-group from children to adults. The main manifestation is a gap in memory for past events that may cover minutes or years. There is a recent increase in incidence, perhaps because of more awareness and newer therapeutic approaches that address traumatic childhood memories. The diagnosis is made with caution in those who may claim symptoms to avoid accountability for personal actions.

At a Glance 13-2 Types **of Dissociative Amnesia**

Localized amnesia: Usually occurs within hours after incident

Selective amnesia: Retention of overall identity, but fragments are forgotten

Generalized amnesia: Inability to recall any aspect of one's life

Continuous amnesia: Inability to recall any aspect of identity, both past and present

---

Just the Facts

The person with amnesia usually appears alert and may give no indication to observers that anything is wrong.

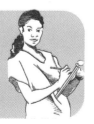

Just the Facts

Using the mental mechanism of dissociation can change our ability to look at ourselves and our actions objectively and prevent us from making positive changes in our behavior.

Case Study: Displaced Guilt

Elizabeth is a 23-year-old married mother of 2-year-old twin boys who has been diagnosed with dissociative amnesia. Despite her ability to state her first name, she is unable to recall her last name or that she has a husband and family. Her husband, Seth, tells the nurse that 3 weeks prior to the onset of the symptoms Elizabeth was in a car accident in which the other vehicle involved was thrown into the path of a semi-truck. The mother and two children who were passengers in the vehicle were killed on impact. Seth states that Elizabeth is unable to recall any details of the accident or recognize him or the twins as familiar. She has been spending most of her days sitting in the porch swing. She has not attempted to care for the boys or to interact with them since the accident. Seth is crying and afraid she will never come back to them.

How are Elizabeth's symptoms characteristic of localized dissociative amnesia?

_____

How would you initiate a therapeutic relationship with Elizabeth?

_____
_____

How can the nurse help Seth to cope with his present situation?

_____
_____
_____

Mind Jogger

How would the nurse initiate a therapeutic relationship with the client who is experiencing amnesia?

Dissociative Fugue

Dissociative fugue is demonstrated by the inability to recall some or all of a person's past or identity, accompanied by the sudden and unexpected travel of the person away from home or place of employment. The person often assumes a new identity in the new geographic location. Travel may include simple short trips for a few hours or days, or more extensive travel across many miles over a period of weeks or months. The person usually does not demonstrate outward indications of a psychologic problem and adapts to a new social setting without being noticed.

Common Signs and Symptoms. Although these people forget their name, family, and where they live, they seem to remember things unrelated to their identity, such as how to drive a car or how to read. When they suddenly return to their former self, they are unable to remember the time of the altered identity or fugue itself. This escape from their identity is usually caused by a traumatic event that has resulted in severe psychologic stress, none of which they are able to remember. Most cases of fugue are seen in adults and occur during times of disaster or periods of environmental or personal chaos when there is an actual threat of death, injury, or loss. It is important to recognize that this type of dissociation may also occur in people who are trying to avoid a legal, financial, or unwanted personal situation. This is referred to as **malingered fugue** and is especially relevant in forensic or criminal activity.

Most cases of this disorder resolve rapidly with treatment, although some resistant amnesia can persist for an extended period of time. The extent and length of the fugue may result in a loss of employment or severely disrupt marriage and family relationships.

Mind Jogger

How might dissociative fugue be compared with manipulative behavior?

Just the Facts

Persons who emerge from dissociative fugue states, confused and frightened by their strange and unfamiliar surroundings, are often picked up by law enforcement authorities.

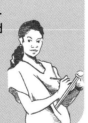

At a Glance 13-4 Associated Signs and Symptoms of Dissociative Fugue

- Inability to recall some or all of one's past or identity
- Sudden travel away from home
- Assumption of a new identity
- Mood swings
- Anxiety
- Grief
- Shame or guilt
- Suicidal behaviors

Incidence and Etiology. Few people have actually been diagnosed with dissociative fugue. However, its prevalence may increase during times of extremely stressful events such as wartime or the massive human and physical losses seen as a result of the terrorist attacks of September 11, 2001.

Just the Facts

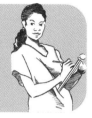

Most incidents of dissociative fugue are brief—hours or days—with most people experiencing full recovery.

Dissociative Identity Disorder

In dissociative identity disorder (formerly known as multiple personality disorder), two or more distinct identities or personalities are present in the same person. These identities alternate in assuming control of the person's behavior. In addition, there is an inability to recall important personal information that cannot be explained as simple forgetfulness. People with this disorder are unable to connect various aspects of their identity with the past and the present, resulting in fragmentation of the original personality. It is believed that people with severe sexual, physical, or psychologic abuse during childhood are predisposed to the development of this disorder. The young child is confronted with an intolerable traumatic event at a time when the psychologic defenses are inadequate to deal with the anxiety. The child dissociates the event and feelings associated with the memory, resulting in the split of the personal identity.

Common Signs and Symptoms. The dissociated part of the personality takes on characteristics of its own. This subpersonality learns to deal with feelings and emotions that could overwhelm the primary personality. Each personality character may appear as if it has a distinct personal history, self-concept, identity, and name with its own memories, behavior patterns, and social relationships that are evident when that personality is in control. These behavior patterns may include aggression, sexual promiscuity, pleasure seeking, or childlike fearfulness. Only one personality is manifested at a time, with one of them usually being dominant during the course of the illness. Psychiatrists refer to this main personality as the "host" person. This primary or host personality usually assumes the person's given name and is passive, dependent, self-blaming, and depressed; it is often the personality that seeks treatment. The host is unaware of the other states during their dominance, but the others may be aware of each other to some extent. The alternate identities usually emerge in a pattern and are often in conflict and critical of the others. The changing of one personality to the other usually occurs very abruptly and is referred to as the **switching process.** This switch is most often triggered by psychosocial stress and may be preceded by behaviors such as rapid eye blinking, facial changes, changes in voice and persona, or a sudden break in the continuity of thought processes. The number of identities can range from as few as 2 to as many as 100.

At a Glance 13-5 Fragmented Personality States of Awareness

- Original personality is usually unaware of the alternate personalities.
- Alternate states are aware of the original one and have varying awareness of each other.
- Alternate personality states often display traits that are foreign to the original personality, such as a giddy, extroverted personality in a person who is naturally very shy.

Persons with this disorder have memory gaps for both recent and remote memory. The passive aspects of the personality tend to have less recall, whereas the more hostile and controlling states retain a more complete memory. Sometimes an identity that is not in control will introduce auditory or visual hallucinations to gain control of the conscious state, such as a voice that criticizes the present identity for something they are doing.

Mind Jogger

How would a person with dissociative identity disorder differ from one who has a personality disorder?

At a Glance 13-6 Common Signs and Symptoms of Dissociative Identity Disorder

- Inability to recall relevant personal information
- Inability to associate the identity with the past and present in organized way
- Multiple personality states, switching from one identity to another
- Migraine headaches
- Asthma
- Digestive disturbances
- Nightmares
- Flashbacks
- Hyperactive startle reflex
- Self-injurious behaviors
- Suicidal gestures or acts
- Aggression
- Repetitive abusive relationships

Incidence and Etiology. Adult dissociative identity disorder is diagnosed more frequently in adult women, and women also tend to have more identities than adult men. The disorder tends to run a lengthy and chronic course from symptom recognition to diagnosis, with the average onset during the early school years. The disorder is less pronounced after age 40. People with this disorder often report a history of severe physical and sexual abuse, particularly during childhood. There is some question that these memories may be distorted, especially if the trauma occurred during periods when imaginary and fantasy play is considered normal. Many times, however, the abuse is validated by actual evidence such as scars from the trauma.

Depersonalization Disorder

Depersonalization disorder is marked by a persistent and repetitious feeling of being detached from one's mental thoughts or body without the presence of disorientation. The person has a feeling of not recognizing himself or is unsure about his personal information and identity. The person may sense that his body is imaginary, in an altered state, or disappearing.

Common Signs and Symptoms. People who actually have this disorder are socially dysfunctional because of the intensity imposed by the feelings of detachment. In **derealization,** the person perceives the external environment as unreal or changing. He or she may see other people as mechanical but be able to recognize the illogical nature of these feelings. There may also be accompanying anxiety, panic, depression, or obsessive and somatic complaints. The person may perceive an unusual change in the size or shape of objects or people may seem unfamiliar and mechanical. People may not seek treatment until adolescence or early adulthood, although symptoms may have been present since childhood. The condition tends to be chronic with recurrent brief episodes related to traumatic or stressful events in the person's life.

Incidence and Etiology. The prevalence of this as a chronic disorder is unknown. It is estimated that perhaps half of all adults may have experienced a single brief episode of depersonalization, usually precipitated by severe stress or life-threatening situational experience.

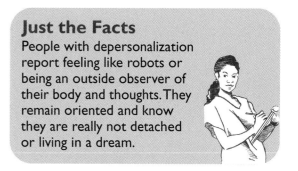

Just the Facts
People with depersonalization report feeling like robots or being an outside observer of their body and thoughts. They remain oriented and know they are really not detached or living in a dream.

Application of the Nursing Process

Nursing Assessment

During the diagnostic process, any physical condition that could produce the symptoms of amnesia and dissociation must be ruled out. These conditions include head injury, epilepsy, brain disease, pharmacologic side effects, or substance abuse. Psychotic disorders such as schizophrenia must also be ruled out. Psychologic tests are used to further evaluate the authenticity of the symptoms. A clinical interview is included to ascertain any significant childhood or adult trauma.

Along with a physical assessment, a baseline psychosocial assessment is done to deter-

---

At a Glance 13-7 Common Signs and Symptoms of Depersonalization Disorder

- Feelings of detachment from one's body or thoughts
- Inability to recognize oneself or personal information
- Anxiety or panic
- Depression
- Somatic complaints
- Obsessions
- Perceptual changes of size or shape
- People seem unfamiliar and mechanical

mine behavioral alterations such as disorientation, level of anxiety, amnesia, any depression, and the extent to which functioning in the social and work environment is affected. It is important for the nurse to describe the client's behavior and verbalized statements because clients with dissociative disorders can present ambiguous pictures or personalities to various staff members as a manipulative means of causing conflict.

Nursing Diagnoses

Once assessment data are obtained, nursing problems are identified. Common nursing diagnoses used to address problems seen in clients with dissociative disorders include:

- Altered thought processes, related to memory loss and repressed trauma
- Sensory perceptual alteration, related to depersonalization and view of self
- Personality identity disturbance, related to childhood trauma or more than one personality state
- Self-care deficit, related to mechanical trancelike state or aimless wandering
- Ineffective individual coping, related to repressed memories and issues, loss of identity, or travel away from home
- Anxiety, related to repressed traumatic events or loss of identity
- Risk for violence, related to self-destructive behaviors
- Family coping ineffective, related to loss of identity

Expected Outcomes

The ultimate goal of the therapeutic process is to help the person integrate the fragmented personalities into one identity. Extensive psychotherapy is used to help clients retrieve repressed ideas and memories. The process includes the planning of nursing outcomes that are anticipated with the implementation of nursing interventions to address the nursing problems. The timeframe in which a realistic

expectation can be anticipated for symptom resolution differs with the type of dissociative disorder. Expected outcomes for the client may include:

- Associate memory deficit with past stressful events
- Recover memory deficits and develop improved coping mechanisms to deal with stressful events
- Verbalize reality-based perception of environmental stimuli in stressful situations
- Verbalize understanding of multipersonality states and the need to consolidate all the personalities into one
- Perform self-care activities independently
- Demonstrate more adaptive coping methods in response to stressful situations
- Verbalize feelings and identify positive effective ways of managing fear and anxiety
- Verbalize understanding of personality conflict in dissociative state
- Demonstrate self-control over behaviors toward self and others

Expected outcomes for the family may include the following.

- Verbalize realistic expectations for client's behavior and treatment process
- Demonstrate support of the client and of the family unit

Nursing Interventions

The nurse must first establish a trusting and supportive therapeutic relationship with the client. It is important to use active listening and communication techniques that encourage verbalization of feelings, conflicts, and information regarding the traumatic events that led to the current dissociative state. This process assists the client to develop personal insight and an awareness and understanding of the self and behaviors that are self-defeating and damaging, along with alternative plans for behavioral changes. Clients need encouragement and support to achieve control over their anxiety and previous dissociative response to those situations that trigger the symptoms. People with these disorders are overwhelmed with fear of not knowing or being out of control.

Other interventions include:

- Encourage the client to keep a daily journal of thoughts and feelings.
- Develop a contract between the client and staff for dealing with self-destructive behaviors.
- Promote a safe environment to protect the client from self-injury or injury to others.
- Assist the client in developing effective coping skills.
- Model positive and desired behaviors.
- Identify environmental stressors that trigger the dissociative symptoms.
- Decrease anxiety-producing stimuli.
- Use stimuli that stimulate pleasant memories and pleasurable feelings for the client. This assists the client to remember past experiences without the risk of precipitating increased trauma.
- Avoid flooding the client with details of past traumatic events. This may cause the client to regress further into the dissociative state that is serving to protect the person from the emotional pain.
- Help the client to understand that periods of imbalance are to be expected and will decrease as the personal identity is restored.
- Maintain an awareness of behavioral changes that may indicate self-destructive behavior.
- Assist the client to identify alternatives to self-injury such as physical exercise, written methods of expression, or creative art and task-oriented activities, which provide a means of nonverbal expression of thoughts that the person may not be able to verbalize.
- Assist the client to identify the purpose that each subpersonality (dissociative identity disorder) serves in the total personality of the person.
- Identify contributing factors within the family dynamics and the environment.
- Help the family to provide encouragement and reinforcement of positive client behaviors.

Evaluation

During the evaluation process, it is important to note the progress the client has made toward identifying and demonstrating a more adaptive response to stressful stimuli. This step is helpful in decreasing the dissociative response. The client must also come to an understanding of the relationship between the dissociative state and the increased anxiety that is felt as repressed past trauma is triggered by environmental factors. Recalling past traumatic events is crucial to this understanding. In dissociative identity disorder, evaluation centers on the client's acknowledgment of the existence of more than one personality and how these various states function as protection from the anxiety related to traumatic memories. It is also important to note the client's progress toward the ultimate goal of integrating all personalities into a single personality.

Nurses are faced with a challenging and frustrating task of accepting the client's behavior while trying to understand the complex nature of the dissociative states. Providing a safe and trusting environment with acceptance and support allows the client to develop a sense of power and self-control in a consistent, caring milieu with a positive forward progression in the treatment process.

Summary

The dissociative disorders are characterized by an interruption from the conscious acquaintance with identity, personal background, and family history. These disorders are most often seen in people who have experienced severe trauma or abuse. Dissociation is the mechanism that allows the mind to separate these traumatic memories from the conscious awareness. These repressed memories can resurface at any time, usually triggered by environmental factors. The repetition of these thoughts cannot be controlled or prevented by the client when they are occurring.

Dissociative amnesia takes two forms. It may be a localized amnesia that occurs shortly after an incident where the person retains an overall understanding of who he or she is but forgets pieces of the identity picture. The second form is a generalized amnesia in which the whole life span is beyond recall. When the amnesia is accompanied by sudden travel away from home or place of employment with the establishment of a new identity, it is referred to as a dissociative fugue. The person functions in this new location without drawing any attention to the false identity. When the fugue is terminated, the person may return home with no recollection of the events before or during the fugue.

Another type of dissociative disorder occurs when two or more distinct identities or personalities are present in the same person and alternately assume control of the person's behavior. Treatment of an identity disorder may be extensive and focuses on reintegration of the personalities into the original personality.

Depersonalization occurs with a persistent and repetitious feeling of being detached from one's mental thoughts or body. The person retains orientation but is socially dysfunctional because of the intensity created by the feelings of detachment.

The nurse must first establish a trusting and supportive therapeutic relationship with the client. The client is then supported to develop an awareness of the self-defeating behaviors with alternative plans for changing these patterns. Interventions are directed at helping the client to develop a sense of power and self-control toward a predictable and positive outcome.

Bibliography

American Psychiatric Association (2000). *Diagnostic and statistical manual of mental disorders text revision* (4th ed.). Washington, DC: American Psychiatric Association.

Gale Group. (2001). Dissociation/Dissociative Disorders, *The Gale encyclopedia of psychology* (2nd ed.). Available at http://www.nga.org/cda/files/GALENCYC.pdf. Accessed on July 11, 2004..

National Alliance of Mental Illness Factsheet (2000). Reviewed by Maser, J. D. Available at http://www.nami.org/Content/ContentGroups/ Helpline1/Dissociative_Disorders.htm. Accessed on July 11, 2004.

Simeon, D., Guralnik, O., Knutelska, M., & Schmeidler, J. (2002). Personality factors associated with dissociation: Temperament, defenses, and cognitive schemata. *American Journal of Psychiatry,* 159:489–491. Available at http://ajp.psychiatryonline.org/cgi/content/full/159/3/489. Accessed on July 11, 2004.

Varcarolis, E. M. (2002). *Foundations of psychiatric mental health nursing* (4th ed.). Philadelphia, PA: W. B. Saunders.

Student Worksheet

FILL IN THE BLANK

Fill in the blank with the correct answer.

1. An interruption from the conscious knowledge of personal identity and background history is termed _____.

2. When certain memories are removed from conscious awareness, the separated parts are _____ in the unconscious and may resurface at any time.

3. In dissociative identity disorder, the main personality is referred to as the _____ person.

4. The changing of one personality or the _____ process in dissociative identity disorder usually occurs very abruptly and is most often triggered by psychosocial stress.

5. A persistent and repetitious feeling of being detached from one's mental thoughts of body without noted disorientation is referred to as _____ disorder.

MATCHING

Match the following terms to the most appropriate phrase.

a. Acute inability to recall personal information shortly after a traumatic event

b. Persistent feeling of being detached from one's mind or body

c. Seeing the external environment as unreal or changing

d. Sudden travel from one's home setting accompanied by the inability to recall one's past

e. Inability to recall one's past accompanied by unexpected travel to avoid unwanted situation

1. _____ Fugue
2. _____ Localized amnesia
3. _____ Malingering
4. _____ Depersonalization
5. _____ Derealization

MULTIPLE CHOICE

Select the best answer from the multiple-choice items.

1. A woman who claims to be Ryan's biologic sister visits him in his home. She tells him that he has a family in another location. When she asks Ryan why he doesn't come home, he replies, "I'm sorry, but I don't know who you are." Ryan is demonstrating symptoms of:

   a. Derealization
   b. Malingering
   c. Dissociative fugue
   d. Depersonalization

2. Alice has been admitted to the psychiatric unit with a diagnosis of dissociative identity disorder. The nurse observes that during interaction with other clients, Alice is laughing and quite talkative. When the nurse approaches Alice to administer her medications, Alice slumps her shoulders as she looks away with tears in her eyes and says in a childlike voice, "Are you going to hurt me?" The nurse's best response in this situation is:

   a. "You were laughing a minute ago. What happened to Alice?"

   b. "These medications are to help Alice feel better."

   c. "I'll come back later when you feel better."

   d. "Why do you think I am going to hurt you?"

3. Ralph is a client with dissociative amnesia. The nurse has identified a nursing diagnosis of personal identity disturbance. An appropriate expected outcome for this client is:

   a. Client will describe details of traumatic past event.

   b. Client will verbalize understanding of need to integrate personality.

   c. Client will demonstrate an understanding of the role of each personality.

   d. Client will function independently in all self-care activities.

4. The nurse is addressing past memory deficits with a client who has a dissociative disorder. To avoid flooding the client, it is important for the nurse to:

   a. Instruct the client to focus on the current stress factors.

   b. Reorient the client to time, place, and person at each contact.

   c. Observe for cues that the client is ready to revisit the traumatic incident.

   d. Include details of the traumatic events surrounding the memory loss in the first session.

5. A client tells the nurse a rather confusing story of recent events surrounding her symptoms of amnesia. The nurse's best response is:

   a. "You must be very angry that it is difficult for you to remember this."

   b. "You seem to overreact each time you try to talk about this."

   c. "Let me see if I correctly understand what you are telling me."

   d. "We will try this again when you can tell the story like it happened."

SCENARIO 1: "ART'S DISAPPEARANCE"

Art is a 47-year-old division dean of a university extended campus location. He is married and the father of two teenage children. He has been active in campus and community affairs, including assisting with productions of the local amateur theater. Art is scheduled to board an 8:15 a.m. flight to meet a professional colleague in a city 300 miles from his hometown. At 7:00 a.m. the day of his intended arrival, the colleague notifies the university and Art's wife that Art did not arrive on his scheduled flight. When his wife checks with the airport, she is told that her husband never boarded the flight. Art's car is found at the airport with the keys locked inside.

Six months later, investigators have uncovered no clues as to Art's whereabouts or what may have occurred in his disappearance. Several months later, Art walks into his office at the university accompanied by an unfamiliar woman whom he introduces as his wife. It is apparent to the office personnel that he does not recognize them or his previous position in the division office. He states that a young man saw him at a restaurant in a neighboring state and told him about his real identity. Art states he has no recollection of the institution or his family but has come back to this place because he needs to find out the truth about himself. He is voluntarily admitted to the psychiatric unit for evaluation and treatment.

What symptoms indicate that Art is experiencing a dissociative state?

_____

_____

_____

What type of dissociative disorder do Art's symptoms suggest?

_____

_____

How should the nurse approach Art when discussing past traumatic events?

_____

_____

SCENARIO 2: "HOME BUT LOST"

Phillip has just arrived in his hometown after recovering from shrapnel wounds received during military action in Iraq. He is brought to the emergency room after he is found wandering on a boat dock incoherent and bleeding from his wrists. When asked his name, it is obvious that he has no recollection of his identity or what he was doing on the pier. However, when he is asked about recent events in his life, he states he attended class at the high school the day before. When Phillip's family is located, they tell the nurse that Phillip is 26 years old and has not attended high school in 8 years. Once his lacerations are treated, Phillip is admitted to the psychiatric unit with a diagnosis of dissociative generalized amnesia.

What feelings may be responsible for Phillip's attempted suicidal acts?

_____

_____

Why is it important to obtain information from the family about Phillip's likes, dislikes, activities, or hobbies?

_____

_____

What is the purpose of reintroducing things and people from his past that represent pleasant experiences for him?

_____

_____

Why is it important not to flood Phillip with information about his recent past in Iraq?

_____

_____

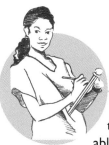

LEARNING OBJECTIVES

After learning the content in this chapter, the student will be able to:

1. Demonstrate an understanding of substance dependence and abuse.

2. Describe etiologic factors that contribute to substance abuse.

3. Discuss the term *codependency* and its relationship to substance abuse.

4. Assess the client with substance intoxication and withdrawal symptoms.

5. Identify nursing diagnoses common to clients with disorders related to chemical dependency.

6. Determine expected outcome criteria for the client in the acute withdrawal phase and the recovery period of substance-abuse disorders.

7. Plan effective nursing interventions to address the detoxification phase and the recovery period of treatment in chemical dependency.

8. Identify evaluation criteria to determine the effectiveness of the treatment intervention.

9. Describe treatment goals for teaching the client and family steps toward long-term sobriety.

CHAPTER 4

Substance-Related Disorders

KEY TERMS

Addiction
Blackout
Codependent
Craving
Delirium tremens
Enabling
Inhalants
Relapse
Substance
Substance abuse
Substance dependence
Substance intoxication
Tolerance
Wernicke-Korsakoff syndrome
Withdrawal
Withdrawal syndrome

Substance Use, Abuse, and Addiction

The term **substance** is used in reference to any drug, medication, or toxin that shares the potential for abuse. According to the National Council on Drug Abuse, the economic cost to society in the United States alone is estimated at over $250 billion. There has been a continuous pattern of consistent increases in this amount in the past 20 years.

Addiction is a physiologic and psychologic dependence on alcohol or other drugs of abuse that affects the central nervous system in such a way that withdrawal symptoms are experienced when the substance is discontinued. Drug abuse and addiction can result in serious health problems that in turn invoke enormous cost to the health care system in the way of treatment, detoxification, and rehabilitation programs. With the surging incidence of HIV infection, AIDS, and other diseases, the expense of prevention, research, and treatment has soared to new levels. Society is additionally burdened by drug-related criminal behaviors that involve both the participation in usage or sale of drugs and the violence associated with the drug industry. The cost of arrest and incarceration in drug-related crimes has risen steadily in the past decade. In addition, there is the cost of lost jobs and families who, as a result of these behaviors, are reduced to dependence on welfare and other subsidiary means of support. Finally, the number of premature deaths attributed to drug abuse enlarges this picture to include not only financial losses but human lives shortened as a result of the detrimental nature of substance use and abuse.

Substances are grouped by the *DSM-IV-TR* into 11 classes (see At a Glance 14-1). In addition to these categories, a class of polysubstance dependence is also recognized. Prescription drugs and over-the-counter medications, originally intended as harmless treatment, can also become part of the web of addiction. For most people who use pain relievers, CNS depressants, or stimulants as prescribed, the risk is small. However, when these drugs are used in ways other than that intended by the physician, the risk for addiction exists. Symptoms of substance-related disorders usually appear at higher dosages and usually disappear as the dose is decreased or the drug is discontinued. Medications included in this category by *DSM-IV-TR* are seen in At a Glance 14-2.

At a Glance 14-1 Substance Classifications Recognized by *DSM-IV-TR*

- Alcohol
- Amphetamines (or similarly acting sympathomimetics)
- Caffeine
- Cannabis
- Cocaine
- Hallucinogens
- Inhalants
- Nicotine
- Opioids
- Phencyclidine (PCP)
- Sedatives, hypnotics or anxiolytics

Exposure to toxins and other chemical substances can result in a mental disorder as well. Toxic substances that may cause substance-related illness include those listed in At a Glance 14-3.

Volatile substances such as gasoline and paint, if used for the purpose of intoxication, are referred to as **inhalants.** The most common symptom associated with these toxic substances are alterations in cognitive functioning or mood, which usually resolve over a period of weeks or months once exposure is terminated.

At a Glance 14-2 Classifications of Drugs That May Cause Substance-Related Disorders

These classifications include, but are not limited to:

- Anesthetics
- Analgesics
- Anticholinergics
- Anticonvulsants
- Antihistamines
- Antihypertensives
- Antimicrobials
- Antiparkinson agents
- Cardiovascular medications
- Chemotherapeutic agents
- Corticosteroids
- Gastrointestinal medications
- Muscle relaxants
- Over-the-counter medications such as sleep aids, antihistamines, decongestants, weight loss agents, gastrointestinal aids, and pain-relief drugs
- Nonsteroidal antiinflammatory drugs

At a Glance 14-3 Toxins and Other Chemical Substances

- Heavy metals (lead, aluminum, iron)
- Pesticides (nicotine)
- Nerve gases
- Carbon dioxide
- Ethylene glycol (antifreeze)

Theoretical Approaches to Substance Use and Abuse

Why does a person advance down this path of self-destruction? There are several theoretical approaches to explain causation and motivational factors leading to drug abuse and dependence.

Genetics and Family Influences. Social learning involves the effects of modeling, imitative, and identification behaviors that begin at an early age. Children of substance-abusing parents are at a greater risk for substance abuse and subsequent problems because of both genetic and environmental factors. There is an apparent link between heredity and the development of substance-use disorders. Studies show this tendency to be especially true for alcoholism, where the risk for alcohol abuse is increased by 50% in first-generation relatives of alcoholics. Research also shows that the younger a person is when drug usage begins, the greater the probability that it will progress to abuse and dependency. Chaotic home environments and association with peers who engage in drug-related behaviors also increases the likelihood that this will occur. This scenario is often accompanied by weak parent–child attachment with ineffective parenting and hostile, troubled relationships.

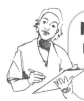

Mind Jogger
How would a strong solid family system aid in reducing the risk of adolescent drug use?

Peer Pressure. Adolescence is a time when new things are exciting and pressures to conform to peer pressure is at its highest. Teenagers may get involved with illicit drugs for various reasons, and experimentation is common. They often do not see the connection between their present actions and the consequences these actions may impose. Teenagers with a family history of substance abuse, those who are depressed or have low self-esteem, and those who feel like a misfit among the crowd are at particular risk for developing a drug problem. Adolescents tend to perceive the drug-using behavior on the part of family, peers, and community as an endorsement of drug usage.

Environmental Stress Factors. Stressful situations increase the need for coping strategies to manage the resultant anxiety, which is usually the excuse or reason the person uses to justify the repeated use of the substance. Stress is cited as a major factor in the initiation and continued use of alcohol and other drugs. It is a significant factor when the person relapses and returns to a pattern of self-destructive behaviors.

Chronic Physiologic Disease. Addiction or dependency is also described as a chronic disease in which there are changes in brain chemistry that bring about the perceived need to continue usage of the drug. It is suggested that herein lies the reasoning that one substance is often replaced with another as the individual travels the path to dependency. The brain cells have become adapted to functioning with the substance or substances and cannot function properly without it for long. The drug must be continued to avoid symptoms of withdrawal.

Personality Characteristics. Dependency cannot be discounted as a component of the personality in people who abuse drugs. The

need to depend on an external force to provide a sense of self is reflected in the form of a weak self-esteem and an inability to define values and boundaries for behavior. Conformity and blending into the social drug culture result in the substance taking control of the person's existence. The person is painfully aware of the dependency on the drug to fulfill a need for affection and power. Most people who abuse drugs have difficulty expressing feelings and may release these explosively as the drug diminishes their ability to control them. Feelings of emotional isolation and a low frustration tolerance are further indicators of the need to borrow a feeling of strength and security from an external substance.

Codependency—A Family Disease. Codependency is a multigenerational pattern of coping mechanisms that lead to self-defeating behaviors. This state evolves from a transmission of family dynamics in which the person is discouraged from feeling or expressing needs, leading to suppressed anger and emotional pain. People in this situation often mistake feelings of control within the family as security and learn to tolerate and excuse the maladaptive behavior. This tolerance results in adjustment to the circumstances and the appearance of normalcy to the outsider.

A theoretical approach based on the family systems model proposes that substance abuse is a family disease in which members either are drug users or **codependent,** and that these factors are interrelated in a way that enables or feeds the problem. Families often display defensive actions that in a way normalize and excuse the behavior of the drug user, and thus unintentionally increase the likelihood that the abusive pattern will continue.

Codependent people tend to feel a responsibility for the drug user's problem and internalize a form of guilt for the behavior of that person. As a result, they continue to do everything possible to sustain the relationship and are unable to recognize the detrimental effects of the codependency on their own physical and mental health. This pattern of either con-

Just the Facts

Determinants of Our Sense of Self

External control

Primary motivation is acceptance by others

Will compromise values under peer pressure

Depends on external source of strength (other people, drugs, activities)

Internal Control

Acts on clearly defined self-chosen beliefs and convictions

Accepts responsibility for decisions and consequences of those choices

Recognizes and is willing to act on the need for change

sciously or unconsciously helping the maladaptive behavior to continue is referred to as **enabling.** The enabler commonly makes excuses or lies to others about behaviors related to the substance abuse. They may also cover up financial and legal problems out of a false sense of responsibility. Social events may be avoided because of shame or fear of ramifications related to the drug use, such as questioning or abusive language and actions. Codependent people deny their own needs while living and doing for another what they need to do for themselves. The passive nature of enablers is seen as they silently comply with the choices and decisions of the user even though they may not agree with them. This yielding behavior allows the user to maintain a perceived sense of control over the dependency and provides a false permission for the addiction to continue.

Despite attempts to protect the user from the consequences of substance abuse, the enabler often feels powerless and, in all actuality, is controlled by the person with whom he or she is codependent. Enablers are caught in a cycle of thinking they are helpless to change the situation because to stop these actions would bring greater disaster. Rigid, inflexible family rules predispose the codependent person to a feeling of being trapped in this dysfunctional situation.

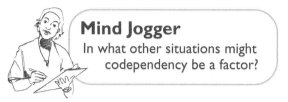

Mind Jogger

In what other situations might codependency be a factor?

Substance Use Disorders

Substance Dependence

Substance dependence is defined by *DSM-IV-TR* as a maladaptive pattern of substance use leading to clinically significant impairment or distress. The main symptom of dependence is a set of physiologic, cognitive, and behavioral indications that the person continues to use the substance regardless of the adverse substance-related problems he or she may be experiencing. There is a pattern of repeated substance use that can lead to tolerance, withdrawal, and compulsive drug ingestion. Use of any drug except caffeine has the potential for a diagnosis of substance dependency.

Common Signs and Symptoms. Specific criteria must be present for 1 year for a diagnosis of dependency to be assigned. To understand these requirements, we must first understand what is meant by the cluster of indicators seen in dependency. Almost all people using a substance to this degree experience **craving** or a strong inner drive to use the substance. **Tolerance** develops through continued use as the brain adapts to repeated doses of the drug with a declining effect as the drug is taken repeatedly over time. This results in the need to use greater amounts of the substance to obtain the same effect. The tolerance may be varied in degree depending on the drug involved and its effect on the central nervous system. Substantial levels of tolerance may develop with heavy drug use that would be lethal to a person who does not use drugs. In people who smoke cigarettes, a habit of 2 to 3 packs per day indicates a tolerance to nicotine that would produce toxic effects in the nonsmoker. High blood levels of a drug without obvious symptoms of intoxication often signify tolerance.

A maladaptive change in behavior or **withdrawal** occurs as the blood or tissue concentrations of a substance decline in a person who has engaged in heavy prolonged use of the substance. Once these unpleasant symptoms occur, the person is likely to seek relief by reingesting the substance. This cycle typically begins on awakening and continues throughout the day. The pattern of compulsive use is demonstrated as larger amounts of the substance are taken over a more extensive period than was intended. The person may indicate a desire or attempt to decrease the substance use but is unsuccessful in these efforts. Much time and energy is devoted to planning activities necessary to obtain the substance. What once may have been valued and enjoyable time spent with family, friends, and colleagues in recreational activities is surrendered to substance use. Even though the person may have recurrent physiologic and psychologic ill effects from drug usage, it continues. This failure to refrain from using the substance is the key symptom used in diagnosing substance dependency. The presence of tolerance and withdrawal pose a higher risk for medical problems and relapse rate.

Just the Facts

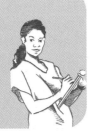

Cluster of Indicators in Substance Dependence
Craving
Tolerance
Withdrawal
Compulsive use

At a Glance 14-4 Associated Symptoms of Substance Dependence

- Substance taken in larger amounts over longer period than was intended
- Persistent desire or unsuccessful efforts to control substance use
- Much time is spent in pursuit of obtaining the substance
- Important activities are given up because of substance use
- Use is continued despite negative problems experienced related to drug use

Nicotine. Although not considered a maladaptive drug by most users, nicotine is included in the *DSM-IV-TR* substance category for dependence. The health dangers related to cigarette smoking are well publicized, with warning labels related to these health hazards printed on all tobacco products. Nicotine dependence can develop with use of all forms of tobacco (cigarettes, cigars, chewing tobacco, snuff, and pipes). The nicotine content of tobacco, added to the repetitive nature of its use, contributes to its ability to produce rapid dependence. Tolerance to nicotine is demonstrated by a more intense effect the first time it is used without producing adverse effects such as dizziness or nausea. People often use nicotine to relieve or avoid symptoms of withdrawal early in the morning or after prolonged periods where use of the drug is not permitted. Those who spend a considerable amount of time using the substance are considered chain-smokers. The most common signs of dependence are tobacco odor, cough, excessive skin wrinkling, and chronic pulmonary disease. Tobacco use markedly increases the risk of lung, oral, and other cancers and increases the risk for cardiovascular and cerebrovascular conditions. Nicotine use usually begins in the early teens, and about 95% of those who continue to smoke become daily users.

Nicotine withdrawal symptoms are experienced within 24 hours of cessation or reduction in usage. Symptoms include a depressed mood, insomnia, irritability, frustration, anxiety, decreased concentration, restlessness, bradycardia, and increased appetite with weight gain. These symptoms usually peak in intensity between the first and fourth days with considerable improvement by 3 to 4 weeks. The hunger and weight gain may persist for 6 months or more.

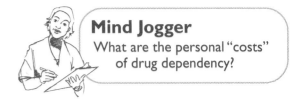

Mind Jogger
What are the personal "costs" of drug dependency?

Phases of Chemical Dependency. Although there are many proposed theories about the etiology or cause for chemical dependency, research is ongoing to help us understand this condition. An estimated one third of hospital admissions are alcohol related, although the incidence of alcohol as a contributing factor in motor-vehicle accidents, falls, trauma, and other disorders may not always be readily apparent. Chemical dependency is a destructive and progressive process from the first use of a chemical to the far end of the harmful decline.

Most people who become chemically dependent do not intend to become alcoholics and drug abusers. They start with a need to belong, to escape, or to experiment, unaware of the destructive process ahead. Chemical dependency is a progressive and predictable continuum of symptoms that increase in severity and frequency. There are four phases that occur from the first use of a chemical to the eventual dependency with continued use.

In phase one, or first use, a mood of euphoria is experienced, and the user learns that the chemical can provide a temporary escape or altered emotional state each time it is used. The user learns to control the effects by regulating the amount of substance and prioritizing the opportunities to use it.

During phase two, the person experiences hangover effects and starts to feel guilty for behaviors related to use of the substance. A need for the drug may develop, leading to tolerance and increased use to obtain the same effect. The person's friends and companions may change to a group who approve of and indulge in similar drug-related behaviors.

As the user enters phase three, a dependent lifestyle begins, with periods in which control over substance use is lost. The person can no longer predict the outcome and

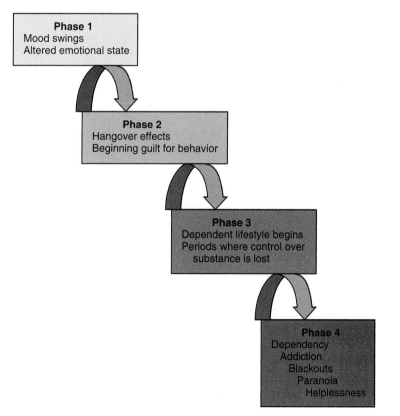

FIGURE 14-1. Phases of chemical dependency.

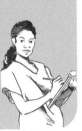

Just the Facts

Blackout is a form of amnesia for events that occurred during the drinking period (e.g., client does not remember conversations or activities engaged in during the time of drinking).

begins to engage in behaviors that compromise his or her values. As the substance assumes control, insight is lost and a revolving cycle begins in which the drug use becomes the priority.

In phase four, the user demonstrates dependency or addiction with periods of blackout, paranoia, and helplessness. Engaging in the acquisition of the substance is no longer seen as a social activity, but as survival.

The characteristic warning signs that exist in the series of events leading to chemical dependency are described in At a Glance 14-5.

Substance Abuse

The primary indication of **substance abuse** is a maladaptive, recurring use of a substance accompanied by repeated detrimental effects as a result of the continued use. This problem

At a Glance 14-5 Warning Signs of Chemical Dependency

Early	Uses chemical to relax in social situation
	Avoids situations where drugs/alcohol will not be available
	Is preoccupied with drugs and their usage
	Has occasional blackouts (periods in which person cannot remember drug use)
	Experiences personality change during substance use
Dependency	Shows increase in tolerance
	Denies drug problem—hides drug use from others
	May switch to other chemical use
	Neglects and loses friends
	Blames others for problems—projection
	Has increased craving
	May have aggressive behaviors with drug use
	Has physical withdrawal symptoms when use is interrupted
	Consumes unpredictable amounts of substance
	Neglects nutritional needs
Chronic	Shows irreversible physical damage (liver, brain, and other medical problems)
	Has decreased tolerance
	Has severe withdrawal symptoms
	Feels persistent remorse
	Has drug-related arrests
	Has delirium tremens (DTs)
	Hallucinates
	Has seizures
	Death may occur

must persist over a period of 1 year to meet the diagnostic criteria for a diagnosis of abuse.

Common Signs and Symptoms. Unlike that for dependency, the criteria for substance abuse do not include tolerance, withdrawal, or compulsive use. Abuse does include the devastating physical effects of the drug, as well as the social, legal, and interpersonal hazards of prolonged substance use. Although abuse is more common in people who may have recently initiated drug usage, a person can continue to have the adverse consequences of drug usage without becoming chemically dependent.

Incidence and Etiology. Drug or substance abuse results in repeated absences from work, school, or home with repeated poor performance in these areas because of hangover effects. The incidence of abuse is more common in episodic substance use, such as when the person becomes intoxicated on a weekend or at a particular event. There tends to be an increase in encounters with disciplinary authorities as a result of abuse-related behaviors (e.g., arrests for disorderly conduct, public intoxication, driving while intoxicated, suspension or expulsion from school, involvement of child protec-

tive services). Despite the persistent negative personal and interpersonal problems that result from repetitious abuse of the substance, the person does not abstain from continued use.

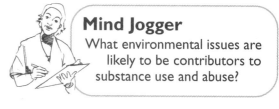

Mind Jogger
What environmental issues are likely to be contributors to substance use and abuse?

Substance-Induced Disorders

Substance Intoxication

Substance intoxication is the development of a reversible pattern of behavior caused by recent ingestion of a substance. This syndrome is clinically seen as maladaptive behavioral and psychologic changes that are related to the effects of the substance on the central nervous system.

Common Signs and Symptoms. These symptoms, which include belligerence, a labile mood, impaired thinking and judgment, and impaired functioning in the social or work setting, appear shortly after use of the substance and are unrelated to any other medical condition. The most common changes that occur with intoxication involve disturbances in the areas of perception, sleep-wake cycle, attention, concentration, thinking, judgment, psychomotor activity, and interpersonal relationships. Some symptoms are common to the abuse of several drugs, whereas others may be indicative of specific drug use. The major groups of substances are listed in At a Glance 14-7 with symptoms related to intoxication involving each group of drugs.

Substance Withdrawal

The essential symptom of the **withdrawal syndrome** is the development of a substance-

---

At a Glance 14-6 Signs and Symptoms of Substance Abuse

- Maladaptive recurring use of a substance
- Episodic binges of substance use
- Recurrent substance use in physically hazardous situations
- Hangover effects
- Substance-related encounters with law enforcement officers
- Suspension or expulsion from school
- Substance-related family and marital difficulties
- Symptoms that do not meet criteria for substance dependence

specific maladaptive change in behavior. The behavior is accompanied by physiologic and cognitive symptoms caused by the reduction or cessation of heavy and prolonged substance use. These effects cause significant disruption and impaired functioning at all levels. Withdrawal is recognized as a disorder for all substances addressed in the section on intoxication.

Common Signs and Symptoms. The signs and symptoms of withdrawal usually develop within several hours to a few days after drug cessation and vary with the substance involved. They are listed in At a Glance 14-7.

Incidence and Etiology of Substance-Induced Disorders

There is a strong association between familial predisposition and the substance-related induced disorders. Children of a person with substance-related disorders are also more likely to develop substance-related problems. There is some evidence that genetics may determine the variances in the doses necessary

At a Glance 14-7 Substance-Related Information

Intoxication	Withdrawal	Substance-Related Information	Signs and Symptoms of Associated Disorder
Alcohol			
Drug-related maladaptive behavior, odor on breath or clothes, slurred speech, incoordination and unsteady gait, difficulty focusing with glazed appearance of eyes, very passive or very argumentative manner, memory impairment, poor concentration, stupor	Autonomic response (diaphoresis, increase in pulse rate), tremors— "shakes" (24-48 hours after cessation), insomnia, nausea and vomiting, easily startled, irritable, flushed face, hallucinations Auditory (buzzing, ringing, clicking, voices) Visual (people, animals, insects) Tactile (insects, spiders crawling) Psychomotor agitation, increased anxiety, grand mal seizures, delirium tremens	Tends to loosen inhibitions Most common cause of preventable birth defects Devastating effects on health Alcohol equivalents (1 oz spirits = 5 oz; glass of wine = 12 oz beer) Legal level of intoxication— 0.08% to 0.10% in most states (5-6 drinks) Average age for first use is 12 years of age Examples: Beer, wine, bourbon, scotch, gin, vodka, rum, tequila, liqueurs Common substances containing alcohol that may be used by dependent people to satisfy craving (liquid cough or cold preparations, mouthwash, isopropyl rubbing alcohol, nail polish remover, cologne, aftershave, extracts used in food)	Increased risk of accidents, violence, suicide Criminal behaviors Absenteeism Wernicke-Korsakoff syndrome Delirium tremens

continues

At a Glance 14-7 Substance-Related Information (Continued)

Amphetamines

Dilated pupils, dry mouth and nose, halitosis, lip-licking, tachycardia or bradycardia, hypertension or hypotension, nausea and vomiting, perspiration, chills, weight loss, difficulty staying still, excessive activity, confusion, seizures, dyskinesias

Fatigue, vivid unpleasant dreams, insomnia or hypersomnia, increase in appetite, increased or decreased psychomotor activity, dysphoric mood, anhedonia (inability to find pleasure in previously enjoyed activities) and drug craving, marked symptoms "crashing" often follow intense period of use (speed-run)

Can be smoked, snorted, orally ingested, or injected

After smoking or injecting, user experiences intense rush or "flash" that lasts a few minutes (described as pleasurable by user)

Snorting or smoking produces euphoria, but not intense rush

Snorting produces effects within 3-5 minutes, oral within 15-20 minutes

May take episodic (intense drug use separated by periods of nonuse) or daily

Intensive high-dose called "speed runs" or "binges"— usually by injection

Tolerance for methamphetamine occurs within minutes—users try to maintain the high by binging on the drug

Ice smoke is odorless—leaves a residue that can be resmoked—high for 12+ hours

Toxic effect on the brain

Methamphetamine

Hyperthermia, violent behavior, anxiety, confusion, insomnia, paranoia, auditory hallucinations, mood disturbances, delusions, out-of-control rages

No physical symptoms reported. Chronic user may experience depression, anxiety, fatigue, paranoia, aggression, and intense craving for the drug

May be extensive long term damage to dopamine-producing cells

See Amphetamines

continues

At a Glance 14-7 Substance-Related Information (Continued)

Intoxication	Withdrawal	Substance-Related Information	Signs and Symptoms of Associated Disorder
Marijuana (Cannabis)			
Sclera of eyes appear inflamed, increased appetite, dry mouth, tachycardia, loud rapid talking with bursts of laughter, loses train of thought easily, strong odor on breath or clothing, distorted sense of time, short-term memory impairment, impaired judgment and perception, negative developmental effects (youth), sleepiness, stuporous	Physical and mental lethargy, anhedonia, depression, anxiety, hallucinogen-like mental effects, paranoid ideation	Most widespread and frequently used illicit drug Long-term use can lead to loss of ambition and purpose Teens who smoke are 8 times more likely to use marijuana Average age for first use is 14 years of age Marijuana available today can be 5 times more potent than that 20 years ago Street names—joint, weed, pot, grass, Mary Jane, Texas tea, hay, stick, MJ, locoweed… Hashish— hash, bhang, ganja, charas, Sweet Lucy	Euphoria Inappropriate laughter Grandiosity Sedation Lethargy Impaired short-term memory Delayed mental processing Impaired judgment Distorted sensory perception Impaired motor function Anxiety Dysphoria Social withdrawal Conjunctival redness Increased appetite Dry mouth Tachycardia
Cocaine			
Increasing difficulty to abstain from use, need for frequent dosing for "high"—(short half-life), tachycardia or bradycardia, dilated pupils, runny nose, chronic sinus problems, nosebleed, nausea or vomiting, weight loss,	Fatigue, vivid unpleasant dreams, insomnia or hypersomnia, increased appetite, psychomotor increase or decrease, delusions, hallucinogens (auditory and tactile/coke bugs), mood changes including depression, suicidal ideation, irritability, anhedonia, attention disturbance, craving on seeing any white powder	Crack is the powerfully addictive smokeable form of cocaine Give temporary illusion of enhanced power and energy As elevated mood fades— depression occurs Use during pregnancy causes miscarriages, stillbirths, or dependent babies Can lead to permanent vegetative or zombi-like state	Paranoid ideation Aggression Anxiety Weight loss Rambling speech Headache Ringing in the ears (tinnitus) "Coke bugs" tactile hallucinations Auditory hallucinations

continues

blood pressure changes, perspiration, chills, changes in psychomotor activity, muscle weakness, chest pain, respiratory depression, cardiac arrhythmias, confusion, seizures, dyskinesias, coma

Over a million Americans, age 12 and over, are chronic users
Common names: Coke, flake, snow, dust, happy dust, girl, cecil, blow, crack

Erratic behavior
Social isolation
Mood changes
Suicidal ideation
Irritability
Anhedonia
Emotional swings
Inattentiveness

Hallucinogen/Club Drugs

Extremely dilated pupils, blurred vision, warm skin, diaphoresis, body odor, mood and behavior changes, distorted sensory perception, tachycardia, tremors, incoordination, unpredictable flashbacks (reexperiencing perceptual symptoms similar to those experienced during previous usage—may include geometric forms, peripheral-field images, flashes of color, intensified colors, images left suspended in path of moving object, afterimages or shadows, halos around objects), perceptual disturbance and impaired judgment (may cause accidents or attempts to fly from high places)

Flashbacks—persisting perception disorder

Drugs such as LSD (acid) or "designer" drugs such as ecstasy (MDMA)
Used as "raves" or "trances" at clubs and bars
Many are tasteless, colorless, and odorless—undetectable in beverages
May be administered to person without his or her knowledge
Other drugs—club names: Acid, cubes, big D, angel dust, hog, peace pill, Mesc, Ecstasy (XTC, Adam, Georgia Home Boy, Businessman's trip, serenity)
Ketamine-K (Special K, Cat Valium) Veterinary anesthetic used as liquid applied to marijuana or tobacco/powder for sniffing
Rophypnol (Roofies, Roche, Forget-me) Illegal but similar to Valium
Methamphetamine (Meth, Speed, Ice, Glass, Crystal, Crank)
LSD (Acid, Blotter, Cubes, Dots, L, Sugar)

Mood swings
Fearfulness
Anxiety
Feelings of going insane
Perceptual disturbance
Impaired judgment
Increase in blood sugar
Increase in cortisol hormones

continues

At a Glance 14-7 Substance-Related Information (Continued)

Intoxication	Withdrawal	Substance-Related Information	Signs and Symptoms of Associated Disorder
Inhalants (sometimes called "poppers") Nitrous Oxide			
Odor of paint, glue, etc., on breath or clothes, runny nose, watery eyes, poor coordination, drowsiness or stupor, possession of bags or rags with dried solvents, discarded pressurized aerosol containers (i.e., whipped cream, hair spray, paint), glue-sniffer's rash around nose or mouth, conjunctival irritation, coughing, dyspnea, sinus discharge, slurred speech, blurred vision, lethargy, muscle weakness, depressed reflexes, tremors, euphoria	Clinically meaningful withdrawal syndrome has not been established.	Known by street names as huffing, sniffing, and wanging Many first-time users have serious respiratory problems and permanent brain damage Types: Volatile solvents such as paint thinners, degreasers, gasoline, varnish Aerosols such as hair spray, vegetable oil spray, lighter fluid, whipped topping Gases such as ether, nitrous oxide, propane Nitrites Glue, nail polish remover Liquid paper Among first drugs children use—as many as 6% use by 4th grade Methods: Inhalant-soaked rag stuffed into mouth Sniff substances sprayed into paper or plastic bag Inhale from balloon filled with substance High is quick leading to repeated use that may cause death by suffocation or cardiac arrest	Confusion Belligerence Aggression Apathy Impaired judgment and social functioning Hallucinations Delusions Perceptual changes Dizziness Visual disturbances Unsteady gait Tremors Euphoria Glue-sniffer's rash Redness of the eyes Respiratory distress with rales/rhonchi Coughing Sinus discharge Headache Weakness Gastrointestinal disturbances Slowed psychomotor response Stupor Cardiac arrhythmias Death ("sudden sniffing death")

continues

At a Glance 14-7 Substance-Related Information *(Continued)*

Opiods (includes heroin and morphine derivatives)

Drowsiness, lethargy, slurred speech, constricted pupils, nonreactive to light, scars on inner arms (injecting), memory and attention impairment	Anxiety, restlessness, irritability, fever, muscle aches in back/legs, increased sensitivity to pain, nausea and vomiting, lacrimation/rhinorrhea, dilated pupils, sweating, diarrhea, yawning, insomnia, craving/drug-seeking behavior	Use during pregnancy causes miscarriages, stillbirths, and dependent babies Sharing needles currently leading cause of HIV and hepatitis B/C Common names: Harry, horse, Miss Emma, Schoolboy, lords, dollies, perkies, T's, Big O, black stuff	Initial high followed by dysphoria Apathy Incoordination Impaired judgment Drowsiness Slurred speech Inattention Memory lapse Constricted pupils Respiratory depression Death

Phencyclidine (PCP)

Unpredictable behavior, violence Mood swings, disorientation, fear, terror Nystagmus (constant involuntary movement of eyeball) Poor coordination, ataxia, strange gait, rigid muscles, dilated pupils, masklike facial appearance, decreased response to pain, decreased sensory perception, hypertension, tachycardia, hyperacusis, (abnormal sensitivity to sound), seizures and coma	Peak effects—2 hours after oral use Mild—resolve after 8-20 hours Severe—several days Psychotic disorder may persist for weeks Dependence on other substances will complicate the withdrawal		Inability to control emotions Anxiety Rage Aggression Panic Flashbacks Disorganized thinking Hyperthermia Hypertension Seizures Nystagmus Hypertension Needle tracks Hepatitis HIV disease Delirium Psychotic symptoms Catatonic posturing Coma

continues

At a Glance 14-7 Substance-Related Information (Continued)

Intoxication	Withdrawal	Substance-Related Information	Signs and Symptoms of Associated Disorder
Sedative, Hypnotic, or Anxiolytics			
Slurred speech, inco-ordination	Sweating, pulse greater than 100		Maladaptive be-havior change
Seems intoxicated but without odor	Increased hand tremors, insomnia, nausea and		Labile mood
Flat affect, unsteady gait, impaired at-tention and mem-ory, nystagmus, stupor and coma	vomiting, hallucinations, psychomotor agitation, anxiety, and grand mal seizures		Impaired judg-ment and func-tioning
			Inappropriate sexual behavior
			Aggression
			Slurred speech
			Unsteady gait
			Nystagmus
			Impaired mobility and coordina-tion
			Tachycardia
			Tachypnea
			Hypertension
			Hyperthermia
			Diaphoresis
			Tremors
			Insomnia
			Anxiety
			Nausea
Caffeine			
Recent consumption in excess of 250 mg (more than 2-3 cups brewed cof-fee)	Headaches		Sensory alter-ations
			Anxiety
			Agitation
Restless, nervous-ness, excitement, insomnia, flushed face, diuresis, and gastrointestinal complaints			Restlessness
			Sweating
			Flushed face
			Diarrhea
			Cardiac arrhyth-mias
			Gastrointestinal discomfort

continues

At a Glance 14-7 Substance-Related Information *(Continued)*

Ingestion of more than 1 g per day may cause muscle twitching, rambling thoughts and speech, cardiac arrhythmias, tachycardia, increased activity levels and agitation.

Anabolic Steroids*

Hallucinations, grandiose feelings of euphoria and unusual power, increased aggression, anxiety, and paranoia Restlessness, nervousness, complaints of heart palpitations	Wide mood swings ranging from violent or homicidal episodes known as "roid rages" to depression	Testosterone-based drug Can stop growth prematurely and irreversibly in adolescent Usually taken in megadoses up to hundreds of milligrams per day (dosage for medicinal purposes is 1-5 mg/day). May "stack" steroids with stimulants, antidepressants, pain killers, and other drugs May "cycle" or take drugs for 6-12 weeks, stop for several weeks, and start another cycle (believe they can escape detection by doing this). Used by most to enhance appearance—causes rapid weight gain. Shotgunning—taking steroids intermittently Tapering—slow decrease in usage Bulking up—increase muscle mass with steroids Ergogenic—performance enhancing Plateauing—drug is ineffective Roid rage—uncontrolled outbursts of anger, frustration, combativeness

continues

At a Glance 14-7 Substance-Related Information *(Continued)*

Intoxication	Withdrawal	Substance-Related Information	Signs and Symptoms of Associated Disorder
Nicotine			
Dizziness and nausea with early use	Depressed mood, insomnia, irritability, frustration, anxiety, difficult concentration, restlessness, bradycardia, increased appetite with weight gain		
Tobacco odor on breath, hair, clothes			
Cough, chronic pulmonary disease			
Excessive skin wrinkling			
Risk of lung and oral cancers			
Risk of cardiovascular and cerebrovascular disease			

to produce intoxication in different people. Because of their smaller body mass and slower body metabolism, women tend to become intoxicated more easily than men.

Substance-Specific-Related Disorders

Each substance is associated with one or both of the substance-induced disorders highlighted in At a Glance 14-7. Alcohol, amphetamines, cocaine, inhalants, cannabis, and hallucinogens all have the potential of causing the psychoactive symptoms. Although the ingestion of caffeine can produce effects on the central nervous system, no psychoactive manifestations are associated with this substance. The substances are also associated with some or all of the mental disorders listed in At a Glance 14-8.

At a Glance 14-8 Other Substance-Related Conditions

- Delirium
- Amnesic disorder
- Psychotic disorder, with delusions
- Psychotic disorder, with hallucinations
- Mood disorder
- Anxiety disorder
- Sexual dysfunction
- Sleep disorder

Alcohol-Related Disorders

Alcohol is the most commonly used brain depressant in most cultures and the cause of considerable associated physiologic problems and sometimes death. Ninety percent of adults in the United States have used alcohol to some degree, but most people are able to moderate their drinking and avoid related problems.

Common Signs and Symptoms. The use of alcohol is associated with a significant increase in the risk of accidents, violence, and suicide. In people with antisocial personality disorder, there is also an increase in the incidence of related criminal acts. An increase in absenteeism from work, job-related accidents, and decreased employee productivity are commonly linked to alcohol.

In addition, chronic use of alcohol can result in an encephalopathy and psychosis known as **Wernicke-Korsakoff syndrome.** This is a nutritional disease of the nervous system found in alcoholics, caused primarily by thiamine and niacin deficiency. Significant cerebral deterioration and actual brain cell death occur with chronic and permanent impairment. With Wernicke's encephalopathy and Korsakoff's psychosis, there is progressive memory loss and disorientation with emotional lability and apathy, weakness, and fatigue.

Alcohol-induced delirium, or **delirium tremens** (DTs), is a state of profound confusion and delusions along with all of the usual withdrawal symptoms that are seen within a short period following cessation of alcohol use. The episode generally ends after several days of insomnia and rigorous activity when the person falls into a deep sleep. On awakening, the person is coherent but without memory of the events during the delirium. The delirium may last from 72 to 80 hours, during which there is a 20% fatality rate.

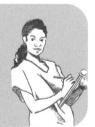

Just the Facts

The development of seizure activity during delirium tremens is a life-threatening situation and must be considered a medical emergency.

Incidence and Etiology. Alcoholism is prevalent across all educational and socioeconomic levels. Women tend to develop a higher blood alcohol concentration because of their lower body water, higher percentage of body fat, and slower metabolic rate and thus may be at greater risk for subsequent liver damage than men. Alcohol abuse and dependence is more common in men. Women are reported to start drinking at a later age than do men, but dependence progresses more rapidly in women.

There is a strong familial pattern of alcohol-related problems, with an estimated 40% to 60% of occurrences thought to be genetically linked. Environmental factors account for the remainder. (See previous discussion on etiologic factors.)

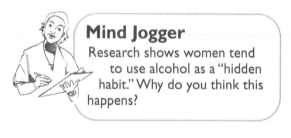

Mind Jogger

Research shows women tend to use alcohol as a "hidden habit." Why do you think this happens?

Amphetamine-Related Disorders

The amphetamine and amphetamine-like substances include both those sold on the illegal market and those that may be obtained by prescription for the treatment of obesity, attention-deficit/hyperactivity disorder, and narcolepsy. Most of the effects of these drugs are similar to those of cocaine, although the risk for inducing cardiac arrhythmias and seizures is lower.

Common Signs and Symptoms. The psychoactive effects of most amphetamine-like substances last longer than those of cocaine, and the stimulating effects on the autonomic nervous system may be more potent. Paranoid ideation, hallucinations, and intense anger with aggressive behavior and threats are commonly associated with amphetamine or methamphetamine use. The person may develop mood changes, weight loss, and malnutrition. It is common for users of amphetamine to also use alcohol and benzodiazepine antianxiety drug agents to calm the jittery feelings caused by the stimulant.

Incidence and Etiology. The pattern of amphetamine usage fluctuates by geographic location, with a greater concentration in heavily populated areas. The peak use of these drugs is between 26 to 34 years of age. High school students represent about 16% of users. Chronic use often leads to decreased effectiveness. Some move on to other addictive substances, whereas others decrease or stop using amphetamines after 8 to 10 years.

Caffeine-Related Disorders

Caffeine is found in many different sources including coffee, caffeinated soda, tea, over-the-counter pain relievers, cold remedies, anti-drowsiness aids, and weight-loss agents. Chocolate and cocoa have a lower caffeine content than the other sources listed. There is no link between the intake of caffeine and a clinical picture that meets the criteria for substance dependence or abuse. There is evidence that caffeine intoxication and withdrawal may be clinically significant.

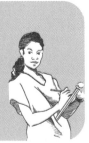

Just the Facts

The average consumption of caffeine in the United States is approximately 500 mg/day. Intake in excess of 10 grams can cause grand mal seizures, respiratory failure, and death.

Common Signs and Symptoms. Mild sensory alterations, such as ringing in the ears or flashing lights, have been reported by those who are heavy users. Physical symptoms from excessive intake may include anxiety, agitation, restlessness, sweating, flushed face, and diarrhea. There are some reports of cardiac arrhythmias and gastrointestinal discomfort.

Incidence and Etiology. The use of caffeine and caffeine-related products is seen across all cultural groups. Consumption is much greater in Sweden, Norway, Denmark, Great Britain, and other European countries. Intake tends to decrease with age and is greater in men than in women. Caffeine is used more among those who smoke or use alcohol and other substances. The prevalence of caffeine-related disorders is unknown.

Cannabis-Related Disorders

Cannabis or marijuana (bhang) is derived from the cannabis plant and is used widely in the form of rolled cigarettes. Although usually smoked, marijuana may be taken orally mixed in tea or food. The cannabinoid chemicals present in the plant are primarily responsible for the psychoactive effects.

Common Signs and Symptoms. The essential features include a "high" feeling followed by euphoria, inappropriate laughter, grandiosity, sedation, lethargy, impaired short-term memory, delayed mental processing, impaired judgment, distorted sensory perceptions, and impaired motor function. There may be accompanying anxiety, dysphoria, or social withdrawal as the use increases. Within 2 hours after marijuana use, there is conjunctival redness, increased appetite, dry mouth, and increased heart rate.

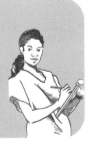

Just the Facts

Cannabis drug effects usually last 3 to 4 hours. Because the drug is fat-soluble, the effects may be detected in the urine for 7 to 10 days and up to 4 weeks in heavy users.

Cannabis is often used with other substances such as alcohol, cocaine, and nicotine. It can also be mixed and smoked with opioids, PCP, or hallucinogenic drugs. In people who use high doses, regular use commonly results in depression, anxiety, and irritability, with psychoactive effects similar to those of the hallucinogens. High use can also result in severe anxiety or panic attacks, as well as episodes of paranoid delusional thinking or depersonalization. Chronic cannabis use is associated with weight gain, sinusitis, pharyngitis, bronchitis with persistent cough, and emphysema. It should be noted that cannabis or marijuana smoke contains larger amounts of carcinogens than tobacco, contributing to the potential for cancer.

Incidence and Etiology. The cannabis drugs are the most widely used illicit psychoactive substance in America. The highest prevalence is seen in 18- to 34-year-olds. Surveys show that around 40% of adolescents have used marijuana. It is not known how many reported cases of cannabis-related disorders exist.

Cocaine-Related Disorders

Crack cocaine is the most common form of cocaine used in the United States today. It is easily vaporized and inhaled, making the onset of effects particularly rapid. Cocaine has extremely potent euphoric effects, which increases the potential for dependence after the drug has been used for a very short time. An early sign of dependence is that the person is unable to resist using the drug when it is available. Because of the 30- to 50-minute half-life of the drug, the user must use the drug frequently to maintain the "high." This short effect and the craving for more lead users to spend thousands of dollars in a short time, with devastating personal and financial consequences. Most people with dependence have signs of tolerance and withdrawal at some point.

Common Signs and Symptoms. Common mental and physical complications of chronic cocaine use are paranoid ideation, anxiety, and weight loss. There may be rambling speech, headache, ringing in the ears, and tactile ("coke bugs") and auditory hallucinations. The withdrawal symptoms are likely to enhance craving and the likelihood of reusing the drug. Because of its powerful effects on the central nervous system, it is common to see erratic and aggressive behaviors. Mood changes such as depression with suicidal ideation, irritability, anhedonia, emotional swings, and inattentiveness are also seen. The substance takes over the person's life to the point of social isolation.

Incidence and Etiology. Most data that have been collected are based on usage patterns rather than disorders. The actual percentage of those who use or abuse cocaine and have diagnosed disorders is not known. Cocaine use is seen in all races and socioeconomic, age, and gender groups. Although the overall prevalence of cocaine use in the United States has decreased, the highest rate increase in 2003 was in 18- to 25-year-olds. There is a tendency for men to be more commonly affected than women.

Hallucinogen-Related Disorders

Hallucinogens are usually taken orally, although injection does occur. Tolerance to the euphoric and psychedelic effects of these substances develops rather quickly, but there is no clear documented evidence regarding a withdrawal pattern that falls into the criteria for a disorder. However, most users continue to use hallucinogens despite knowledge of the adverse effects, such as memory impairment, panic reactions, or flashback episodes ("bad trips") that may occur during drug intoxication.

Common Signs and Symptoms. Under the influence of a hallucinogenic drug, the person may display mood swings, fearfulness, anxiety, and feelings of going insane or dying. Many of these drugs have stimulant effects similar to those of amphetamine intoxication. The perceptual disturbances and impaired judgment seen in toxic episodes or flashbacks may result in fatal accidents such as users believing they can fly and subsequently jumping from a building or bridge. Associated physiologic changes include increases in blood glucose and cortisol hormones. LSD intoxication is usually confirmed through urine sampling.

Incidence and Etiology. Use of and intoxication with hallucinogens usually begins during adolescence. Younger users may experience more intense emotional states as a result of the drug effects. Use is shown to be three times more common in men than women. There was an increased incidence of use in the United States during the years 1960 to 1970. Despite a decline following this period, it is reported that there was a slight increase in use during the late 1990s. Hallucinogens are used most by individuals between the ages of 26 and 34 years. Environmental factors, along with the personality and expectations of the person using the drug, may contribute to the decision to use these substances.

Inhalant-Related Disorders

Most drug compounds containing nitrous oxide that are inhaled can produce psychoactive effects. Tolerance is reported with heavy use, although withdrawal patterns that meet the criteria for an assigned disorder have not been documented. Because inhalants are inexpensive, legal, and easily accessible, they tend to be used over a longer time. This may result in the person spending more time recuperating and giving up important social, occupational, or recreational activities. Substance use often continues despite the person's awareness of both physical and psychologic problems caused by the chemicals.

Common Signs and Symptoms. Behavioral or psychologic changes include confusion, belligerence, aggression, apathy, and impaired judgment and social functioning. Hallucinations, delusional thinking, and perceptual changes may develop during periods of confusion and intoxication. These changes are usually accompanied by dizziness, visual disturbances, unsteady gait, tremors, and euphoria. Higher doses can lead to lethargy, slowed psychomotor response, muscle weakness, and stupor. People who use inhalants usually have an odor of paint or solvent on their breath or clothing with a residue "glue sniffer's rash" evident around the nose and mouth. There may be redness of the eyes, respiratory distress, rales or rhonchi, coughing, sinus discharge, headache, weakness, and abdominal pain with nausea or vomiting. Inhalants can cause permanent damage to both the central and peripheral nervous system. Death can occur from cardiac arrhythmias or respiratory failure, commonly referred to as "sudden sniffing death."

> ## Just the Facts
> "Sudden sniffing death" can occur with the use of inhalants as a result of acute cardiac arrhythmias, hypoxia, or electrolyte imbalances.

During adolescence, the use of inhalants may first be noticed because of school-related problems such as truancy, a drop in grades, or dropping out of school. Most adolescents use inhalants under the influence of peer pressure in a group setting. However, heavy usage tends to be a solitary pattern.

Incidence and Etiology. Because of the easy accessibility of these drugs, it is difficult to track the actual number of inhalant users. However, there tends to be a pattern of usage beginning in the 9- to 12-year-old age-group with peak usage during adolescence. It is more prevalent in males than in females.

Over the past 10 years, the prevalence of sniffing glue and aerosols such as whipped topping and spray paint has increased. There is also a rise in reports of lighter fluid inhalation, with a higher incidence in deprived populations, especially in children and adolescents.

Opioid-Related Disorders

Opioid drugs are regularly prescribed treatments and are contained in analgesics, anesthetics, antidiarrheal agents, and cough suppressants. Heroin may be injected or snorted and is the most abused drug in this class. Opioid dependence is evident by compulsive, prolonged self-administration of these substances for no legitimate medical reason. The drugs are usually purchased through illegal channels or by faking medical conditions to acquire multiple prescriptions from different physicians. Health care professionals with opioid dependence may resort to drug diversion in their place of employment or to prescription forgery to obtain the drug (see section on substance abuse by health care professionals).

Common Signs and Symptoms. With opioid intoxication there is an initial "high" followed by apathy, depressed mood, inability to coordinate motor functioning, and impaired judgment. These changes are accompanied by drowsiness, slurred speech, inattention, memory lapses, and pupil constriction. Severe intoxication can lead to respiratory depression, unconsciousness, and death. Opioid dependence is commonly associated with a history of drug-related crimes and unprofessional conduct among health professionals who have access to controlled drugs. Periods of depression are common after repeated use of the drug.

Incidence and Etiology. The incidence of opioid drug use has increased among white middle-class people, especially in women.

There is an increased risk in medical and other health professionals. The prevalence for opioid use tends to decrease after age 40. Heroin use is more common among men, with a 3 : 1 ratio over women. Survey reports from 2003 show the highest rate of heroin use among high school seniors since the 1970s. Use most commonly begins during the late teens or early 20s. Family members of people with opioid dependence typically have an increased incidence of other substance-related disorders or antisocial personality disorder.

Phencyclidine-Related Disorders

Phencyclidine (PCP) is not a difficult drug to obtain and is commonly used several times a week by those with dependence on the substance. Users often demonstrate dangerous behaviors because of lack of insight and judgment under the influence of the drug. Aggressive behaviors such as fighting are a particular problem for PCP use. The drug can be taken orally, injected, or smoked. PCP is the most commonly abused substance of the drug compounds in this category.

Common Signs and Symptoms. Psychologic effects may include inability to control emotions, anxiety, rage, aggression, panic, flashbacks, and disorganized thinking. Medical problems such as hyperthermia, hypertension, and seizures can compound the picture with recurrent PCP use. Other indicators of use may be nystagmus, hypertension, evidence of needle tracks, hepatitis, or HIV disease. Those with substance intoxication may exhibit delirium, psychotic symptoms, catatonic posturing, or coma.

Incidence and Etiology. The prevalence of phencyclidine use is more common in men 20 to 40 years of age. It is reported that about 3% of drug-related emergency room visits and deaths are related to PCP use. The highest percentage of initial use is seen in the 12- to 17-year-old age group.

Sedative-, Hypnotic-, or Anxiolytic-Related Disorders

Sedative, hypnotic, and anxiolytic drugs include the benzodiazepines, the barbiturates, and other sedative agents. All prescription sleeping medications and antianxiety drugs also fall into these categories. These agents are all brain depressants and are particularly lethal when mixed with alcohol. These drugs are available both by prescription and on the illegal street market. The medications with a rapid onset are more likely to be abused by those who obtain them by prescription.

Common Signs and Symptoms. The clinical picture is usually one of maladaptive behavioral and psychologic changes such as mood lability, impaired judgment and functioning, and inappropriate sexual or aggressive behavior. Other indicators may be slurred speech, unsteady gait, nystagmus, and impaired mobility or coordination. Physiologic effects may include tachycardia, tachypnea, hypertension, hyperthermia, diaphoresis, tremors, insomnia, anxiety, and nausea.

Dependence and abuse of these agents is often associated with abuse of other substances such as alcohol, cannabis, cocaine, heroin, methadone, or amphetamines. The sedatives may be used to counteract the adverse effects of the other substances. Habitual users are usually in search of the original feeling of euphoria and take increased doses trying to achieve this end. Accidental overdose and acute respiratory arrest that result in death are not uncommon.

Incidence and Etiology. Most people take these drugs as directed by their physician for legitimate medical reasons with no intent of misuse. Approximately 6% of those surveyed acknowledge using the drugs illicitly. Those who originally obtained the prescription for medical reasons and have continued to increase doses often justify the continued use by claiming the original symptoms. They often go to multiple physicians in different locations to acquire the prescriptions to continue their habit. Use of this group of drugs to get an intentional "high" is most common among teenagers and young adults in their 20s. The prescription pattern of increasing dosage is more prevalent in the 40 and older age group.

Substance Abuse by Health Care Professionals

Those who work in the health care professions are entwined in a fast-paced and demanding environment. The decision to use alcohol or other drugs as a means of tolerating and coping with the pressure is alarmingly prevalent within the health care industry. There are many who believe that the chaotic and stressful climate in which doctors, nurses, and other health care providers work leads some to give in to the relief that the drugs offer. The easy accessibility of sedative-hypnotic, anxiolytic, and opioid drugs to those who work in health care professions has also contributed to the number of drug-impaired health care workers. Most of them do not start using a drug with the intention of abusing. However, once the cycle of abuse or drug diversion begins, the person is often powerless to control the need for the substance and dependence takes over.

Professional ethics and practice standards of these groups and a personal set of values are the reasons why most people in the health-related fields refrain from ever falling into this trap. Most health care workers are able to provide care that includes medication administration with integrity and professionalism. To address the numbers of health care workers who fail in keeping these standards, many states have formed professional help groups for impaired health professionals. These groups work closely with professional licensing boards to develop guidelines by which the person may seek and receive treatment. There are very strict and specific compliance rules and regulations governing the status of the license to practice in these situations. The stipulations as to whether the person may or may not return to practice varies with the situation. The license may be suspended and reinstated once the requirements for treatment have been proven, or the license may be revoked.

Application of the Nursing Process

Nursing Assessment

When assessing the client who abuses substances, it is first important to remember that underneath the surface of denial and rationalization are the feelings of fear, insecurity, anx-

---

Case Study: Suspicious Behavior

Judy is a licensed practical nurse who works the day shift in an oncology center. Patrick, a registered nurse who lives across the street from her, works the night shift on the same unit. He often works with only one night off and fills in for other nurses who want time off. His wife stays home with their five children, three of whom are under the age of 6 years. Judy has noticed that for the past few weeks, Patrick has been less social and more distant when she tries to talk to him. He seems so tired and sluggish, sometimes his speech is even slurred in the morning during shift report. There have been several times that Judy has asked him to complete charting that he leaves undone. She is concerned that maybe he is working too much and mentions the change in behavior to the unit supervisor.

The unit supervisor asks Judy if she has been giving more unit doses of injectable morphine to the unit patients. She states that the unit supply of morphine has been refilled almost daily for the past few weeks. Judy states that the majority of the patients with increasing doses are on PCA (patient-controlled analgesia) pumps and that she is administering about the same number of single injections each day. When they check the sign-out register for controlled drugs, they note that most of the injectable doses are being given during the night shift. Some of the doses are signed out for patients who have PCA pumps who would not be receiving routine single doses of the drug. Judy senses that she and the unit supervisor are thinking the same thing.

What are the indicators for a problem in this situation?

_____

_____

What symptoms does Patrick demonstrate that may explain the increased need for stock refills?

_____

_____

What factors may have led to Patrick's situation?

_____

_____

At a Glance 14-9 The Impaired Nurse or Health Care Provider

Clues—Drug-Related Problems	When to Report
Alcoholic	
Moody and irritable	At least two people witness smell of alcohol on breath, hair, or clothing
Unkempt appearance	
Numerous excuses for behavior	A positive blood alcohol level
Smell of alcohol on breath or hair	Displays a pattern of poor nursing judgment or repeated medication errors
Excessive use of mouth fresheners	
Social isolation	Slurred speech, falling asleep, or staggering while on duty
Slurred speech, motor incoordination	
Bloodshot eyes	DWI while driving to work or on duty (home health)
Flushed face	
Drug-impaired	
Rapid mood swings or changes in performance	Positive urine drug screen result for which a legitimate prescription cannot be produced
Social isolation	
Frequent breaks or use of bathroom	Falling asleep at work, staggering gait, or slurred speech
Repeatedly volunteers for extra shifts, overtime	
Offers to give medications for other nurses	Forgetfulness, poor performance, frequent errors
Consistently signs out for vial or ampoule of controlled drugs so wasting is necessary	Drug diversion evidence
Discrepancies in signing for controlled substances and on medication record	Giving drugs without doctor's order
Patients complain of ineffective pain medication	Signing out drugs to discharged or deceased patients
Always wears clothing with long sleeves	

iety, and low self-esteem. Some people who are frightened by the effects of the substance or their behaviors while under the influence of the substance may present voluntarily for treatment, whereas others are reprimanded to treatment subsequent to a substance-related arrest. If the person enters the hospital for another medical reason and is a substance user, withdrawal may become an issue. The assessment process should be directed toward identifying the type of substance the person has been using, the amount and frequency of use, the method of administration, and the length of time the substance has been abused. The nurse should also take note of any suicidal ideation or intent, along with the presence and character of any withdrawal symptoms. Knowledge of the withdrawal symptoms for the various substances can help the nurse recognize and report their occurrence. If the client is an alcohol user, it is important to ask about amount consumed, how often the drinking occurs, and the time of the most recent drink. Remember that most substance abusers underreport the amount they ingest. The client's motivation for treatment is cru-

Mind Jogger

How might a drug user employ a surface attitude of sincerity and willingness to change as a manipulative means toward discharge?

cial to the outcome. Reason for admission is often a determining factor in the client's willingness to comply with the terms of the treatment contract. If the client is seeking relief from the substance-related problems with a sincere recognition of the drug problem, an expectation of success is more realistic.

A description of current chemical use is obtained, including how much, how often, when use began, any attempts to decrease or discontinue using the substance, and any previous treatment. The CAGE questionnaire is often used to screen for alcohol dependency. CAGE is an acronym that includes the following questions:

1. Have you ever felt you should **C**ut down on your drinking?
2. Have people **A**nnoyed you by criticizing your drinking?
3. Have you ever felt **G**uilty about your drinking?
4. Have you ever had a drink first thing in the morning (**E**ye-opener) to steady your nerves or get rid of a hangover?

A positive answer to two or more of these questions is indicative that the client abuses alcohol. This information is reported to the treating physician. It is also important to determine why the client is seeking treatment. As the nurse interacts with the client during this initial interview, a therapeutic trusting relationship can be established in which the client is accepted and respected for who he or she is at the present time. Long-term recovery is often marked by periods of **relapse,** or the reoccurrence of substance using behavior after a significant period of abstinence. The nurse should refrain from judging the client or referring to this as failure. The nurse acts as a role model to demonstrate more effective problem-solving and coping skills. Active listening is used to embrace the person beneath the substance and to offer concern and support for the efforts to gain control over his or her life.

A baseline physical and emotional nursing assessment is done to determine admission status and provide a baseline from which to determine progress toward an expected outcome.

Nervous System
- Orientation
- Level of consciousness (LOC)
- Coordination, gait
- Short- and long-term memory (any difficulty following commands)
- Signs of depression or anxiety
- Tremors or decreased reflexes
- Pupils (constricted or dilated)
- Complexion (ruddy or pale, petechiae)

Cardiovascular and Respiratory
- Vital signs
- Peripheral pulses
- Dyspnea on exertion
- Abnormal breath sounds (an alcoholic client is susceptible to aspiration while intoxicated)
- Arrhythmias
- Fatigue
- Peripheral edema

Gastrointestinal
- Nausea or vomiting
- Changes in weight or appetite
- Time of last meal
- Signs of malnourishment
- General nutritional status
- Color and consistency of stool

Integumentary
- Location, size, and characteristics of any skin lesions
- Needle tracks or scarring on arms, legs, fingers, toes, under the tongue, or between gums and lips

Emotional Behavior
- Affect
- Rate of speech
- Suspiciousness, anger, agitation
- Occurrence of hallucinations, blackouts
- History of violent episodes
- Support system: Is anyone present with the client? How do they interact with each other? Are they willing to be involved in the treatment of the client?

At a Glance 14-10 Potential Problems Resulting from Substance Dependence

Nursing Diagnosis	Related Risk Factors
Risk for injury	Impaired judgment
	Increase in risk-taking behaviors
	Substance withdrawal
	Seizures
	Delirium
	Flashbacks
	Anger and agitation
Anxiety	Withdrawal symptoms
	Anticipated abstinence
Altered nutrition	Inadequate nutritional intake
	Impaired absorption
	Money used for drugs instead of food
	Drug chosen over food
Fluid volume deficit	Secondary nausea and vomiting
Ineffective individual coping	Reliance on drug to solve problems
	Loss of family, income, job
	Excessive and ineffective denial of problem
	Underlying fears
Altered health maintenance	Drug-impaired health status
Noncompliance	Resumption of drug use after period abstinence
Social isolation	Dysfunctional interpersonal relationships
Powerlessness	Dependence on drug
	Inadequate coping skills
	Dysfunctional family system
	Negative role models
Self-esteem disturbance	Self-destructive drug-related behaviors
	Weak underdeveloped ego
Sensory perceptual alteration	Hallucinations, withdrawal syndrome
Sleep pattern disturbance	Drug interference with REM stage of sleep cycle
Risk for violence toward self and others	Decreased inhibitions and inability to control anger
Knowledge deficit	Drug effects and withdrawal process

Nursing Diagnosis

Once the assessment data have been collected, the nurse determines problems that are created as a result of the substance dependence and its effect on the person's ability to function in activities of daily living. Potential nursing diagnoses applicable to the client with substance abuse or dependence are included in At a Glance 14-10.

Expected Outcomes

During the acute stage of withdrawal, the client needs physical and psychologic support to return to a more stable state of health. Detoxification is usually accomplished within 7 days. Once the drug is out of the system, the person may experience sleeping and eating difficulties along with varied levels of irritability and anxiety. The nurse should remember that the substance user without the drug is a person who is hungry, angry, lonely, and tired, whose mind and body will want the drug. During this stage of treatment the nursing goals will be to:

- Promote safety and protection of the client.
- Promote adequate food intake to restore nutritional balance.
- Promote and maintain fluid and electrolyte balance.
- Promote a restful sleep pattern.
- Decrease anxiety and promote relaxation.
- Stabilize vital signs and general physical state.
- Prevent seizures.

Following the withdrawal period, the nurse will contribute to the long-term treatment goals. Efforts are directed to help the abuser live a full and productive life as a member of society without the use of the substance. Expected outcomes that address the planning strategies for continued sobriety and abstinence from drug use are that the client:

- Identifies the drug as a problem and takes ownership of the problem
- Identifies changes in lifestyle that are necessary
- Acknowledges responsibility for own behavior and recognizes the association between the substance and personal problems
- Verbalizes understanding of substance abuse and dependence as an illness requiring continued treatment and support
- Identifies alternative coping mechanisms to use in response to stress instead of the substance
- Demonstrates increased feelings of self-worth by verbalizing positive statements about self
- Demonstrates efforts at positive change with interdependence on others and living one day at a time
- Begins to develop or reestablish a support system with family, employer, and non–substance-using friends

- Identifies available social support systems and how to access them
- Continues to abstain from substance use
- Verbalizes understanding of illness and the recovery process
- Demonstrates willingness to participate in a group recovery treatment program

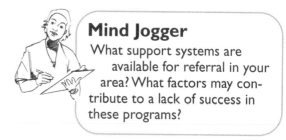

Mind Jogger

What support systems are available for referral in your area? What factors may contribute to a lack of success in these programs?

Nursing Interventions

Planned interventions during the acute withdrawal state are directed toward controlling the symptoms of withdrawal without oversedating the client. Benzodiazepines are usually the drug of choice for alcohol detoxification, starting with a relatively large dose with daily reductions until withdrawal is complete. Multivitamin therapy and thiamine replacement therapy are used to prevent neuropathy and encephalopathy from chronic alcohol use (Wernicke-Korsakoff syndrome), because chronic alcohol users are usually deficient in thiamine and niacin. Antabuse (disulfiram) is a long-term alcohol abuse treatment that inhibits alcohol ingestion by producing severe adverse effects if alcohol is ingested. Symptoms may include diaphoresis, flushing, throbbing headache, palpitations, severe nausea and vomiting, weakness, dyspnea, and hypotension. Severe cases may result in coma, cardiac or respiratory arrest, and death. Additional anti-convulsants may be ordered if seizure activity is not controlled by the benzodiazepines. Antiemetic agents may also be used to control symptoms of nausea and vomiting.

Opiate withdrawal symptoms can be minimized with clonidine (Catapres) in a detoxification setting. This agent lowers blood pressure, so it is essential to monitor vital signs closely during the withdrawal period. This approach is not as effective as using an opioid substitute, but the benefit is that it is nonaddicting and can keep the client opiate free so other therapies can be initiated. Methadone is typically the opioid substitute used in heroin withdrawal maintenance programs. It is a chemical relative of heroin and is taken once daily by mouth to prevent symptoms of heroin withdrawal and to reduce craving for the drug. The daily dose is titrated over 2 weeks to a maintenance dose. The client may be in a maintenance program for up to 2 to 4 years. A longer-acting drug called orlaam (LAAM) can be taken three times weekly and is used in some situations. In addition, the regimen for opioid withdrawal may include a muscle relaxant, antianxiety agent, and an anticholinergic for abdominal cramping.

Nursing interventions toward expected outcomes during acute substance withdrawal include:

Potential for Injury

- Remove hazardous articles and furnishings.
- Seizure precautions every 15 minutes.
- Assess for hypoglycemia and electrolyte imbalance.
- Observe for respiratory depression, arrhythmias.
- Identify and reduce seizure precipitating factors.
- Monitor medication levels.
- Initiate and administer withdrawal sedation.

Neurologic–Cardiovascular Compromise

- Determine level of intoxication and withdrawal stage.
- Reorient as necessary.
- Provide a quiet and safe environment.
- Monitor vital signs every 1 to 2 hours during first 3 to 4 days of withdrawal.
- Monitor neurologic signs every hour until stable, then as needed.
- Provide education about substance effects on body.

Nutritional Alterations

- Provide high-protein, high-vitamin (B and C) diet.
- Provide pleasant and positive mealtime environment.
- Provide frequent, small feedings with between-meal high-nutrient snacks.
- Encourage oral hygiene.
- Provide free access to alternative nutritious beverages.
- Offer bedtime snacks.
- Restrict caffeine intake.
- Teach client importance of nutritional balance.
- Record intake and output.
- Weigh daily.

Anxiety, Fear, Hopelessness

- Approach client in calm, reassuring, and nonjudgmental manner.
- Encourage expression of feelings.
- Reinforce client's value as a person.
- Listen actively.

Noncompliance and Denial of Illness

- Educate about illness and addiction process.
- Listen to client's reasons for noncompliance.
- Discuss importance of following treatment plan.
- Help to identify alternatives to maladaptive coping strategies.

Social Isolation and Ineffective Individual Coping

- Initiate a therapeutic one-on-one relationship.
- Encourage client to talk about himself or herself.
- Demonstrate appropriate role-modeling behaviors.

- Help client to identify reasons for social isolation.
- Help client to set realistic interaction goals
- Teach problem-solving skills.
- Encourage participation in all group activities.
- Refer to therapist, counselors, and treatment programs.
- Refer to social services or community support services.
- Refer family members to Al-Anon or Al-Ateen as appropriate.

Evaluation

The evaluation process will depend on the anticipated outcome. Acute withdrawal outcomes are achieved when the client no longer

Just the Facts

Interventions for the Person Who Is Inhaling or Huffing

Use a calm approach—do not excite or argue with the person (can become aggressive).

Try to determine what substance was used (aerosol cans, bags, rags can provide clues).

Keep person calm in a well-ventilated environment (may have respiratory difficulty).

Avoid stimulation (can cause hallucinations or violence).

Get help for the user as quickly as possible.

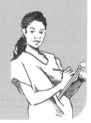

At a Glance 14-11 Alcoholics Anonymous, Al-Anon, Narcotics Anonymous: Hope and Help for Drug Abusers and Their Families

Alcoholics Anonymous (AA) is an international fellowship of men and women who have a drinking problem. There are no age or education requirements. Anyone may attend open AA meetings, but only those with a drinking problem may attend closed meetings. Members share their experiences, provide anonymity to each other, and meet together to attain and maintain sobriety. AA is a program of total abstinence. Members stay away from one drink, one day at a time. Sobriety is maintained through sharing experience, strength, and hope through meetings and the Twelve Steps for recovery from alcoholism.

The purpose of Al-Anon is to help families and friends of alcoholics recover from the effects of living with the problem drinking of a relative or friend. Al-Ateen is a recovery program for young people and is sponsored by Al-Anon members. The only requirement for membership in these groups is that there be a problem of alcoholism in a relative or friend.

Narcotics Anonymous (NA) was started from the AA concept for those for whom drugs have become a major problem. Membership is open to all drug addicts, regardless of the particular drug or combination of drugs used. When this group was formed, the word "addiction" was substituted for "alcohol" to reflect the disease concept of addiction. One of the keys to the success of this group is the therapeutic value of addicts working with other addicts, sharing their successes and challenges in overcoming active addiction. The Twelve Steps and Twelve Traditions of NA are the core principles of the recovery program.

Web Sites:
  http://www.alcoholics-anonymous.org
  http://www.al-anon.org
  http://www.na.org

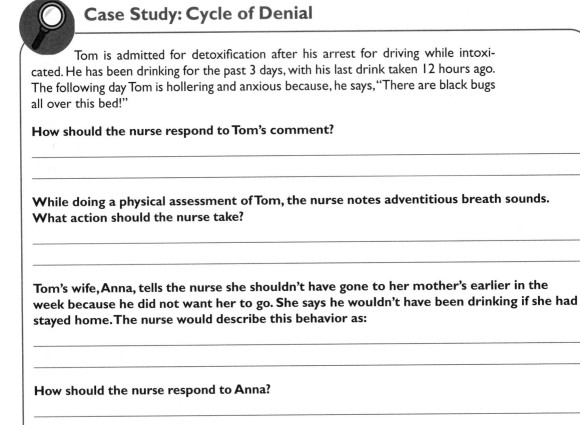

Case Study: Cycle of Denial

Tom is admitted for detoxification after his arrest for driving while intoxicated. He has been drinking for the past 3 days, with his last drink taken 12 hours ago. The following day Tom is hollering and anxious because, he says, "There are black bugs all over this bed!"

How should the nurse respond to Tom's comment?

_____

_____

While doing a physical assessment of Tom, the nurse notes adventitious breath sounds. What action should the nurse take?

_____

_____

Tom's wife, Anna, tells the nurse she shouldn't have gone to her mother's earlier in the week because he did not want her to go. She says he wouldn't have been drinking if she had stayed home. The nurse would describe this behavior as:

_____

_____

How should the nurse respond to Anna?

_____

_____

How can involvement in an Alcoholics Anonymous treatment program benefit Tom? What is essential to Tom's success at sobriety?

_____

_____

exhibits any signs or symptoms of substance intoxication or withdrawal and has sustained no injuries during the detoxification period. As the client gains insight into the illness and expresses a willingness to admit and take responsibility for his or her own substance problem, the treatment process can become a meaningful step toward a positive recovery phase. Acceptance of this responsibility is the first step toward a drug-free existence. Relapse is common, and recovery is an ongoing process of commitment toward a goal of abstinence.

Summary

Substance abuse and dependency are among the most preventable of the mental disorders. Yet millions of people continue to use

At a Glance 14-12 Sources of Information on Drug Abuse and Treatment

Al-Anon Family Group
National Referral Hotline
800-344-2666
Alcoholics Anonymous (AA)—Worldwide
475 Riverside Drive
New York, NY 10115
212-870-3400
Drug Abuse Information and Treatment Referral Line
800-662-HELP; Spanish 800-66-AYUDA
Narcotics Anonymous and Nar-Anon Family Group
Nationwide Referral Line: 202-399-5316
National Council on Alcoholism and Drug Dependence
12 West 21st Street
New York, NY 10010
800-622-2255 or 800-475-4673
http://www.ncadd.org
National Institute on Drug Abuse
6001 Executive Blvd., Rm. 5213
Bethesda, MD 20892
300-443-1124
http://www.nida.nih.gov or
   http://www.drugabuse.gov
National Clearinghouse for Alcohol and Drug Information
1-800-729-6686
http://www.health.org

and abuse drugs each day, with alcohol being the drug most often abused by Americans. The destructive nature of substance abuse is the very reason that prevention becomes a component of health care programs on drug use.

Substance use disorders are divided into 11 categories by *DSM-IV-TR*. These substances include prescription and over-the-counter drugs, abuse of which is showing a steady increase. There are perhaps underlying symptoms precipitating the unmonitored overuse of these drugs without an awareness of the potential dangers of this practice. Most symptoms caused by abuse of these drugs will subside as the drug dosage is decreased or discontinued. Toxins and other chemicals used with the intent of intoxication also fall into this group of disorders. Volatile substances such as gasoline or antifreeze are referred to as inhalants when used for this purpose.

There are various theories regarding why substance abuse and dependence occurs. Observational learning of maladaptive coping tools such as drugs are embraced in the minds of youth who grow up in homes where drug use is a common occurrence. The urge to conform to the group is also considered a major reason for the growing use of drugs by the adolescent population. Addictive behaviors demonstrate a generational pattern, supporting the theories of genetics and codependency. Addiction is also seen as a chronic disease that weaves a physical and mental web of destruction around its victim.

The substance-use disorders include substance dependence and abuse. A diagnosis of substance dependence is assigned when the criteria of craving, tolerance, and withdrawal symptoms are present. As tolerance develops, the substance is usually ingested in larger amounts over a longer period than was intended by the user. Efforts at controlling the drug use are futile, and increasingly more time is spent in acquiring the drug. The person relinquishes a stable and productive family and social life to the power of the drug. Despite the negative results of this pattern of living, drug use continues. Intoxication and withdrawal symptoms may vary with the particular substance, although some have similar effects. With substance abuse, the person experiences all the devastating physical effects of the drug but does not demonstrate tolerance withdrawal or compulsive use. There tends to be instances during substance use when behaviors lead to negative social, legal, and interpersonal encounters. Despite these repeated drug-related problems, the person does not abstain from continued use.

Substance-induced disorders include various conditions that are directly related to the effects of the substance. Although the drug groups share some commonalities, some associated features are specific for an individual substance. All of the drugs except caffeine are associated with psychoactive symptoms classifying them as mind-altering drugs.

Nursing assessment is first directed toward obtaining data regarding drug use that is then used for planning interventions for a safe withdrawal phase. The detoxification phase will leave the abuser free of the drug with the potential to confront the drug problem. The first step in recovery is for the person to admit that a problem exists. Involvement in chemical dependency treatment programs requires this initial recognition and willingness to make changes toward a lifestyle of continued abstinence. Success is often dependent on participation in a recovery group such as AA, where participants support each other in their continuing efforts at abstinence. Relapse is common in the long-term treatment process. Cognitive and behavioral changes along with lifestyle alterations that encourage a drug-free existence are necessary in the long road to recovery.

Bibliography

Alcoholics Anonymous World Services, Inc. (2004). *Twelve steps and twelve traditions.* Available at http://www.alcoholics-anonymous.org/default/en_about_aa_sub.cfm?subpageid84&pageid=13. Accessed on July 11, 2004.

American Academy of Child and Adolescent Psychiatry (AACAP) and National Institute of Drug Abuse (2000). Drugs and teen substance abuse. Available at http://www.focusas.com/SubstanceAbuse.html. Accessed on July 11, 2004.

American Psychiatric Association (2000). *Diagnostic and statistical manual of mental disorders text revision* (4th ed.). Washington, DC: American Psychiatric Association.

Enoch, M.A., & Goldman, D. (2002). Problem drinking and alcoholism: diagnosis and treatment, *American Family Physician, 65*(3), 441–450.

McCrady, B.S., and Epstein, E.E. (1999). *Addictions, A comprehensive guidebook,* New York, NY: Oxford University Press.

National Institute on Alcohol Abuse and Alcoholism (2001). Frequently Asked Questions on Alcohol Abuse and Alcoholism. Available at http://www.niaaa.nih.gov/faq/faq.htm. Accessed on July 11, 2004.

National Institute on Drug Abuse (2001). Facts about inhalant abuse, *NIDA Notes,* 14(6). Available at http://www.nida.nih.gov/NIDA_Notes/NN99Index.html#Number6. Accessed on July 11, 2004.

National Institute on Drug Abuse (2002). Research Report Series—Prescription Drugs: Abuse and Addiction. Available at http://www.nida.nih.gov/ResearchReports/ResearchIndex.html. Accessed on July 11, 2004.

National Institute on Drug Abuse (2003). Marijuana Abuse. Available at http://www.nida.nih.gov/ResearchReports/marijuana/PDF. Accessed on July 11, 2004.

Stewart, K.B., and Richards, A. B., (2000). Recognizing and managing your patient's alcohol abuse, *Nursing 2000, 30*(2), 56–59.

Swift, R.M. (2001). "Opioid dependence—Cocaine dependence," *Pharmacology Update,* Center for Alcohol and Addiction Studies.

Student Worksheet

FILL IN THE BLANK

Fill in the blank with the correct answer.

1. The term _____ is used in reference to any drug, medication, or toxin that has the potential for abuse.

2. Volatile substances such as gasoline or paint are referred to as _____ when used for the purpose of intoxication.

3. _____ is a strong inner drive to use a substance.

4. When repeated doses of a drug are used with a declining effect as the brain adapts to continued use, the user has developed a(n) _____ to the substance.

5. Negative behavioral changes with physiologic and psychologic alterations are characteristic of _____.

6. A person who enables drug-using behavior by accepting responsibility and guilt for the user is said to be _____.

7. Three early warning signs of chemical dependency include _____, _____, and _____.

8. Signs and symptoms of withdrawal usually develop within _____ after drug cessation.

9. Delirium tremens is _____.

10. A nutritional disease of the nervous system caused by a thiamin and niacin deficiency found primarily in alcoholics is _____.

MATCHING

Match the following terms to the most appropriate phrase.

a. Shakes

b. Denial

c. Thiamine

d. Codependence

e. Withdrawal

f. Tolerance

g. Benzodiazepine

h. Anhedonia

i. Nystagmus

j. Anxiety

k. Depressant

1. _____ Action of alcohol

2. _____ Controls seizures during withdrawal

3. _____ Early symptom of alcohol withdrawal

4. _____ Inability to find pleasure in previously enjoyed activities

5. _____ Not admitting to having a drug problem.

6. _____ Reason for morning drinking

7. _____ Overly responsible behavior

8. _____ Develops as brain adapts to repeated use of drug with declining effects

9. _____ Marked symptoms of "crashing" following intense period of substance use

10. _____ Vitamin used in treatment of alcohol dependence

11. _____ Constant involuntary movement of eyeball

MULTIPLE CHOICE

Select the best answer from the multiple-choice items.

1. The nurse is assessing hourly vital signs on a client in acute alcohol withdrawal. The client's blood pressure and pulse were recorded as 132/68, 78 at 2200; 138/72, 84 at 2400; 148/86, 90 at 0200; and 160/94, 94 at 0400. Which of the following actions would the nurse initiate?
   a. Increase fluid intake to 3000 cc in the next 12 hours.
   b. Initiate interventions for fall precautions.
   c. Obtain a clean catch urine specimen.
   d. Notify the physician.

2. Jeff is admitted to the psychiatric unit with a blood alcohol level of 0.30%. He is disoriented with slurred speech and a staggering gait. Which of the following assessments by the nurse is correct regarding this client?
   a. He has symptoms of intoxication.
   b. He has developed a tolerance to alcohol.
   c. He is experiencing alcohol withdrawal.
   d. He is probably using more than one substance.

3. Ronald tells the nurse he is not an alcoholic. He states he drinks "two or three beers" with his buddies every day after work and maybe one or two after he gets home. He says, "I can handle it. I've never missed work because of it." Which of the following mechanisms is Ronald using to deal with his problem?
   a. Denial
   b. Projection
   c. Displacement
   d. Rationalization

4. While the nurse is assessing a client to be admitted for treatment of alcohol dependency, the client says, "I suppose you think I am just another drunk." The nurse's best response to this statement would be:
   a. "We treat many people who have the same problem you do."
   b. "Why do you think you are a drunk?"
   c. "At least you are being honest about it."
   d. "We are most concerned that you receive treatment for your problem."

5. Emma is a licensed nurse who is admitted for treatment of prescription drug (oxycodone and lorazepam) dependency. Which of the following attitudes by the nursing staff would be considered an enabling behavior?
   a. Helping her to identify the issues in the nursing environment as the result of the drugs and not the cause of her drug habit.
   b. Agreeing that the staff shortages and increasing pressures at work may have led to her drug-using behaviors.
   c. Supporting her as she acknowledges that this treatment is required by the State Board of Nursing.
   d. Encouraging her to participate in a drug-related support group.

6. The nurse is assessing a client who has been admitted from the emergency room after several days of inhaling spray paint. In addition to the odor of paint and a sinus discharge, which of the following symptoms would this client display?
   a. Dilated pupils, masklike facial appearance, nystagmus
   b. Constricted pupils, drowsiness, attention deficit
   c. Lip-licking, nausea and vomiting, dyskinesia
   d. Coughing, dyspnea, watery eyes

7. A 59-year-old client is admitted to the psychiatric unit with a diagnosis of chronic alcoholism and Wernicke-Korsakoff syndrome. Which of the following will be included in this client's treatment plan?
   a. Methadone maintenance program
   b. Patient teaching in stress management
   c. Thiamine and niacin vitamin supplements
   d. Fifteen-minute interval suicide precautions

8. Rex has been admitted to the detoxification unit with a diagnosis of methamphetamine dependence. Which of the following is most necessary for Rex to remain drug-free after detoxification?
   a. Understanding how the drug is affecting him
   b. Admission that he has a drug problem
   c. Moving to a new geographic location
   d. Becoming involved in a community activity center

9. Andy is being examined in the emergency room after police aborted his attempt to jump from a 10-story building. His urine sample tests positive for LSD. Which of the following adverse effects is Andy most likely experiencing?
   a. Illusion
   b. Temporary insanity
   c. Perceptual changes
   d. Delirium tremens

10. Which of the following drugs has the potential to be detected in a urine sample for up to 4 weeks?
    a. Cannabis
    b. Cocaine
    c. Alcohol
    d. Inhalant

SCENARIO: NOWHERE ELSE TO TURN

Frank is a 37-year-old unemployed mechanic who has been admitted for evaluation and treatment of polysubstance abuse with opioid and alcohol dependency. Following a motor vehicle accident while "wiped out" on cocaine and alcohol, Frank is voluntarily admitting himself for detoxification. He has been using heroin, cocaine, and alcohol constantly for the past week. He is unable to remember where he has been or how long it has been since his last meal. He states he has a $200 to $300 a day drug habit and drinks at least a six-pack of beer daily. He admits to doing many "bad things" to acquire the drugs. He is divorced and has not seen his three children in more than 2 years.

How would the nurse approach Frank on admission?

_____

_____

What questions would be important to ask Frank?

_____

_____

Frank states the last time he injected heroin and cocaine was 24 hours ago, shortly after which the accident occurred. He has had two previous admissions to treatment programs, but has not been successful in maintaining his abstinence. What criteria for substance dependency does Frank's case demonstrate?

_____

_____

_____

The nurse assesses Frank's affect as appropriate and his mood as anxious and dysphoric. He remains isolated in his room with the curtains drawn. He states he is having some abdominal cramping and his legs are "knotting." He denies craving at this time but says his skin feels like it is "crawling." What nursing diagnoses would the nurse assign to Frank's symptoms?

_____

_____

_____

_____

The physician orders methadone tablets for the next 72 hours. The rationale for giving this medication is:

_____

_____

How does Frank's behavior indicate symptoms of withdrawal?

_____

_____

What other nursing interventions are important for Frank during the detoxification process?

_____

_____

Frank tells the nurse, "I have nothing to live for anymore." How should the nurse respond?

_____

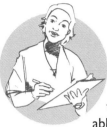

LEARNING OBJECTIVES

After learning the content in this chapter, the student will be able to:

1. Describe signs and symptoms that characterize anorexia nervosa and bulimia nervosa.
2. Identify etiologic factors in the development of severe disturbances in eating behaviors.
3. Assess indications of eating disturbances in the client with an eating disorder.
4. Formulate nursing diagnoses and anticipated outcomes for clients with eating disorders.
5. Plan effective nursing interventions for behaviors associated with abnormal eating patterns.
6. Define evaluation criteria to determine effectiveness of planned interventions.

Eating Disorders

KEY TERMS

Anorexia nervosa
Binging
Bulimia nervosa
Compensatory methods
Purging

The Relationship Between Food and Self-Image

In a multicultural society where an abundance and variety of foods and established eating habits are fundamental to everyday life, it is customary to plan events and family happenings around food. In addition, the fast-paced "eat and go" phenomenon has made fast food a multibillion dollar industry. While food is certainly enticing to the mind and essential for the body, nutrition and dietary intake can also become a factor in the treatment of eating disorders. Numerous "dieting" approaches are advertised and sold as quick-fix remedies to curb an increasing trend in obesity. Although obesity is considered a medical condition with many health risks and possible contributing psychologic factors, according to *DSM-IV-TR,* it has not been established that obesity is consistently associated with a behavioral or psychologic syndrome. In the midst of a society in which the image of an "ideal" physique and appearance is associated with glamour and popularity, the desire to conform to this standard is set in motion. When "thin is in," the perceived need to conform often overshadows sensible and nutritionally safe food intake. People that have a preoccupation with obesity, weight reduction, and nutritional intake have a difficult time distinguishing between realistic ways of controlling weight and body image and what constitutes a severe disturbance and often a dangerous pattern of eating behaviors.

Eating Disorders

Research indicates that the incidence of eating disorders is related to genetic predisposition along with environmental risk factors. The exact cause, however, is unclear, with social, psychologic, and physiologic issues all contributing to the clinical challenge of understanding and treating the problem. People with these disorders have in common the misperception that individual self-worth is related to shape and weight and the ability to control them. Other symptoms tend to evolve out of this irrational thinking. As we discuss the disorders associated with eating patterns, you will gain an understanding of how food and its relationship to the view that a person has of self can become a negative and menacing threat to life.

Anorexia Nervosa

Anorexia nervosa is characterized by an individual refusal to maintain the least essential normal body weight. The *DSM-IV-TR* describes the person as "intensely afraid of gaining weight," and demonstrating a "significant disturbance in the perception of the shape or size of his or her body." Although the term "anorexia" means a loss of appetite with nervous origin, the absence of appetite is not used to describe this disorder. The primary symptom is the maintenance of subnormal levels of weight for age and height. When the disorder develops during childhood or adolescence, the problem may be seen as a failure to advance in a growth pattern rather than in weight loss. The guidelines suggest that for the diagnosis of anorexia nervosa to be assigned, the person should fall below 85% of the normal body weight for that person's age and height. Other specific criteria suggest a body mass index equal to or below 17.5 kg/m^2. These criteria must be viewed with the person's body build and that of other family members in mind.

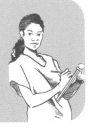

Just the Facts

Anorexia nervosa is characterized by an intense fear of gaining weight and refusal to maintain body weight that is normal for height and age.

Common Signs and Symptoms. In people with this disorder, weight loss is usually accomplished by reducing total food intake to only a few foods, with a drastic exclusion of both overall caloric intake and essential nutrients or food groups. In addition, the person may attempt increased weight loss through **purging** (i.e., self-induced vomiting or excessive use of laxatives and diuretics) and increased compulsive exercise. The person with anorexia nervosa has an extreme fear of gaining weight or "becoming fat" that is not relieved by weight loss. This fear may actually intensify as weight loss accumulates.

A distorted view of body weight and shape is exhibited. Some people may see their body as being "fat," whereas others may realize they are thin, but see certain body areas such as the buttocks, arms, abdomen, or thighs as too fat. They may use methods such as repeated weighing, measuring of body parts, or viewing themselves in a mirror to reinforce their perceived self-image. The person's self-esteem is dependent on body shape and size. Weight loss is seen as a major accomplishment of self-control, whereas weight gain is viewed as a failure. Distorted thinking is also seen in repeated denials of the dangerous medical implications of this condition (see At a Glance 15-1). An indicator of physiologic dysfunction in a female who is menstruating is decreased levels of pituitary hormones (FSH and LH) and ovarian estrogen secretion, which result in amenorrhea, or the absence of menstrual periods. Most of the physical conditions can be reversed as weight returns to normal.

At a Glance 15-1 Associated Medical Conditions of Anorexia Nervosa

Decrease in WBC
Anemia
Osteoporosis
Metabolic disturbances
Malnutrition
Constipation
Dry skin
Swollen salivary glands
Subnormal body temperature
Dehydration
Impaired kidney function
Dental problems
Elevated liver enzymes
Decreased thyroid functioning
Low levels of sex hormones (estrogen/testosterone)
Lethargy
Lanugo on trunk, face, upper arms, and shoulders
Calluses on dorsal hand surface (from inducing vomiting—Russell's sign)
Arrhythmias, cardiac arrest, and death

There are two subtypes that indicate whether the individual behaviors include purging or binge eating. The restricting type includes those whose weight loss is effected through dieting, starvation, or excessive exercise. The second subtype involves those who regularly indulge in binge eating, purging, or both. Most people with anorexia nervosa who engage in binge eating also follow these episodes with purging methods.

Other symptoms seen in people with this disorder include a depressed mood, social withdrawal, irritability, insomnia, swollen joints, lethargy, and a decreased libido. The person loses bone mass, and vital signs can dip to dangerously low levels, sometimes leading to cardiac arrest and death. Symptoms of depression may be secondary to the effects of starvation and lack of nutrition to body cells. The person with anorexia nervosa

Just the Facts

An indicator of physiologic dysfunction in the woman with anorexia nervosa who is postmenarche is the presence of amenorrhea.

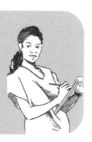

also exhibits an obsessive preoccupation with thoughts related to food. They may hoard food items or collect magazines and recipes related to food. Many actually prepare tasteful meals for their families but do not actually consume any portion of the food themselves. Some consider this a psychologic response to the body's undernourished state.

Just the Facts

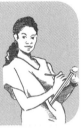

Anorexia nervosa most often begins between the ages of 13 and 18 years, with women accounting for more than 90% of the cases.

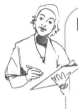

Mind Jogger

Considering their distorted view of self and compulsive need for perfection, in what type of occupational situations might the person with an eating disorder be employed?

At a Glance 15-2 Common Signs and Symptoms of Anorexia Nervosa

- Reduced total food intake and nutrition
- Purging
- Compulsive exercise
- Obsessive preoccupation with food
- Intense fear of becoming fat, not relieved by weight loss
- Distorted view of body weight and shape
- Self-esteem dependent on shape and size
- Weight loss seen as accomplishment
- Denial of potential medical problems
- Amenorrhea (female)
- Possible binge eating
- Lethargy
- Depression and decreased libido
- Social withdrawal

Incidence and Etiology. Anorexia nervosa most often begins between the ages of 13 and 18 years, with more than 90% of the cases occurring in women. It is rare in women over the age of 40.

Symptoms commonly follow stressful life events, such as starting high school, moving to a new location, sexual abuse, or traumatic family relationships. Clients with this disorder are typically well-educated, coming from middle- to upper-income families. Early appearance is one of a loving, cohesive family with model compliant, obedient, and perfectionist children who aim to please parents and teachers. However, further evidence usually reveals unresolved family conflicts with inconsistent patterns of overprotective and rigid parenting in which the child remains in a dependent state. The eating disorder may be a desperate attempt by the adolescent to separate from the family system, in particular, from a dominant and overcritical mother.

People with this disorder are often shy, quiet, orderly, and oversensitive to rejection with heightened feelings of inferiority, self-imposed guilt, and unreasonable expectations for perfection. A misperceived inability to overcome this lack of self-worth and value is addressed by an attempt to gain control of their lives by exercising control over their body. A sense of worth and value becomes intertwined with the ability to shed pounds. The image seen in the mirror is not necessarily compatible with the image seen in the distorted thinking of people with anorexia. They believe that their need for autonomy and control of self is demonstrated by controlling what they eat, which is ultimately their body image. They have a distorted view of their

Mind Jogger

How might the unmet needs of the person with anorexia nervosa be seen in terms of Erikson's theory of psychosocial development (see Chapter 6)?

body and perceive weight gain as a lack of control over themselves and failure to meet their unrealistic self-standards.

> ### Mind Jogger
> How might the peer pressure of adolescence contribute to this sense of value and appearance?

Bulimia Nervosa

The characteristics of **bulimia nervosa** are binge eating with repeated attacks to the self and self-induced destructive methods to prevent weight gain. Subgroups include both purging and nonpurging types, depending on the use of the methods and regularity of their use. The behaviors must occur at least two times a week for a period of 3 months to meet the *DSM-IV* diagnostic criterion.

Binging is defined by *DSM-IV-TR* as eating in a discrete period of time (usually less than 2 hours) an amount of food that is definitely larger than most people would eat under similar circumstances.

Common Signs and Symptoms. There is a seeming lack of control or inability to stop eating during a binge episode. The type of food consumed varies, but typically is an indulged craving for high-calorie, sweet, or carbohydrate foods such as pastry, ice cream, cake, or pizza. The person with bulimia usually consumes more calories on a binge than those without the disorder consume in an entire meal. Clients are usually ashamed of their eating problem and attempt to hide their symptoms. Rapid hidden consumption of food is typical with continued eating despite an uncomfortable feeling of fullness. Binging usually follows a depressed mood state, individual stressors, periods of strict dieting, or negative self-talk about body image. The binge may temporarily relieve the dysphoric state; however, increased depression and self-

dislike quickly emerge after the episode. A continued pattern of binge eating results in an impaired ability to refrain from indulging in the binge or to stop it once the eating begins.

> ### Just the Facts
> Bulimia nervosa is characterized by repeated self-induced destructive methods to prevent weight gain resulting from binge eating, with a seeming lack of control over the eating episode, and purging by self-induced vomiting, overuse of laxatives, diuretics, and excessive exercise.

The second primary symptom of this disorder is the repeated use of inappropriate and risky methods of preventing weight gain. The most commonly used method is induced vomiting after the binge. Purging is used by most people who present for treatment of the eating disorder. The person may feel a temporary sense of relief after the vomiting, both physically and psychologically, indicating a dis-

> ### At a Glance 15-3 Associated Medical Conditions of Bulimia Nervosa
>
> - Loss of dental enamel—teeth appear ragged and "moth-eaten"
> - Increased dental caries
> - Swollen salivary glands
> - Calluses or scars on dorsal surface of hand
> - Menstrual irregularities
> - Constipation
> - Rectal prolapse
> - Tears in esophageal or gastric mucosa
> - Electrolyte imbalances
> - Metabolic alkalosis (loss of stomach acid) or metabolic acidosis (frequent diarrhea)
> - Gastric distress or bleeding
> - Kidney failure

torted view of success in preventing weight gain. Purging is usually easily induced after repeated stimulation of the gag reflex by inserting fingers or other flat objects into the pharynx. A smaller percentage of people use laxatives, diuretics, or enemas as **compensatory methods,** but these are usually used in addition to induced vomiting. Fasting for a period of time may also be used in combination with excessive exercise to alleviate the guilt felt after binging. The person may engage in exercise during inappropriate times in unusual places regardless of any medical contraindications.

At a Glance 15-4 Common Signs and Symptoms of Bulimia Nervosa

- Binging with inability to stop eating
- Craving for high-calorie or sweet foods
- Consumption of many calories in a binge
- Shame over eating problem
- Attempts to hide food consumption
- Depression
- Negative self-image
- Repeated use of induced vomiting
- Use of laxatives, diuretics, or enemas
- Normal weight for age and height with little fluctuation
- Outward preoccupation with food
- Stashing of food
- Associated personality and anxiety disorders
- Inadequate interpersonal skills

Incidence and Etiology. The client with bulimia nervosa is typically within a normal weight range for height and age. Behaviors center on a dissatisfaction with body size and shape that leads to an outward preoccupation with dieting and limited food intake but with little or no alteration in weight or appearance. The person may sneakily stash food or make excuses for spending extended time in the bathroom, usually after consuming a large amount of food. Many with bu-

limia nervosa have symptoms of depression, borderline personality disorder, anxiety and panic disorders, or post-traumatic stress syndrome. Substance abuse is also common, with some affected individuals engaging in theft and forgery. Social skills are inadequate, and interpersonal relationships suffer from the person's lying and hidden behaviors. The disorder usually follows a chronic pattern, with most cases lasting for an average of 5 to 10 years.

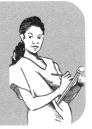

Just the Facts
Those with bulimia are more aware of their own eating disorder and more distressed by the symptoms than those with anorexia.

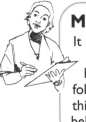

Mind Jogger
It is said that the person with bulimia replaces anxiety felt before the binge with guilt following the binge. How might this lead to other self-abusive behaviors?

Application of the Nursing Process

For clients with anorexia nervosa, the goals of treatment revolve around reversal of the restrictive or maladaptive patterns of eating and thinking about food. Individual planning is also centered on the reestablishment of healthy eating habits. Physical problems often correct themselves as weight is regained and normal nutritional intake is consistent. In addition to these issues, treatment of the client with bulimia nervosa also includes a focus on relinquishing the behaviors of binging and purging as normal eating patterns are restored. Cognitive-behavioral psychotherapy addresses the psychologic issues of both disorders.

With the anorexic client, family therapy focuses on modifying the family dynamics to allow recovery to occur. Inclusion of the family in the treatment plan and counseling sessions assists family members to see how the maladaptive behaviors of the family are intertwined in the client's eating behaviors. The client must confront dysfunctional thoughts and irrational beliefs about self-image and food in realistic terms. Behavior therapy may involve a reward contract in which privileges are exchanged for increased food intake. Gradual increase in caloric intake may also be used to help the client overcome the fearful avoidance of food. Antidepressant medications (e.g., fluoxetine, nortriptyline, olanzapine, and mirtazapine) may be used in combination with psychotherapy. In some cases, antianxiety medications (e.g., lorazepam or chlorpromazine) may be useful to relieve anxiety associated with treatment.

In the client with bulimia nervosa, therapy is designed to help the person take a self-inventory of eating, binging, and purging behaviors. Education is provided about healthy nutritional habits along with efforts to reorganize the maladaptive thinking related to food, body-image, and personal achievement. Behavioral methods include a means of exposing the person to foods that invite binging, but the action is prevented. With repeated exposures, the person gradually becomes less fearful of the foods that previously initiated the compulsive behavior. Anxiety-reducing relaxation techniques are used to decrease the need for compensatory action and introduce preventative strategies. Family therapy may help clients whose family dynamics are a contributing factor, but it has not been found to be as effective as in the client with anorexia nervosa. Antidepressant medications have been used successfully for clients with bulimia nervosa when combined with psychotherapy. Fluoxetine and desipramine are commonly used with careful monitoring for side effects.

Nursing Assessment

Many people with eating disorders deny their problem and maintain their maladaptive eating patterns for several years before treatment is sought, often by concerned family members. Behaviors such as binging and purging by the person with bulimia nervosa are done in secret and may not be detected until more objective symptoms are noted. It is difficult to gain insight into the problem unless it is viewed from the client's perspective. The attitude and approach of the nurse when assessing the client, whether in an emergency room or other clinical situation, is essential to gaining the trust of the client. Many people with eating disorders are ashamed of their behaviors and may want to divulge the magnitude of their problem, but may refrain because of negative or blocking statements made by the nurse. The nurse must examine his or her own feelings about food, dieting, and body image to maintain an objective view of the client's situation.

Information about dietary intake and eating patterns should be gathered with caution to avoid questions that may infer that the client has an eating disorder. Questions that ask how often the client induces vomiting after eating or inquire about feelings after binge eating would imply that a problem exists. A nonconfrontational and nonjudgmental approach is important to convey caring, compassion, and willingness to understand the extent of the client's problem. Because they are usually supersensitive to criticism and frustration, it is best to avoid asking clients questions that can be misinterpreted in this context. Use of active listening and open-ended techniques will aid in encouraging the client to communicate freely.

Other data to be collected include any reports of insomnia or fatigue, increased feelings of anxiety, and intolerance to cold temperatures. Any changes in bowel elimination or decreased urine output should be determined because they relate to laxative or diuretic use. Assess the body for general signs of inadequate nutrition, increased hair growth, brittle dry nails or skin, and erosion of tooth enamel. Look for abrasions or calluses on the back of the hands related to induced purging.

Nursing Diagnosis

Because the effects of eating disorders may affect several body systems, outcome planning based on the individual assessment is necessary. The following nursing diagnoses that encompass the usual problems encountered in the care of clients with eating disorders are suggested.

- Altered nutrition: less than body requirements related to eating patterns and excessive exercise
- Altered bowel elimination: constipation or diarrhea related to laxative abuse and inadequate dietary intake
- Altered oral mucous membranes, related to frequent vomiting
- Body image disturbance, related to misperception of weight and shape
- Coping, ineffective individual related to situational crisis
- Anxiety, related to feelings of hopelessness and lack of control
- Denial, ineffective related to behaviors that are detrimental to health
- Family process alteration, related to family dynamics and defined individual boundaries
- Fluid volume deficit, related to vomiting, diarrhea, diuretic or laxative use
- Posttrauma response, related to sexual or physical abuse
- Powerlessness, related to lack of insight into self-destructive behaviors and irrational thinking about food and body image

- Social isolation, related to psychologic barriers and concealing behaviors

Expected Outcomes

Initial treatment is focused on decreasing the client's anxiety, stabilizing the weight loss pattern, and normalizing eating patterns. Outcomes for the client may include:

- Verbalizes decreased fear and anxiety related to weight gain and inability to maintain control
- Consumes adequate nutritional intake to meet appropriate body requirements for height and age
- Verbalizes importance of appropriate eating pattern
- Verbalizes understanding of events or thoughts that precipitate anxiety
- Ceases engaging in self-destructive behaviors (binge eating or purging)
- Participates in activity level appropriate for health maintenance

In addition to goals that address the physiologic aspects of the disorders, the anticipated outcomes for the client as related to the psychologic disturbances may include:

- Verbalizes rational thinking processes and view of body image
- Expresses understanding of relationship between symptoms, distorted thinking, and behaviors
- Discusses present health problem with health care team members
- Identifies ways to maintain a healthy means of weight control
- Identifies family roles and boundaries, and modifies them as indicated
- Identifies strengths and makes positive self-statements
- Demonstrates improved interpersonal skills in social setting

In addition, the client's family should be able to verbalize an understanding of the relationship of dynamics to the client's disorder.

Nursing Interventions

The nurse may have multiple roles in working with a client who has an eating disorder. In addition to meeting the physiologic needs of the client, the nurse may also function to provide psychotherapeutic interventions that include teaching, counseling, and being a group leader. Formulating a plan of care for the client with an eating disorder should include the following actions:

- Initiate behavior modification plan with privileges and restrictions based on food intake and weight gain.
- Weigh client daily before breakfast using same scale.
- Maintain a strict intake and output log.
- Monitor status of skin and oral mucous membranes.
- Stay with client during meals and at least hour following food intake.
- Restrict time for meals to 30 minutes to reduce focus on food and eating.
- Remind client that tube feeding may be employed if nutritional status deteriorates.
- Monitor amount and time of activity level.
- Monitor vital signs on a regular basis.
- Establish a trusting relationship conveying caring, concern, and compassion.
- Use a firm and supportive approach to eating and related behaviors.
- Encourage the client to verbalize feelings of fear and anxiety related to achievement, family relationships, and intense need for independence.
- Help the client to achieve realistic view of his or her body by measurements and comparisons to norms for height and age.
- Assist the client in setting practical limits on expectations for self-standards.
- Promote independent decision making as appropriate to establish a sense of control.
- Provide ways to reinforce the client's strengths and positive attributes.
- Encourage family to participate in education regarding connection between family processes and the client's disorder.
- Encourage participation in group and social role-play activities.
- Avoid discussions that focus on food and weight.
- Role model appropriate ways of dealing with environmental stressors.
- Explore with the client ways of increasing autonomy and assertive behaviors.

Evaluation

Evaluation will focus on the established anticipated outcomes for the individual client. Normal weight for height and age and normal laboratory values and vital signs, with absence of previous abnormal physical findings, will demonstrate a successful health status outcome. Psychotherapeutic progress is seen as the client embraces a realistic self-image and sets reasonable expectations and standards for achievement. An improved sense of control over self and coping skills to confront environmental stressors with self-confidence will result in a more positive self-esteem. As the guilt and shame over previous behavior is released, the client is able to recognize the relationship between food, eating patterns, and the ill-fated journey of the disorder. It is also important to evaluate family interaction patterns and progress of the client toward autonomy and independent decision making. Follow-up counseling and support toward continued abstinence from previous unhealthy behaviors is indicated in view of the high incidence of relapse. Referrals to support groups are helpful to reinforce treatment outcomes and prevent a return to maladaptive eating habits.

Summary

Research indicates that both genetics and environmental risk factors play a role in the chances that a person may develop an eating disorder. The exact cause is not known, but there are many social, psychologic, and physiologic issues that contribute to the clinical picture.

Anorexia nervosa is characterized by an individual refusal to maintain sufficient body weight above 85% of the normal values for height and age. There is an accompanying disturbance in the person's perception of his or her body shape and self-image. Weight loss in this disorder is usually accomplished through a reduced food intake of calories and nutrients. Self-induced vomiting and excessive use of laxatives may be used to further prevent weight gain. An intense fear of becoming fat feeds the distorted view the person has of his or her body weight and shape. If purging and/or binging are not a part of the disorder, it is referred to as the restricting type, which includes weight loss accomplished through dieting, starvation, or intemperate exercise.

Research demonstrates that many clients with anorexia nervosa come from families with unresolved conflicts of parent–child relationships, often with the client in the clutches of an overindulgent and controlling mother. A sense of worth becomes entwined in the ability to lose weight because the client's distorted thinking associates control of self with control over what is eaten.

Bulimia nervosa is characterized by binge eating (i.e., eating in a short period of time an amount of food larger than most people would normally eat in the same situation). Despite an uncomfortable feeling of fullness, the person is unable to stop eating. After the binge, there is usually a feeling of shame and effort to hide the symptoms. The client with bulimia nervosa is typically within a normal weight range for height and age. However, distorted thinking centers on a dissatisfaction with body size and shape that leads to an outward preoccupation with dieting. Despite the limited food intake, there is little change in the person's outward appearance.

Treatment methods focus on reversing the restrictive or maladaptive patterns of eating and thinking about food and reestablishing healthy eating habits. Psychotherapy may employ education about healthy nutritional habits, behavioral methods and contracting, group therapy, and especially cognitive therapy to reorganize the maladaptive thinking related to food, body image, and personal achievement.

The attitude and approach of the nurse is paramount to establishing a trusting relationship in which the client is willing to participate in treatment. To gain insight into the problem, it is important to hear the symptoms and perception of the illness from the client's perspective. As the client is able to release the shame and guilt over previous behaviors, there is a restored ability to recognize the relationship among food, eating patterns, and the eating disorder.

Bibliography

American Psychiatric Association (2000). *Diagnostic and statistical manual of mental disorders text revision* (4th ed.). Washington, DC: American Psychiatric Association.

Behavioral and personality traits identify patients with eating disorders. *Psychol Med* 2001; 31: 635–645. Available at http//www/psychiatrymatters.md/international/news/2001/week_23/day_1. Accessed on July 11, 2004.

Fairburn, C. G., & Harrison, P. J., (2003). Eating disorders. *Lancet,* 00995355, 2/1/ 2003, *361* (9355). Psychology and Behavioral Sciences Database Collection.

Harvard Mental Health Letter, 10575022 (Feb 2003). "Anorexia nervosa–Part I," (19),*8.* Psychology and Behavioral Sciences Database Collection.

Harvard Mental Health Letter, 10575022 (Mar 2003). "Anorexia nervosa–Part II," (19),*9,* Psychology and Behavioral Sciences Database Collection.

Orbanic, S. (2001). Understanding bulimia, *American Journal of Nursing, 3* (101).

Student Worksheet

FILL IN THE BLANK

Fill in the blank with the correct answer.

1. The client with anorexia nervosa demonstrates a disturbance in the _____ of the shape and size of his or her body.

2. The person with anorexia nervosa accomplishes the pattern of extreme weight loss by a drastic reduction in both _____ and _____.

3. The anorexic client sees weight loss as a major accomplishment of _____, whereas weight gain is seen as _____.

4. The adolescent search for autonomy is often seen in the client with anorexia who makes a desperate attempt to separate from a(n) _____ parent.

5. The person with bulimia nervosa usually consumes more _____ on a binge than a person would normally eat in the same situation.

6. _____ is used by most persons with bulimia to achieve a temporary sense of relief after a binge.

7. The client with bulimia nervosa is typically within a normal _____ for height and age.

8. Behavior modification interventions include _____ and _____ based on food intake and weight gain.

9. When caring for the client with an eating disorder, the nurse restricts meal time to _____ to reduce the focus on food and eating.

10. It is important for the nurse to _____ healthy and appropriate ways of dealing with environmental stressors.

MATCHING

Match the following terms to the most appropriate phrase.

a. Absence of menstrual periods.

b. Privileges are exchanged for increased food intake.

c. Self-induced vomiting or use of laxatives.

d. Use of laxatives, diuretics, or enemas, and induced vomiting to prevent weight gain.

e. Eating a large amount of food in a short time with inability to stop.

1. _____ Purging

2. _____ Binging

3. _____ Reward contract

4. _____ Amenorrhea

5. _____ Compensatory methods

MULTIPLE CHOICE

Select the best answer from the multiple-choice items.

1. The nurse is assessing a 17-year-old who is being evaluated for anorexia nervosa. Which of the following data would suggest this diagnosis?
   a. Periodic patterns of weight gain and loss over the past year
   b. Refusal to talk about the subject of food and nutritional planning
   c. Extreme weight loss from self-imposed restricted food and nutrient intake
   d. Periods of overeating and self-induced vomiting with no change in weight pattern

2. While implementing nursing interventions for the client with an eating disorder, it is important for the nurse to:
   a. Provide opportunities for independent decision making.
   b. Confront the client with the absurdity of his or her distorted thinking.
   c. Use an approach that conveys a sense of concern and sympathy.
   d. Encourage client to talk about the caloric value of various food items.

3. Medications that have been found to be effective in combination with psychotherapy to address the symptoms related to bulimia nervosa are:
   a. Antithyroid
   b. Antidepressant
   c. Anticholinergic
   d. Beta-adrenergic blockers

4. Kate is a 20-year-old teacher who has admitted herself for treatment of bulimia nervosa. Which of the following statements is most appropriate for the nurse to make in the initial approach to Kate?
   a. "Why would you want to lose weight when you look so good already?"
   b. "I just don't understand why you make yourself vomit after you eat."
   c. "Tell me about the last time you did binge eating and what you did afterward."
   d. "Would it not be easier to go on a weight-reduction diet instead of hurting yourself?"

SCENARIO: CASSIDY'S SECRET

Cassidy is a 23-year-old college graduate recently married to Stan, a promising young banking associate. Stan has brought Cassidy to the outpatient clinic after he found her unresponsive when he arrived home from work. Cassidy is 5 feet 8 inches tall and weighs 101 lbs. Stan states he knew she was on a crash diet during the months prior to their wedding but had no idea her weight loss was a serious problem. He relates that during their courtship she often found ways to avoid eating and would spend countless hours working out in the university gym. As he reflects on the past few years, Stan says that Cassidy often described herself as fat, even though she seemed to get thinner. He mentions that her college roommate told him Cassidy wasn't eating right, but he thought it was just the stress of finishing school. Stan tells the nurse that Cassidy is the oldest of three children from a single-parent family. Her mother worked many hours and left Cassidy to manage her two younger brothers. He says that she would often express ambivalent feelings about her mother, stating that her mother "needed" her but did not care about her. During family occasions, Cassidy's mother would show outward affection for her daughter and state how proud she was of her.

Cassidy is pale, thin, and somewhat emaciated, with sunken cheeks and dry mucous membranes. She hesitates to open her mouth, which when examined reveals numerous dental caries and brownish stained enamel. Cassidy states that she started self-induced vomiting when she was 9 years old. She had started getting "pudgy" and her mother told her she was going to be fat if she didn't stop eating. She also states that her mother told her she could keep herself from gaining weight by making herself vomit after she ate. Her mother told her she had been doing this for years to try to lose weight, but never seemed to change in size. Cassidy says she binges on things like pie, chocolate, and banana splits, after which she purges with vomiting and laxatives. She admits to taking as many as 8 to 10 laxative pills at a time to feel relief from the guilt she feels over her food intake and to ensure weight loss after the binge. She works out for as much as 4 hours daily at the gym to compensate for the food she eats. Cassidy relates a feeling of shame for her eating problem and is embarrassed that Stan has now found out the secrets she has tried so hard to conceal.
What approach should the nurse employ to help Cassidy at this point?

_____

_____

How do Cassidy's symptoms indicate an eating disorder?

_____

_____

Cassidy is diagnosed with anorexia nervosa and admitted for stabilization of her physical symptoms and for treatment to address the psychologic issues underlying her eating problem. Cassidy expresses sadness because she and Stan want to have a baby, but she is afraid that her behavior will hurt her chances of having a normal pregnancy. What factors related to an eating disorder may affect the issue of pregnancy?

_____

_____

How can the nurse help Cassidy to view her self-image in a positive way excluding body appearance and weight?

_____

_____

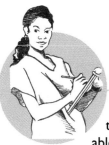

LEARNING OBJECTIVES

After learning the content in this chapter, the student will be able to:

1. Define human sexuality and various modes of sexual expression.

2. Describe signs and symptoms of the psychosexual disorders.

3. Identify etiologic factors in the development of a sexual disorder.

4. Perform an unbiased nursing assessment of the client with a sexual disorder.

5. Formulate nursing diagnoses and outcomes to address problems common to clients with these disorders.

6. Plan selected nursing interventions to address the needs of the client with a sexual disorder.

7. Describe evaluation methods for determining the effectiveness of planned interventions.

8. Discuss current treatment available for people with a sexual dysfunction disorder.

Sexual Disorders

KEY TERMS

Exhibitionism
Frotteurism
Necrophilia
Paraphilia
Pedophilia
Sexual dysfunction
Sexual masochism
Sexual orientation
Sexual sadism
Sexuality
Telephone scatologia
Transvestic fetishism
Voyeurism
Zoophilia

Human Sexuality

Sexuality is described as an innate part of human dynamics integral to our development throughout the life cycle. It is the blend of physical, chemical, and psychologic functioning characterized by our gender and sexual behavior. The manner in which our parents and other adults interact with us during early psychosexual developmental periods is instrumental in the formation of a wholesome adjustment and attitude toward our body and our feelings about sexuality. This adjustment as a child leads to a healthy self-image and satisfying adult sexual relationships that respect the rights of others. The expression of sexual feelings is demonstrated throughout our life in various individual ways. It is important for the nurse to develop a self-awareness of his or her attitudes and beliefs toward sexual issues that may hinder the effective care of any client. This allows the nurse to be a client advocate, to present factual information about sexual development, and to promote an understanding of these human needs for all age-groups.

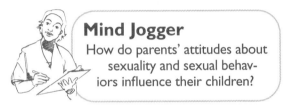

Mind Jogger
How might the nurse's attitude toward sexuality affect his or her ability to initiate a therapeutic relationship with the client?

An individual preference or sexual attraction is referred to as one's **sexual orientation.** These modes of sexual expression fall into several categories. Heterosexuality is a sexual preference for members of the opposite sex. This is generally accepted as the usual attraction and is necessary for procreation of the species. Homosexuality is a preference for members of the same sex, whereas a bisexual orientation is an attraction to members of both sexes. Although the issue of sexual orientation continues to be one of debate and contro-versy, a healthy view of human sexual development and sexuality is a prerequisite to a healthy and satisfying sexual exchange between two people. A sexually intimate and fulfilling relationship is mutually satisfying for both partners. It must be emphasized that the feelings toward sexuality and sexual intimacy experienced by the adult are significantly affected by the feelings experienced as a child during early developmental years.

Mind Jogger
How do parents' attitudes about sexuality and sexual behaviors influence their children?

Categories of Psychosexual Disorders

The psychosexual disorders include all mental alterations that prevent a person from functioning in a normal healthy relationship within societal norms. The *DSM-IV-TR* addresses these disorders under the categories of sexual dysfunctions, paraphilias, and the gender identity disorders.

Sexual Dysfunctions

Sexual dysfunctions are identified by abnormal sexual desire and psychophysiologic changes that accompany the sexual response cycle. These disturbances cause marked discomfort and anxiety leading to troubled interpersonal relationships.

Just the Facts
Sexual dysfunctions are characterized by a disturbance in sexual desire or response that results in marked anxiety and interpersonal difficulties.

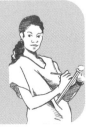

A sexual dysfunction can occur during any phase of the sexual response cycle or is characterized by pain associated with sexual intercourse. Phases of the response cycle consist of the desire to have sexual activity; subjective pleasures and physiologic changes of excitement; peaking or sexual pleasure in orgasm; rhythmic release of sexual tension; and resolution or relaxation together with a general sense of contentment. A dysfunction in one or more of these phases is characterized by the degree of persistent or recurrent symptoms, the quality of sexual stimulation involved, and the level of distress indicated by the person. The problem may be present over the person's lifetime or may be acquired after a period of normal functioning and response. The dysfunction may be related to a particular set of circumstances or a problem that exists with some or all types of stimulation, situations, or partners.

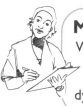

Mind Jogger

What situation or circumstances within a relationship might lead to a sexual dysfunction?

Common Signs and Symptoms. Sexual dysfunction is a comprehensive term that covers a variety of different situations. To understand how vital assessment is to understanding the problem, let us first look at the characteristics of each type of dysfunction:

Sexual Desire Disorders. Hypoactive sexual desire disorder involves a low sexual interest with little motivation to engage in sexual activity. There is an absence of sexual fantasies with little frustration when the opportunity for sexual contact is not available. Occasionally, the decreased desire in one partner can reflect an increased need in the other partner.

Just the Facts

Medications such as antihypertensives, antipsychotics, antidepressants, anxiolytics, and anticonvulsants can cause hypoactive sexual desire disorder.

Sexual Aversion Disorder. Clients experiencing sexual aversion disorder have a dislike for and avoidance of genital sexual contact with a sexual partner. Anxiety, fear, or disgust may be present when sexual contact is attempted. This lack of pleasure usually leads to significant psychologic distress.

Sexual Arousal Disorders. In women with sexual arousal disorders, there is a reoccurring inability to attain or maintain adequate excitement response and vaginal lubrication to complete sexual activity. This results in painful intercourse and avoidance of sexual encounters.

In men, the continued inability to attain or maintain an erection until completion of the sexual act denotes an arousal disorder. In some situations, there is an inability to attain an erection anytime during intercourse. With others, the erection is accomplished but is lost on penetration or during the activity.

Orgasmic Disorders. Women with orgasmic disorders experience a persistent delay or absence of orgasm following normal sexual activity. This may affect the person's body image, self-esteem, or satisfaction in the relationship. The disorder tends to be more prevalent in younger women during early sexual experiences. Once a female learns how her body reaches orgasm, it is uncommon for her to lose the ability to achieve a climax.

Men may feel aroused at the beginning of the sexual act but lose pleasure in the activity and fail to achieve orgasm. In other situations, the problem is premature ejaculation, in which there is recurrent onset of orgasm and ejaculation with minimal stimulation. The ejaculation occurs before the man is ready to do so. Age, type of sexual stimulation, and any prolonged abstinence from sexual activity can contribute to this problem.

Sexual Pain Disorders. Dyspareunia is genital pain in women associated with sexual intercourse. This may be superficial, or it may only occur during deep penetration. Vaginismus is the repeated occurrence of involuntary perineal muscle contractions that prevent penetration of the vagina. This is more common in younger women or those with a history of sexual abuse or trauma.

Sexual Dysfunction Due to a General Medical Condition. There are a variety of conditions that can lead to a sexual dysfunction. Medical conditions and prescription medications that can directly affect sexual functioning are listed in At a Glance 16-1. A person's unfamiliarity with medications or medical situations that interfere with sexual response or performance may prevent the problem from being recognized.

Sexual dysfunction can also occur as a result of substance use. Depending on the substance used, the physiologic effects may include decreased desire and arousal, inability to achieve orgasm, or sexual pain.

Incidence and Etiology. People frequently deny the need for treatment of sexual dysfunctions or are unaware that treatment may be available. The person often avoids the issue, adding to the resulting interpersonal friction and disturbance within his or her relationship. Some may be reluctant to discuss sexual problems with health care workers, or in other cases, the problem may be reported by a spouse, partner, or friend. Other contributing factors could be a lack of understanding about anatomic functioning and effective sexual stimulation techniques. Because sexual desire is a mind and body process, a person's past experiences can sabotage the arousal and re-

---

At a Glance 16-1 Medical Conditions and Medications That May Contribute to Sexual Dysfunctions

Localized diseases: Endometriosis, cystitis, vaginitis, uterine prolapse, pelvic inflammatory disease, testicular disease, genital injury or infections, atrophic vaginitis

Systemic diseases: Hypothyroidism, diabetes mellitus (most common in men), adrenal cortical malfunction, pituitary dysfunction, hypogonadal secretions, hypertension, arteriosclerotic cardiovascular disease

Peripheral/CNS disorders: multiple sclerosis, spinal cord injury, neuropathy, brain lesions, muscular dystrophy

Other: Prostatectomy complications, oophorectomy without hormone replacement therapy, mastectomy, chemotherapy, and radiation

Medications:
- Alcohol
- Anticholinergics
- Antidepressants
- Antihypertensives
- Antipsychotics
- Barbiturates
- Benzodiazepine
- Calcium-channel blockers
- Digitalis
- Dilantin
- Diuretics
- Flagyl
- Lithium
- Marijuana
- Opiates
- Oral contraceptives

---

sponse cycle. This inhibition to arousal can arise from deep psychologic fears or feelings of guilt and shame associated with the sexual act.

Studies show that for people between the ages of 18 and 59, most sexual dysfunction is related to orgasm, hypoactive sexual desire, and arousal problems in women. Erectile dysfunction in men tends to increase after age 50,

Case Study: "Nail in His Shoe"

Esther and Martin have been happily married for more than 30 years. Martin states their sexual relationship has been very good and satisfying for most of that period. Recently, however, Martin has been experiencing impotence and a decrease in his sexual drive. He feels he is letting his wife down and is becoming depressed. Rather than feeling like a failure, he has become distant and the relationship is deteriorating. Martin adds that this is just another "nail in his shoe." He states the doctor can't seem to get his blood pressure under control and has added another drug. He feels defeated and worthless.

What factors might be contributing to Martin's sexual dysfunction?

_____

_____

_____

What further information should the nurse obtain from Martin?

_____

_____

_____

_____

_____

_____

What information should be provided for Martin regarding his medication?

_____

_____

_____

_____

In addition to medication adjustment, what other type of treatment may be needed for Martin and his wife?

_____

_____

_____

whereas premature ejaculation tends to be most prevalent in younger men.

Paraphilias

The **paraphilias** include those sexual behaviors involving unusual objects, activities, or situations that may impose clinically significant anxiety or problems in social, occupational, or other areas of functioning.

Common Signs and Symptoms. These disorders include intense, sexually arousing fantasies, urges, or behavior with nonhuman objects that may cause suffering or degradation to the person or his or her partner, to children, or to nonconsenting adults over a period of at least 6 months. For some, these activities are required for erotic arousal and are consistently included in each sexual encounter. For some disorders, the acting out of the fantasy or urge causes the person marked distress. If the paraphilic act causes injury to a partner, as in sexual sadism or pedophilia, the person may be arrested and incarcerated. In other instances, the person may be referred to treatment after some unusual behavior has brought the person in contact with law enforcement. The person with this type of disorder may use the services of a prostitute to obtain a partner with whom sexual fantasies can be performed. Some may secure employment in settings where contact is made with the desired stimulus for arousal (e.g., a *pedophile* may work in a daycare center or with a scout troop, or a *fetishist* may create displays of women's underclothing). Others collect articles, books, videos, and pictures that represent their particular sensual obsession. Not all people express anxiety or discomfort with their disorder despite being viewed by society as having a perverted and unacceptable character. Others will experience significant guilt and anguish over their unacceptable sexual functioning and desire for degrading activity. Symptoms of depression or a coexisting personality disorder may be present.

> ## At a Glance 16-2 Common Signs and Symptoms of Sexual Dysfunction
>
> - Decreased sexual desire
> - Dislike and avoidance of sexual activity
> - Lack of sexual arousal in women
> - Failure to achieve or maintain erection during sexual act in men
> - Failure to achieve orgasm during intercourse
> - Premature ejaculation in men
> - Pain during intercourse
> - Involuntary perineal muscle contractions preventing vaginal penetration
> - Medical conditions or medications that interfere with sexual functioning
> - Sexual inhibition related to use and abuse of substances

The individual disorders are categorized and described based on the particular symptom or feature exhibited. (See At a Glance 16-2.) There are several common characteristics of these compulsive sexual behaviors that tend to interfere with the ability of the person to form intimate relationships. A conflicting sense of powerlessness and hidden anger create a state of internal anxiety. The person responds to this inner turmoil with a compulsive need to carry out the aversive sexual acts. The person may act to fill a void or to escape the stressful situation with or without recognition of the sexual dysfunction. An attempt is made to overpower another human being, which offers a challenge to get away with the forbidden. People who commit sexual offenses receive a charge from seduction, conning, or intimidation of another to achieve their goal. Values are self-centered and power oriented, with secrecy offering an advantage and source of control. There is frequent use of denial and rationalization as the person attempts to justify the behavior by concealing both the problem and the shame experienced as a result of the actions. Despite arrest, serious penalties, or reprisal, the sexual acts tend

At a Glance 16-3 Categories of Paraphilias

Exhibitionism	Focus is on exposure of genitals to a stranger; this may include masturbation, often with no further attempt at sexual activity with that person. The surprise or shock observed during the exposure is often part of the stimulus for arousal.
Fetishism	Use of inanimate objects (fetish) such as women's lingerie, shoes, or negligee with sexual activity involving these objects. Contact or view of the apparel is usually required for orgasm.
Frotteurism	Activity that involves touching or rubbing contact with a non-consenting person. Men often carry out the behavior in an area where a crowd or dim lighting will obscure the action. Activity will involve rubbing of the genitals against a woman's thigh or buttocks or fondling these areas while fantasizing intimacy with the woman.
Pedophilia	Sexual activity with a prepubescent child 13 years of age or younger. The person with the disorder must be at least 16 years of age or older, and the child must be at least 5 years younger than the perpetrator. Victims are of both genders, although a preference is often displayed by the behaviors. Activities may involve undressing the child, exposure and masturbation in front of the child, touching and fondling, performing oral sex acts on the child, or penetration of the mouth, vagina, and anus with fingers, foreign objects, or penis.
Sexual masochism	Recurrent stong sexual urges, behaviors, or sexually stimulating fantasies involving the actual act of being beaten, bound, humiliated or otherwise made to suffer. These acts may be fantasized or the urges may be enacted during sexual encounters. Acts may include physical restraint, blindfolding, paddling, whipping, electric shock, cutting, or humiliating with human urine or feces. Forced cross-dressing may occur. Hypoxyphilia is a dangerous form of masochism that involves oxygen deprivation by noose, plastic bag, chemicals, or other means of causing peripheral vasodilation that can result in accidental death.
Sexual sadism	Person receives sexual excitement from observing psychologic or physical suffering by the victim. While relishing the terror inflicted, the perpetrator receives additional satisfaction from the accompanying feelings of complete control over the victim. Whether consensual or inflicted, it is the suffering by the victim that causes the sexual arousal.
Transvestic fetishism	Cross-dressing by a man in women's clothing. Sexual arousal is the result of fantasies where he imagines himself as a woman (autogynephilia). The man usually keeps a collection of women's garments with preference for certain items for arousal.

continues

At a Glance 16-3 Categories of Paraphilias (Continued)

Voyeurism	Act of visual observation (window-peeping) of a stranger undressing, naked, or engaging in sexual behavior without the victim's knowledge. The act is done to achieve sexual arousal with orgasm achieved by masturbation. Generally, no further sexual contact is pursued.
Telephone scatologia	Obscene phone calls that lead to sexual arousal.
Necrophilia	Sexual arousal by physical contact or sexual relations with a deceased human or animal.
Zoophilia	Arousal by sexual contact with animals.

to continue with no attempt to control them. The person usually experiences a weak sense of self, accompanied by a feeling of deception and self-dislike for the dual standard portrayed by their behavior. These feelings are reinforced by the subsequent exclusion and isolation from the acceptable and lawful standards of society.

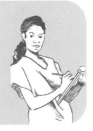

Just the Facts

Sexual abuse of a child is defined as sexual activity imposed upon a child by an adult with greater power, knowledge, and resources.

Mind Jogger

What factors do you think contribute to the high relapse rate of sexual offenders?

Incidence and Etiology. Sexual disorder conditions are not often seen in the clinical setting, nor do people typically seek treatment for them on their own. Treatment for these disorders is most commonly connected to entanglements with law authorities over sexual offenses, pornography, and possession of paraphernalia associated with the acts.

Recognition is sometimes complicated by the fact that certain types of behavior are more acceptable in some cultures than in others. Paraphilias are most prevalent among men and are rarely diagnosed in women. The disorders tend to be chronic and lifelong, although the behaviors may subside with age.

Exhibitionism and fetishism are usually evident by late adolescence and tend to be chronic. Frotteurism is most common from age 15 to 25, with a gradual decrease in events as the person ages. Acts of sexual sadism tend to increase in severity over time and will most likely continue until the person is apprehended by the law. Voyeurism is usually present before age 15 and tends to be chronic.

The perpetrator who exhibits pedophilia usually portrays the actions to the child as "educational" or "enjoyable," and the child often receives threats or warnings of harm if anyone is told of the indiscretions. The child responds to this bribery and secrecy with a sense of guilt and confusion over the forced seductive sexual acts and submission to the perverted passions of the adult. Forced to accept something distasteful and painful, the child develops feelings of powerlessness, helplessness, and rejection by those who ironically should be their "protectors." Perpetrators victimize their own children, those within the family system, and strangers. These acts are considered criminal behavior by a civilized society and are punishable by the law. This disorder usually begins in adolescence and tends to be chronic in nature.

Just the Facts

Common characteristics of the adult who was sexually abused by a parent (incest) as a child are a basic lack of trust, low self-esteem, a poor sense of identity, little or no pleasure in sexual activity, and promiscuity.

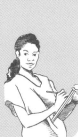

At a Glance 16-4 Common Signs and Symptoms of Paraphilias

- Intense, sexually arousing fantasies, sexual urges, or behaviors involving nonhuman objects
- Sexual behavior involving suffering or humiliation of self or partner that is sexually exciting to the person
- Sexual urges and behaviors that involve children or a nonconsenting partner
- Exposure of the genitals to an unsuspecting stranger
- Touching or rubbing against a nonconsenting person
- Cross-dressing
- Observation of an unsuspecting person who is naked, undressing, or engaging in sexual activity

Gender Identity Disorder

For a diagnosis of gender identity disorder to be assigned, the person must have a strong and persistent cross-gender identification and insist that he or she is, or has the desire to be,

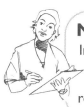

Mind Jogger

In what ways might a person demonstrate nonconformity to the assigned gender role of society?

of the other sex. The person must also have continual discomfort with his or her sexual role. Unlike nonconformity to the stereotype of a boy or girl, the disorder includes a profound problem in the person's sense of sexual identity.

Common Signs and Symptoms. People with gender identity disorder are usually preoccupied with a desire to live as a member of the opposite sex. They may, to varying degrees, adopt the dress, habits, and appearance of the alternate sex. This behavior usually leads to social isolation, particularly in the adolescent who is subjected to teasing and distress by peers. Relationship difficulties result and functioning may be impaired.

In boys, cross-gender identification is shown by a preoccupation with feminine activities. They exhibit a preference for dressing in female clothing and enjoy play that is characteristic of girls, such as playing with dolls or being the "mother" when playing house. They tend to avoid toys and boisterous play that are considered typical for boys. They may express a wish to be a girl and exhibit a dislike for their male genitalia.

Girls usually demonstrate strong negative feelings toward attempts to have them dress or act in a feminine fashion. They usually prefer short haircuts and boy's clothing. They may ask to be called by a boy's name. There is a preference for rough and tumble play with boys, whereas little interest is shown for dolls or activities typical for girls. The girl may exhibit a desire for a penis and a dislike for developing breasts or beginning menstrual periods.

Adults with this disorder tend to be preoccupied with their desire to live as a member of the opposite sex. They may seek ways to adopt the appearance and social role of the other sex through hormonal or surgical means. They are usually uncomfortable in situations where they are functioning as a member of their designated sex.

Incidence and Etiology. Onset of this disorder tends to begin between the ages of 2 to 4 years. Parents typically become concerned when the child enters school if the "phase" of cross-gender interests has not changed. By late adolescence or adulthood, many of those with a childhood disturbance will report a homosexual or bisexual orientation but without an actual disorder. Some people will also have a history of other sexual disorders.

Just the Facts

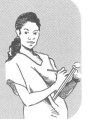

About 75% of boys with a history of gender identity disorder report a homosexual or bisexual orientation as an adult.

At a Glance 16-5 Common Signs and Symptoms of Gender Identity Disorder

- Repetitious statements of desire to be the opposite sex
- Preference for cross-dressing in the young boy or girl
- Strong preference for play and role-play activities typical of the opposite sex
- Fantasies of being the other sex
- Strong preference for playmates of the opposite sex
- Persistent dislike for one's genitalia—wishing to have genitalia of other sex
- Attempts to alter physical secondary sex characteristics of designated sex

Application of the Nursing Process

Nursing Assessment

The nurse can assist in gathering information related to a problem the client may be experiencing with sexual functioning. An interview may be done to assess the particular areas that may be involved (see At a Glance 16-6). All ef-

forts should be made to ensure confidentiality and to respect the private content of the issues being discussed. The client should be encouraged to share feelings and concerns so that appropriate information and treatment can be provided. Referrals for specialized counseling or psychologic treatment may be indicated if medical or drug-related problems are ruled out.

At a Glance 16-6 Interview for Psychosexual Assessment— Sexual Dysfunction

1. Is your present sexual relationship a satisfying one?
2. Tell me about the difficulties you are experiencing in your sexual performance . . .
3. How long has this been a problem for you?
4. Describe any negative sexual experiences you may have had.
5. Do you experience any difficulty with sexual arousal?
6. How often does this occur?
7. Do you have any discomfort with sexual intercourse?
8. What changes do you think might help your sexual relationships?

A multidisciplinary approach is used to cover the full range of sexually deviant behaviors. The assessment consists of a complete social and sexual history, psychosexual and psychologic testing, and physiologic studies of sexual arousal patterns. A psychiatric evaluation may also be performed.

Nursing Diagnoses

Nursing diagnoses that are applicable to all people with sexual disorders may include:

- Sexual dysfunction/sexuality patterns, altered
- Self-esteem, chronic situational low
- Anxiety
- Family processes, altered

- Role or identity disturbance
- Sexuality patterns, altered
- Coping ineffective, person
- Social isolation

Expected Outcomes

Once nursing problems have been assigned, realistic and measurable outcomes are established and the client will:

- Acknowledge and accept responsibility for compulsive and deviant acts without feeling extreme guilt and shame
- Express anger and shame in an appropriate manner
- Refrain from deviant sexual behavior by conscious control of arousal and sexual impulses
- Confront and resolve traumatic developmental issues
- Confront distorted sexual fantasies and thought processes
- Develop an awareness of the feelings and rights of others
- Develop insight into the effect that deviant behavior has on the victim
- Develop more adaptive and effective coping and decision-making skills
- Develop healthy interpersonal and sexual relationships
- Participate and cooperate in a treatment plan to change behavior

Nursing Interventions

It is suggested that there are often traumatic influences in the sexual and emotional development of the person leading up to the onset of the deviant sexual behaviors. Rehabilitation programs focus on cognitive-behavioral, psychodynamic, and trauma-based methods of therapy. Behavioral reconditioning may be used in an attempt to change sexual arousal patterns. A nurturing and caring milieu provides a safe shelter in which the person can acknowledge the past trauma and learn ways to control self-destructive sexual behaviors. Relapse is common during treatment of the paraphilia disorders, and a 12-step program is often initiated in the treatment process. Despite treatment, the perpetrator's personality does not change. Change is only possible when the offender makes a choice to participate in a treatment program. Behavior is directly related to the person's thoughts, so it is only when the person consents to expose inappropriate patterns of thinking and feels self-disgust that rehabilitation can begin. The person must engage in a daily inventory of thought processes and will never reach a point when this is not necessary.

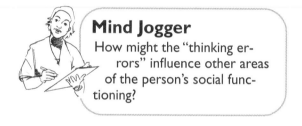

Mind Jogger

How might the "thinking errors" influence other areas of the person's social functioning?

The nurse is integral to planning and implementing the treatment process. Interventions may include:

- Develop self-awareness regarding feelings about own sexuality and relationships (discomfort can be perceived by client as disapproval).
- Initiate a therapeutic relationship using an empathetic and nonjudgmental attitude.
- Encourage the client to verbalize feelings and perception of the sexual problem.
- Utilize communication techniques to guide client to discuss self-esteem and guilt issues.
- Ensure privacy and confidentiality during disclosure and treatment.
- Encourage group and self-help activities with referrals that support rehabilitation.
- Collaborate with mental health team to facilitate behavioral change.
- Report any knowledge of sexual offenses or abuse to appropriate authorities.

Evaluation

Although treatment is not often initiated by people with a sexual disorder, it is essential for the person to develop an awareness of the problem and the stressors that contribute to the dysfunction.

Through an understanding of the consequences of the disorder, the person can identify and work to develop satisfying, acceptable sexual practices with alternative ways of dealing with sexual feelings. It is anticipated that the person will demonstrate a willingness to make changes in patterns of thinking and engage in realistic problem solving.

As the person becomes aware of the underlying motives for his or her actions, a verbalized improvement in self-worth is anticipated. With a reduced level of anxiety and improved coping skills, the person is better equipped to communicate and interact in an appropriate manner. Given the chronic nature of many sexual disorders, it is important that a measure of self-control is evident through active participation in the treatment plan and ongoing demonstration of the desire to handle the situation in a way that results in satisfying and appropriate sexual experiences.

Summary

Human sexuality is a blend of physical and emotional responses that combine to generate our sexual identity and behavior. Sexuality is integral in human development throughout the life cycle. A healthy sexual relationship is one that respects the rights of others and is mutually satisfying for both partners. Through self-awareness of his or her own sexuality, the nurse is able to promote an understanding of sexual needs and responses in the client.

The sexual disorders are classified under the categories of sexual dysfunctions, paraphilias, and gender identity disorders. Sexual dysfunctions may be the result of psychologic trauma, medical problems, or medication side effects. The paraphilia disorders encompass all altered mental processes related to sexual expression that prevent functioning within the laws and morals of society. An identification with our own gender begins at an early age. A resulting sexual orientation develops with an individual preference or mode of sexual expression. A crisis may develop in which the person has difficulty knowing or accepting the identified gender and may feel uncomfortable with his or her body parts.

Deviant sexual behaviors tend to be compulsive and chronic in nature, leading to deceit and denial in an attempt to conceal the problem and avoid reprisal, social isolation, or arrest. Integral in the origin of this behavior is a distorted thinking process. Unable to form intimate relationships, the person attempts to compensate for the anxiety and weak sense of self by performing deviant sexual acts. The acts are compulsive in nature because the person is trying to avoid inner turmoil. Despite attempts to hide the behavior, the person's unconscious demands gratification that can only be satisfied by repetition of the actions.

A multidisciplinary approach is most effective in helping the person with a sexual disorder to confront and change or control the dysfunctional behavior. The quality of nursing intervention for clients with a sexual disorder is dependent on the empathetic and nonjudgmental attitude and approach of the nurse.

Bibliography

American Psychiatric Association (2000). *Diagnostic and statistical manual of mental disorders text revision* (4th ed.). Washington, DC: American Psychiatric Association.

Berkow, R., & Beers, M. H. (1999). *The Merck manual of diagnosis & therapy* (17th ed.). Rahway, NJ: Merck & Co.

Student Worksheet

FILL IN THE BLANK

Fill in the blank with the correct answer.

1. A disturbance in sexual desire or response leading to increased anxiety and interpersonal difficulty is termed a(n) _____.

2. A systemic endocrine disorder that often causes sexual dysfunction in men is _____ _____.

3. Sexual behaviors involving unusual objects, activities, or situations inconsistent with societal laws and standards are referred to as _____.

4. Deep psychologic fears or feelings of guilt and shame associated with the sexual act can lead to a(n) _____.

5. In gender identity disorder, there is a strong and persistent _____ identification along with continual discomfort with one's sexual role.

6. Prior to the onset of deviant sexual behaviors, there are often _____ influences in the sexual and emotional development of the person.

7. Regardless of the required treatment for the person with a paraphilia, the perpetrator's _____ does not change.

8. The person with a paraphilia disorder must expose errors in _____ for rehabilitation to occur.

MATCHING

Match the following terms to the most appropriate phrase.

a. Having sexual activity with a child

b. Enjoyment of inflicting pain during a sexual act

c. Cross-dressing by a man in women's attire

d. Sexual gratification by rubbing against a stranger

e. Intentional exposure of one's genitals in public

f. Unsolicited visual observation of a stranger undressing

g. Sexual arousal using inanimate objects

1. _____ Exhibitionism

2. _____ Fetishism

3. _____ Frotteurism

4. _____ Pedophilia

5. _____ Sexual masochism

6. _____ Transvestic fetishism

7. _____ Voyeurism

MULTIPLE CHOICE

Select the best answer from the multiple-choice items.

1. The nurse is doing patient teaching for a 45-year-old male client newly diagnosed with diabetes mellitus. The client tells the nurse, "I really don't want to talk about my sexual life. That is my business." The nurse can best meet the needs of this client by which of the following responses?

   a. "That is fine if you prefer not to discuss this issue. I will make a note to that effect on your record."

   b. "I understand. I would not want to tell someone about that part of my life either."

   c. "I know it must be difficult for you to talk with a stranger about such a private matter. We can discuss it at a later time."

   d. "We can't help you if you choose not to give us information. There are lots of people with your condition who have problems."

2. The nurse is talking with a 31-year-old female client who is experiencing dyspareunia. Tearfully, the client states her husband "expects me to have sex even though it hurts." Which of the following is the best response for the nurse to make at this time."

   a. "We will be glad to refer you to a counselor who works with victims of sexual assault."

   b. "Tell me more about what happens when you have sexual intercourse."

   c. "After the doctor does a physical exam, we will try to help you with your problem."

   d. "I don't know how you put up with that. It must be very difficult."

3. The nurse is admitting a male client with a diagnosis of polysubstance abuse to the inpatient unit. The client is also a registered sex offender. In establishing a basis for treatment of this client, which of the following nursing interventions is most important?

   a. Using an empathetic and nonjudgmental approach

   b. Warning other clients about his sexual behavior

   c. Separating him from other clients on the unit

   d. Gathering information about his sexual behaviors

4. Josh is a 26-year-old who is mandated by the court to undergo therapy sessions for a charge of sexual indecency with a child. Which of the following will contribute most to success in his treatment process?

   a. Accepts a restriction of supervised-only visits with his son

   b. Allows a parole officer to attend each of his therapy sessions

   c. Admits that he has sexual fantasies about children

   d. Consents to expose the errors in his thinking

5. The emergency room nurse is assessing an 11-year-old girl who has reportedly been sexually abused by her grandfather. Which of the following most likely describes the objective emotional assessment of the child?

   a. Willingness to talk about the incident

   b. Anger toward her grandfather

   c. Fear and withdrawal when touched

   d. Clinging behaviors toward the nurse

SCENARIO 1: PAIN IN DISGUISE

Alex is a 39-year-old unemployed man who is admitted to the inpatient unit after ingesting a number of prescription drugs in a suicide attempt. While doing the initial interview, the nurse is distracted by the client's long finger- and toenails painted in a flashy red color. Shoulder-length red hair encircles distinct attractive facial features accented with modest makeup. As Alex removes his jacket, it is noted he is wearing a shirt with lace, ruffles, and pearl buttons.

What is it important for the nurse to do at this point?

_____

What nursing approach is necessary for Alex to receive the appropriate treatment for his attempted suicide?

_____

What sexual disorder is indicated by the appearance of this client?

_____

Alex tells the nurse he hates himself as he is, that he has felt different all of his life, and wishes he were dead. He states, "The only time I feel real is when I am a woman, but I am only a fraud." What further information should the nurse obtain at this point?

_____

Suggest some ways that Alex might be included in group activities without being a victim. What outcomes are realistic for Alex?

_____

SCENARIO 2: A PROFESSIONAL DUTY

When picking up her child from a daycare center, a nurse observes a 6-year-old boy standing close to a female worker rubbing his genitals against her leg. The worker tells him to go and play, but he continues his behavior. What actions should the nurse take in this situation?

_____

What category of paraphilia does this situation describe?

_____

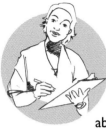

LEARNING OBJECTIVES

After learning the content in this chapter, the student will be able to:

1. Identify etiologic factors most implicated in the development of childhood psychiatric disorders.

2. Describe common signs and symptoms for the various mental disorders in children and adolescents.

3. Perform a nursing assessment of the child with a mental disorder.

4. Formulate nursing diagnoses with expected outcomes to address problems common to clients with these disorders.

5. Plan selected nursing interventions to address the needs of the child and adolescent with a mental disorder.

6. Determine criteria for evaluating the effectiveness of nursing implementation.

7. Discuss current treatment modalities available for the child or adolescent presenting with a psychiatric disorder.

CHAPTER

17

Disorders and Issues of Children and Adolescents

KEY TERMS

Copropraxia

Dyslexia

Echopraxia

Encopresis

Enuresis

Mental retardation

Phonologic

Stuttering

Tic

Disorders of the Child and Adolescent

Although disorders are discussed in this chapter as first diagnosed or occurring during childhood and adolescence, there is no defined line to distinguish between childhood and adult mental disorders. Many disorders diagnosed during adulthood may actually have been present during earlier developmental periods. It is difficult to draw a distinct division between the classifications. There are, however, those disorders that tend to occur first in childhood or adolescence as supported by studies that show as many as one in three children will have one or more mental disorders by the age of 16 years. There is a higher incidence between the ages of 9 and 10 years, with acceleration of the risk by age 16. Anxiety, panic, depression, and substance abuse disorders tend to increase with age, whereas the disorders discussed in this chapter are more common among younger children.

There are numerous genetic and environmental factors that may contribute to the incidence of mental disorders in children and adolescents. The chance of psychiatric symptoms is increased in those with multiple risk factors. Having a first-degree biologic relative with the disorder is the most common underlying predictor of a similar disorder occurring in the child. There is overwhelming evidence that many children who are diagnosed with a psychiatric disorder have a significant family history of mental issues. Environmental factors, including the socioeconomic status of the neighborhood in which the child lives, family income, and educational level of family members, all have an important impact on the child's behavior. It has been shown that youth from families living in extreme or moderately deprived neighborhoods tend to exhibit a significant increase in behavioral problems over those in less deprived areas. Parental divorce in situations where none of the other factors exists can also trigger problems for children and adolescents. When genetic predisposition

and environmental factors are present in the same situation, the risk is compounded. In contrast, it must be said that not all children or adolescents who experience living in underprivileged circumstances develop a psychiatric disorder. Despite the inadequacy of their living conditions, many of these youth grow into well-adjusted, mature, and responsible adults.

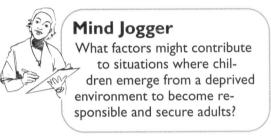

Mind Jogger

What factors might contribute to situations where children emerge from a deprived environment to become responsible and secure adults?

Developmental Disorders

The category of developmental disorders includes those conditions in which the child demonstrates symptoms of deficit before the age of 18 years. They are characterized by performance testing of mentality, skills, coordination, or activity that is substantially below that anticipated for the child's chronologic age and education level. Children with mental retardation fall into this disorder category.

Pervasive developmental disorders (PDDs) are characterized by severe deficits in areas of development including social interaction, communication skills, and behavior. The most common of these conditions is autistic disorder. Although not consistent with a diagnosis of childhood schizophrenia, these conditions can later develop into this disorder.

Mental Retardation

According to *DSM-IV-TR,* **mental retardation** is characterized by intellectual functioning that is significantly below average or an IQ of 70 or below. The onset is earlier than 18 years of age and is accompanied by a decreased ability to adapt to environmental situations. Retardation is further classified as mild, moderate, severe, or profound according to intelligence measurement scales (see At a Glance 17-1).

At a Glance 17-1 Mental Retardation Scale—Consequences

Mild—IQ between 55 and 70	Can lead normal lives Often marry and have children
Moderate—IQ between 35 and 55	Can work at simple jobs Few marry or have children
Severe—IQ between 20 and 40	Usually institutionalized Require much supervision
Profound—IQ below 20 or 25	Institutionalized Most have severe physical and behavior problems

At a Glance 17-2 Signs and Symptoms of Mental Retardation

- IQ of 70 or below
- Decreased ability to adapt to daily living
- Aggression
- Impulsiveness
- Victim of abuse or ridicule
- Decreased societal privileges
- Depression
- Irritability

Common Signs and Symptoms. There is no single set of behaviors that is unique to the child with mental retardation. Some children are passive, serene, and compliant, whereas others may be more aggressive and impulsive in their actions. The aggressive tendencies may stem from the child's inability to communicate in a meaningful way, which leads to frustration. Individuals with this disorder are often taken advantage of by others or become the victims of both physical and sexual abuse. Their functional deficit may also prevent them from access to some opportunities such as educational situations, ability to vote, or driving a vehicle.

Children and adolescents with mental retardation are 3 to 4 times more likely to have a coexisting mental disorder. Because communication is often limited, objective symptoms such as depressed mood, irritability, anorexia, or insomnia may be the basis for determining that an additional problem exists.

Incidence and Etiology. The causes of mental retardation are primarily biologic, psychosocial, or a combination of these factors. Prenatal damage related to toxins, maternal alcohol intake, infections, or genetic abnormalities account for the largest percentage of cases. Birth trauma and childhood illnesses largely account for the remainder of cases. In many individuals, there is no clear cause that can be determined. Children usually are brought for treatment with impaired functioning or the inability to cope with the demands of everyday life. Although the intellectual deficit usually remains unchanged, interventions can provide some improvement of functional life skills in most cases of mild to moderate retardation. Those with mild mental retardation make up about 85% of clients with this disorder. This group can often be educated to approximately the sixth-grade level, in addition to learning the adaptive skills for semi-independent living.

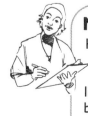

Mind Jogger
How might the presence of a child with mental retardation affect home life or siblings? What adjustments might be necessary as the child reaches school age?

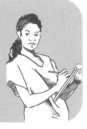

Autistic Disorder

Autistic disorder is characterized by severe abnormal development of the ability to socially interact and communicate with the outside world. Symptoms usually appear before 3 years of age. Children with this disorder are withdrawn and live in a fantasy world with little interest in their environment.

Common Signs and Symptoms. Nonverbal behaviors such as eye contact, facial expression, and gestures used to communicate are profoundly deficient. The child fails to develop age-appropriate peer relationships from lack of either interest or communication skills. The child has a lack of interest in or enjoyment from peer relationships and play activities with other children. Time is occupied with an inflexible and consistent routine of nonpurposeful behaviors and rituals. Children with autism often have accompanying mental retardation, ranging from mild to profound. Verbal skills and the ability to comprehend written words are usually below the level appropriate for the child's age. Children with this disorder may exhibit other behaviors such as hyperactivity, impulsivity, aggressiveness, and inattention to the world around them. The child may demonstrate unusual or exaggerated responses to sensory stimuli, such as screaming when touched, or exhibit a lack of anticipated response to painful stimuli. Some children exhibit a fascination with certain colors, objects, or music. Eating patterns may be stereotyped, such as repeatedly eating the same food. The child may awaken during sleep and engage in rocking movements, head banging, or other self-

injurious behaviors. Mood instability often occurs with sudden outbursts of laughing or crying. The adolescent who is able to understand his or her disorder may experience depression over this mental deficit.

At a Glance 17-3 Signs and Symptoms of Autism

- Lack of responsiveness to others
- Severe impairment in communication
- Repetitive routines
- Do not like to be touched or held
- Withdrawal from social contact
- Unusual responses to environmental stimuli (e.g., head banging, hand flapping, rocking, clinging to inanimate objects)

Incidence and Etiology. The symptoms of autistic disorder are difficult to define in the child under the age of 2 years. Some parents indicate seeing early signs of developmental lag, whereas others report no obvious indicators of a problem. The incidence is fairly uncommon, with approximately 1 reported case per 2,500 individuals, with boys affected 3 to 4 times more often than girls. There is an increased risk of autism in siblings of children with the disorder.

Psychosis

The same diagnostic criteria used for the adult with schizophrenia are used for the child with this disorder. (For more on schizophrenia, see Chapter 12.)

Common Signs and Symptoms. The child with psychosis characteristically exhibits symptoms of hallucinations, delusions, flat affect, disorganized speech, and stereotypical behaviors. There is poor development of intellectual, motor, emotional, and social skills as the child gets older. The child is unable to differentiate real from unreal, often leading to aggressiveness and the inability to tolerate frus-

Case Study: From Martina's World

Martina, a 3-year-old with flaming red hair and bright blue eyes, is admitted to the pediatric unit with asthmatic bronchitis. In addition to her medical condition, Martina has autistic disorder. Martina does not seem aware of the nurse's presence in the room but is intensely occupied with a blue stuffed dog. The nurse is preparing to administer scheduled oral medications to the child. Martina's mother is present in the room.

What approach would help the nurse to establish a trusting relationship with Martina?

_____

_____

What purpose will eye contact serve in helping Martina to communicate with the nurse?

_____

_____

What other behaviors might the nurse anticipate as Martina attempts to deal with her unfamiliar surroundings and activities?

_____

_____

_____

tration. Psychosis further impairs the child's ability to be imaginative or "make believe" in play activities. A lack of interest in others and limited contact with reality result in severely disturbed interpersonal and social relationships. Most individuals who are diagnosed with schizophrenia during childhood will become adults plagued by a chronic psychotic disorder. Treatment plans for the child incorporate various types of psychotherapy along with age-appropriate doses of antipsychotic medications to reduce the psychotic symptoms.

Incidence and Etiology. Schizophrenia is rare in young children, but the incidence increases dramatically during late adolescence. The onset is often associated with stressful events such as starting college or leaving home.

Developmental Coordination Disorder

Developmental coordination disorder is defined as a significant impairment in the development of motor coordination. The problem causes significant functional difficulty for the

At a Glance 17-4 Signs and Symptoms of Psychosis in Children

- Extreme change in usual behaviors
- Social withdrawal
- Disorganized thinking
- Strange mannerisms or talking to invisible objects
- Decrease in academic performance
- Acting-out behaviors

child in school or self-care activities. Other medical conditions such as cerebral palsy or muscular dystrophy can cause similar symptoms and must be ruled out as the cause of the problem.

Common Signs and Symptoms. The child usually demonstrates clumsiness in motor activities with significant delays in developmental milestones such as crawling, walking, running, or dressing. Older children may have problems with motor coordination during play activities or academic skills such as printing or writing. Children with a coordination disorder also may exhibit delays in other developmental areas such as language skills. There may be related fluctuations in mood, behavior, and the ability to interact socially.

At a Glance 17-5 Signs and Symptoms of Developmental Coordination Disorder

- Clumsiness in motor activities
- Delays in developmental milestones
- Lack of motor coordination in play or academic skills
- Delayed language skills acquisition
- Labile mood fluctuations
- Behavior problems
- Deficit in social interaction skills

Mind Jogger

What problems might develop in a daycare environment for a child who has delays or deficits in coordination?

Incidence and Etiology. Developmental coordination disorder is seen in as many as 6% of children between the ages of 5 and 11 years. It is not a life-threatening illness but usually persists over a lifetime. Studies show

an increase in the number of adolescents with this disorder who develop personality disorders, abuse substances, or attempt suicide. If treatment is secured early, however, the prognosis is good.

Learning and Communication Disorders

Learning disorders include situations in which the individual's performance on standardized testing in the skills of reading, mathematics, and written expression are much below the expected norm for that person's age, intelligence level, and educational standing. Children learn to use verbal communication skills and express themselves by observation and listening to those around them. Deficits may be seen in the ability to both interpret and utilize language skills.

Just the Facts
Learning refers to a relatively durable change in behavior or knowledge that is acquired by experience.

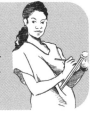

Dyslexia

The most common type of cognitive skill disorder is **dyslexia,** or difficulty in the reading domain. In this disorder, there is a difference between the child's intellectual ability and their success in reading and spelling. Even though these children are of normal or higher intelligence, they may be behind in the level of reading expected for their grade level. The problem seems to stem from an inability to process incoming sensory stimuli with the correct interpretation. The school drop-out rate increases dramatically for children or adolescents with a cognitive learning deficit.

Common Signs and Symptoms. The child with dyslexia usually does not read for pleasure. Spelling and writing by hand may be difficult, with a consistent pattern of letter confusion. Letter reversal is common; for example, "p" may be used for "g" or "b" used for "d." The child often reads from right to left with failure to see similar or different characteristics of words. For instance, instead of seeing "cat" the child sees "tac." There may also be a problem with sounding out words phonetically. Individuals who have difficulty learning may exhibit accompanying signs of discouragement, low self-esteem, and inadequate social skills. Evidence shows that early delays in language development are also associated with communication and developmental coordination problems.

At a Glance 17-6 Signs and Symptoms of Dyslexia

- Deficit in reading or written expression
- Discouragement
- Low self-esteem
- Inadequate social skills
- Increased school drop-out rate
- Delayed language development
- Inadequate communication skills
- Delayed developmental coordination

Incidence and Etiology. A disorder in the reading domain is more frequently seen among boys than girls. Dyslexia is often not diagnosed until the fourth grade or later when reading skills are more complex and increased comprehension is required. The fact that it is normal for some fluctuation to occur in a child's motivation in the academic setting must be considered as well. The quality and number of educational opportunities that are available to the child may also be a factor in the child's progress and skill. Hearing loss or visual impairment must be ruled out as a primary cause of the learning deficit. The prevalence is higher in first-generation relatives of those with learning deficits. Prognosis is good in a large percentage of cases in which diagnosis and intervention are made early in the learning process.

Just the Facts

The way children think about their successes or failures determines what effects these will have on their motivation and attitude toward learning. Children who attribute their failures to a lack of effort may try harder the next time, whereas those who attribute them to a lack of ability often quit trying.

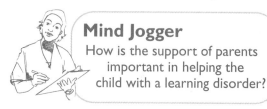

Mind Jogger
How is the support of parents important in helping the child with a learning disorder?

Expressive Language Disorder

Children with expressive language disorder have impairment in both verbal and sign language as evidenced by standardized testing. The language difficulty interferes with the child's performance in school and social functioning. When there is impairment in both the ability to comprehend information being received through the senses and the ability to use verbal language, a diagnosis of mixed receptive-expressive language disorder is assigned.

Common Signs and Symptoms. The child may have limited speech and vocabulary with difficulty learning new words or applying grammar concepts. Children with an expressive disorder usually begin talking later than usual and progress at a slower rate than that which is considered age-appropriate. The child with a mixed language disorder also has a problem in understanding words and sentences that require complex thinking such as cause and effect or comparison of two concepts. There is a decrease in the ability to process incoming sounds or associate and or-ganize words and sentences. The inability to comprehend may be less apparent than the ability to speak effectively. The lack of com-prehension is often seen when the child does not follow commands correctly or respond appropriately to questions. The ability to complete a thought process or follow rules of a game may also indicate the lack of under-standing.

Incidence and Etiology. Children with ex-pressive language difficulty are often younger than 3 years of age when diagnosed. Delays are seen in approximately 10% to 15% of children. This number drops significantly by school age, and most respond well to treat-ment. The incidence of the mixed language disorder is less common, with less than 5% of preschool children having this impairment.

At a Glance 17-7 Signs and Symptoms of Expressive Language Disorder

- Limited speech and vocabulary
- Difficulty learning new words
- Difficulty applying grammar concepts
- Delayed talking
- Slow progress in speech
- Difficulty in understanding words and sentences that require complex thinking
- Decreased ability to process incoming sounds
- Difficulty associating and organizing words and sentences
- Inability to speak effectively
- Lack of comprehension
- Failure to follow commands
- Inappropriate responses to questions
- Inability to follow rules of a game

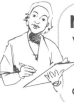

Mind Jogger

What implications might the difficulty in comprehension and expression have for a child who is hospitalized?

Phonologic Disorder

A failure to utilize sounds or articulate sylla-bles intelligibly during speech is the essential feature of the child diagnosed with **phono-logic** disorder. In many cases, the child also has a hearing impairment that contributes to the speech problem.

Common Signs and Symptoms. A com-mon characteristic of this disorder is **stutter-ing**, which is characterized by repetitive or prolonged sounds or syllables that include pauses and monosyllable broken words. Stut-tering causes considerable discomfort for the child in both academic and social situations but may be absent when the child is singing or reading aloud. There may be accompany-ing motor movement such as jerking, twitch-

---

Just the Facts

The following are the structural areas of language:

- Phonemes are the basic sounds of a spo-ken language used in phonics (sounding out to pronounce words).
- Prefixes, suffixes, and root words give meaning to language (e.g., friend, friendly, unfriendly).
- Syntax is a system of rules that specify how words can be arranged into phrases and sentences (grammar) that underlie all language use.

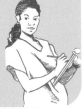

ing, or tremors. Increased levels of anxiety and stress will often initiate the problem, which leads to further anxiety, frustration, and low self-esteem.

> ### At a Glance 17-8 Signs and Symptoms of Phonologic Disorder
>
> - Stuttering in academic and social setting
> - May not be present during singing or reading aloud
> - Motor movement of jerking, twitching, or tremors
> - Increased anxiety
> - Frustration
> - Low self-esteem

Incidence and Etiology. Phonologic problems are more prevalent in men and tend to be mild. The development of a stuttering problem is typically seen between 2 and 7 years of age, with a peak at 5 years. It is seen in less than 2% of children in this age-group, with a prevalence in men.

Behavior Disorders

It is often difficult to distinguish between normal and problematic behavior in a child. Behavior that leads to a disorder is usually more common in a child with a difficult temperament who has intense and negative reactions to the environment. When this behavior interferes with the child's ability to learn or interact with others, it is considered dysfunctional.

Attention-Deficit/ Hyperactivity Disorder

In attention-deficit/hyperactivity disorder (ADHD), a persistent pattern of inattention, hyperactivity, or impulsive behaviors is more

frequently exhibited than would be considered normal for a child of comparable age and developmental level. Some display of these symptoms must be present before the age of 7 years. Many children are diagnosed after the problematic behaviors have been present for some time.

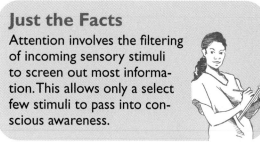

> ### Just the Facts
> Attention involves the filtering of incoming sensory stimuli to screen out most information. This allows only a select few stimuli to pass into conscious awareness.

Common Signs and Symptoms. There may be primary symptoms of inattention, hyperactivity, and impulsive actions. The behavior causes significant difficulty for the child when adapting in home, school, or social settings. There is usually an obvious pattern of disruption and inappropriate functioning as a result of the behavior. The child with ADHD exhibits these behaviors with more frequency than other children of the same mental age and developmental level.

The symptoms of hyperactivity may not be the same at all developmental age levels. Toddlers and preschool children with ADHD usually exhibit more exaggerated activity than other children of the same age. Continual and often destructive physical activity is seen, along with an inability to remain seated for activities such as a television show or storytelling session. In school-age children, these behaviors may be minimized in intensity although fidgeting, noise-making, and other disruptive behaviors increase. The child often gets up from the table during meals or seated activities in the classroom. Although symptoms of the disorder often diminish in late adolescence or adulthood, many continue to exhibit restlessness and difficulty with activities requiring quiet attentiveness or concentration. This results in an unorganized approach to school work and work-related activities with minimal ability to follow through on task-oriented projects. Risk-taking behaviors are common, with little regard for the potential consequences of these actions. Impulsivity, which can occur in any age group, is demonstrated by impatience, the inability to

refrain from interrupting, and discourteously intruding on the rights of others. These children lack the self-control to delay their responses. The impulsive and fearless nature of physical activity often leads to accidental injury and destruction of property. An important point to remember is that it is unusual for the person to demonstrate the same symptoms in all settings, making it necessary to gather information from more than one situation or setting.

Additional symptoms may include a low tolerance or frustration with accompanying temper tantrums, mood changes, low self-esteem, stubbornness, demanding behavior, and poor peer relationships. These behaviors tend to be labeled as willful, leading to conflict within the family and school systems. Family maladjustment and poor parent–child interaction is usually present. These relationships may improve with successful intervention and therapy. The intelligence level of individuals with this disorder ranges from lower than average to gifted.

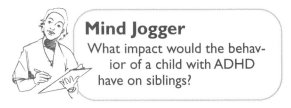

Mind Jogger

What impact would the behavior of a child with ADHD have on siblings?

Incidence and Etiology. ADHD is more commonly seen among first-generation biologic relatives of those with the disorder. In addition, the child's family and school environment along with peer influence also play a part in the development of problematic behavior. Many of these children come from families in which members have a higher incidence of substance abuse and other mental disorders. It is most commonly diagnosed in school-age children, with a higher incidence seen in men. The success of treatment varies, with the largest percentage of children continuing to demonstrate at least one

---

At a Glance 17-9 Signs and Symptoms of ADHD

- Inattention to close detail or careless errors in homework or assigned tasks
- Inability to maintain focus on a task of play activity
- Often seems preoccupied and inattentive to the person who is speaking
- Repeatedly moves focus from one activity to another, failing to follow directions
- Failure to follow a task to completion
- Dislikes tasks that require maintained mental concentration and effort, often avoiding them (e.g., reading, mathematics, mental games)
- Marked disorganization and careless handling or loss of materials necessary to perform a task or complete homework
- Easily distracted by irrelevant external stimuli such as a lawn mower or car honking
- Fidgety and frequent squirming with inability to remain seated when requested to do so
- Difficulty following instructions or taking turns in games or classroom activities
- Excessive and spontaneous talking and interruptions of others at inappropriate times
- Difficulty in playing quietly, appearing as a perpetual wheel in motion
- May engage in potentially dangerous or destructive activity, oblivious to the possible consequences
- Poor parent–child relationships
- Low tolerance to frustration
- Temper tantrums, low self-esteem, stubbornness, demanding
- Poor peer relationships

of the disabling essential symptoms into adulthood.

Conduct Disorder

Conduct disorder is defined as a pattern of repetitive and continuous behavior that either infringes on the basic rights of others or defies the rules of society that would be appropriate for the child's age level. This behavior may have an onset prior to the age of 10 years, with many also having a history of other disruptive disorders. Individuals with adolescent-onset type tend to demonstrate conduct problems in group situations, although their behaviors may be less aggressive.

Common Signs and Symptoms. Children with this disorder demonstrate aggressive actions that result in or threaten harm to other people or animals. They tend to initiate hostile and bullying-type behavior, using threats and fighting with or without weapons that can inflict serious physical injury. They may steal, rape, mug, assault other people, or seriously abuse animals. It is common for these children to lie and "con" by asking personal favors with no intention of repayment. Other behaviors may cause damage or loss of property, such as setting fires or vandalism. The behaviors usually exist in several situations such as the home, school, or community setting. There is usually a pattern starting before the age of 13 years. Defiance of home and family rules and curfews with a pattern of "running away" from home overnight or truancy from school is common.

Preschool children with conduct disorder usually exhibit aggressive behaviors in their home situation and toward other children. They often deliberately destroy other people's property. School-age children continue the deliberate aggressive behaviors, both physical and verbal. In the adolescent, there may also be an early onset of sexual promiscuity, substance use, and physical violence that accompany the earlier behavioral pattern.

Glance 17-10 Signs and Behaviors of Conduct Disorder

- Repeated disruptive and destructive behaviors
- Willful defiance of family rules
- Violation of age-appropriate and societal norms
- Aggressive behavior
- Truancy from school or running away from home
- Sexual promiscuity
- Substance use and abuse
- Vandalism and physical violence
- Cruelty toward animals

Oppositional-Defiant Disorder

Oppositional-defiant disorder is a repetitive pattern of negative, defiant, disobedient, and hostile behavior toward authority figures.

Common Signs and Symptoms. The tendency to argue incessantly with adults, lose their temper, and actively defy or refuse to comply with rules and requests imposed upon them is typical of children with oppositional-defiant disorder. There is a pattern of deliberately acting in a way that annoys others, while blaming others for the behavior. They are usually vindictive, spiteful, and resentful in their interpersonal relationships and usually exhibit resistance to compromise or negotiation with peers or adults. The problematic behaviors may lead to suspension or expulsion from school and frequent encounters with law enforcement officials. There is an increased incidence of sexually transmitted diseases and teenage pregnancy reported in these clients. The tendency for suicidal ideation and suicide attempts increases and may be the factor in seeking treatment.

Parental rejection and neglect with harsh and abusive physical punishment or sexual abuse are often cited as predisposing factors for this disorder. The child may have been re-

At a Glance 17-11 Warning Signs for Suicide Risk in Children and Adolescents

- Verbal threats or behavior hints about suicide
- Decline in quality of schoolwork
- Truancy from school or running away from home
- Sudden withdrawal from friends or family
- Withdrawal from previously enjoyed activities
- Drug or alcohol abuse
- Giving away prized possessions
- Excessive fatigue or physical complaints
- Prolonged expression of sadness or uselessness
- Lack of response to praise or rewards
- Neglect of personal appearance or hygiene
- Unusually rebellious behaviors

moved to a foster or group home situation with a frequent shift in caregivers. Rejection by peers may lead the child to an association with those who engage in delinquent antisocial behaviors, violence, and drug-related activity.

At a Glance 17-12 Signs and Symptoms of Oppositional-Defiant Disorder

- Arguing without compromise
- Willful defiance of rules
- Hostility and anger
- Low tolerance to frustration
- Use of drugs or alcohol
- Physical violence
- Violation of curfews
- Spiteful or vindictive acts

Incidence and Etiology. Oppositional-defiant disorder tends to be more prevalent in preschool children who demonstrate early difficulty with temperament or hyperactivity.

These children have a low tolerance for frustration with frequent angry outbursts and conflict with parents and teachers. It is usually evident before the age of 8 years, with onset not often occurring later than early adolescence. A familial pattern of psychiatric problems is often preexistent in the child. It is also seen more often in families where there is serious marital conflict between parents. A thorough evaluation of the child is important, because many of the behaviors seen in this disorder may normally be seen in children of preschool age through adolescence.

Mind Jogger

What factors in the family and social environment do you think contribute most to the incidence of the conduct disorders? What comparison do you see between these factors and the rate of crimes against society?

Anxiety Disorders

As a child learns to adjust to the world and form a separate identity, many situations create anticipated anxiety or fears that are realistic and normal. The manner in which the child's behavior is viewed and reinforced by others can contribute to an intensified feeling. Reinforcement of the distress felt in these situations also leads to a learned response of excessive and unwarranted anxiety.

Separation Anxiety Disorder

During early childhood development, it is expected that the stages of separation anxiety will be seen in response to new and strange encounters with unfamiliar objects or people. In comparison, the child with separation anxiety disorder experiences excessive anxiety related to separation from home or attachment figures. The disturbance must occur before the age of 18 years and cause significant distress or impairment in functioning for a period of at least 1 month. Symptoms may become evident following a stressful period in the child's life such as starting school, parental divorce, a neighborhood move, or death of a pet or close relative.

Common Signs and Symptoms. The child with this disorder is uncomfortable to the point of misery when separated from the person with whom a love attachment is formed. When the separation is necessary, as in attending school, the child may feel the need to stay in constant touch with the person or be preoccupied with the need to return home. The child may experience somatic complaints such as abdominal pain, nausea and vomiting, or headaches during or before the separation. Excessive worry about the event or of losing the loved ones during a separation may become persistent. There may be a fear of going to sleep without the loved one present or worry that something terrible is going to happen to that person. The degree of anxiety can range from uneasiness to panic and depression. Depending on the age of the child, fears and concerns may vary. The younger child may have fears of the dark, monsters, burglars, fires, water, or other situations that could pose a danger to the family or self. Apathy, sadness, depression, and feelings of being unloved or unwanted are common. These children are often described as demanding of attention, leading to frustration and resentment within the family circle. Treatment is aimed at reducing the anxiety and reinforcing a sense of security in both the child and the family during periods of separation. Although some children are successful in accomplishing these goals, others go on to develop a chronic anxiety disorder, panic disorder, or depression.

Incidence and Etiology. This disorder is more common in children of parents with anxiety or panic disorders. The incidence is fairly common, with approximately 4% of children and adolescents affected by this level of anxiety. The symptoms tend to decrease as the child reaches adolescence.

Tic Disorders (Tourette's Disorder)

A **tic** is defined as a sudden, repetitive, arrhythmic, stereotyped motor movement or verbal speech that occurs before the age of 18 years. There is never a symptom-free period of more than 3 months.

Common Signs and Symptoms. Simple tics may involve such movements as blinking of the eye, wrinkling of the nose, jerking of the neck or shoulder, or grimacing. More complex movements may include hand gestures, contortions of the face, or physical actions such as jumping, retracing steps, hopping, and skipping over lines. Occasionally, the person may assume unusual positions or posturing. **Co,propraxia,** or a sudden ticlike obscene gesture, along with repetitive movements **(echopraxia)** can also occur. Vocal tics are meaningless recurrent sounds such as sniffing, snorting, and throat clearing. More complex behaviors include verbal outbursts of words or phrases, speech blocking, or

---

At a Glance 17-13 **Signs and Symptoms of Separation Anxiety Disorder**

- Severe anxiety about separation from love attachment figure
- Worry about something harmful happening to attachment figure or self
- Refusal to attend school or related activities
- Somatic complaints
- Fear of going to sleep without the attachment figure present
- Apathy, depression, sadness
- Attention-demanding behavior

meaningless changes in tone or volume of speech.

The person with a tic disorder usually experiences an irresistible urge to perform the tic and feels relief once the behavior has occurred. Tics tend to occur in spells that may last from seconds to hours. The severity or frequency of the spells usually changes during the course of the day or as environmental location changes. Some children may be able to suppress tics during a school session, but return to the behavior during recess. Tics generally tend to decrease during sleep or during concentrated activity such as reading or playing the piano. The incidence may increase during periods of stress or demanding and competitive activities. The emotional discomfort, shame, and self-consciousness caused by the behavior may lead to social isolation or personality changes.

> ### At a Glance 17-14 Signs and Symptoms of Tic Disorders
>
> - Eye blinking, wrinkling of nose
> - Jerking of neck and shoulder
> - Grimacing
> - Copropraxia
> - Echopraxia
> - Imitation of body movements
> - Involuntary vocal and verbal utterances
> - Sniffing, snorting, throat clearing

Incidence and Etiology. Tic disorders tend to be genetic. Tourette's disorder tends to occur at an early age, with a prevalence in boys. Many more children than adults are affected with this condition. Tics tend to occur in all cultures and ethnic groups.

Elimination Disorders

Although some cases of elimination problems may be related to physiologic causes, most are psychologic in origin. Learning to control bowel and bladder functions is integral to the growth and development of the child. Problems can arise from the approach or methods used to assist the child in achieving this control, or it may be a delay in development that may resolve with time.

Encopresis and Enuresis

Encopresis is characterized by a repeated passage of feces into inappropriate places such as clothing, trashcans, or the floor. The child with **enuresis** has repeated episodes of urine incontinence during the day or night.

Common Signs and Symptoms. The elimination behaviors are usually involuntary but may be intentional. In encopresis, the child must be at least 4 years of age or have attained normal physiologic control over defecation. The symptoms must occur at least once a month over a period of at least 3 months. The problem of constipation or impaction may stem from either physiologic factors such as ineffective straining or painful defecation or psychologic issues such as anxiety related to place or surroundings at the time the child feels the urge to defecate. In the case of enuresis, the symptoms must occur at least twice a week for at least 3 months to be categorized as a disorder. The child must be at least 5 years of age or have control over urine continence. The symptoms may occur only during the day or night, or both.

Most children with these disorders tend to feel ashamed and embarrassed to the point of

> ### Just the Facts
> Predisposing factors for elimination disorders include delayed or lax toilet training, psychosocial stress, physical abnormalities, medication side effects, and fluid intake.

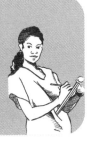

At a Glance 17-15 Signs and Symptoms of Elimination Disorders

- Repeated passage of incontinent feces or urine in inappropriate places
- Feelings of shame and embarrassment
- Social isolation and avoidance
- Psychologic issues related to harsh toilet-training
- Physical factors such as ineffective straining or pain with defecation

social isolation, and they avoid any activities that would predispose them to these feelings.

Incidence and Etiology. Encopresis is only seen in a small percentage of 5 year olds and occurs more commonly in boys. Enuresis is common in as many as 5% to 10% of children in the same age group. The incidence decreases as the child gets older, with most becoming continent by adolescence. Most children with elimination disorders have a first-generation biologic relative who has had the disorder. The risk is much higher for children if one of the parents has a history of either of these problems.

Application of the Nursing Process

Nursing Assessment

The mentally or emotionally disturbed child is usually referred for evaluation and treatment by parents, teachers, other health care professionals, or the judicial system. Parents are often concerned and frustrated with the child's actions and inability to adapt to daily living. To assess all factors that may contribute to the child's disturbed behavior, information is collected regarding the child, the family, and related environmental factors.

These data assist the health care team to determine if there are any relevant extended family issues. It is important that family members be included in identifying areas of concern. Once the family is aware of the existent issues, they are able to reflect on the situation and actively participate in planning strategies necessary to help the child.

Parents, teachers, and other social contacts of the child are the usual sources of information regarding the child's troublesome behavior. A history should include the time at which the problematic behaviors began and any significant occurrences at that time that may have precipitated the symptoms. A thorough physical and emotional assessment is completed. The child's ability to communicate and interact with others is usually assessed and observed using play activities. A thorough assessment is also made of the child's feelings, self-image, distorted thinking, or other subjective symptoms such as abuse, depression, or suicidal ideation. It is not unusual for the child to reveal problems related to familial relationships, such as abuse, that are not divulged or known by others within the family circle. In addition, it is important to assess communication and interaction patterns between family members. Determine the degree to which the child's behavior and actions are disrupting the family functioning or other social settings in which the child participates.

Nursing Diagnosis

Selection of the appropriate nursing diagnoses may vary according to the mental disorder to address the needs of the individual child. This is especially difficult because the child is in a period of constant growth and development, with unpredictable behavior that is influenced by both genetics and environmental factors. Because many of these disorders may overlap and coexist in the same child, planning may identify multiple problem areas. Those problems that can be considered common to all children and adolescents with mental conditions include:

- Risk for injury, related to altered physical mobility or aggressive behavior
- Impaired verbal communication, related to verbal expression or inability to speak or form words and sentences
- Impaired social interaction, related to disruptive or inappropriate behaviors and decreased self-esteem

In addition to those common nursing diagnoses, others may include:

- Self-care deficit, related to cognitive processing or maturity level
- Altered growth and development, related to genetic or environmental factors
- Risk for injury to self, related to neurologic deficits and indifference to the environment
- Personal identity disturbance, related to inability to recognize self as separate being
- Risk for violence, self-directed or directed at others, related to dysfunctional family environment, poor impulse control, or aggressive and self-destructive behaviors
- Coping ineffective: individual, related to low self-esteem, disorganized and maladaptive environment, or immature and inadequate coping strategies
- Coping ineffective: family, related to disruptive or destructive child behavior, and maladaptive family system
- Anxiety, related to unmet needs and dysfunctional social relationships
- Noncompliance, related to low frustration level and negativism
- Sleep pattern disturbance, related to anxiety and fears of separation

Expected Outcomes

Once appropriate nursing diagnoses have been selected, planning includes determining anticipated outcomes toward which the individual client may be able to accomplish progress in re-

solving the identified problems. Realistic timeframes will depend on the individual client and the nature and extent of the problem. Expected outcomes may include the following.

Child or Adolescent:

- Remains free of self-harm and does not harm others
- Establishes effective alternative communication with staff and family
- Chooses and initiates appropriate social interactions with peers
- Demonstrates consistent progress in self-care development toward maximum potential and independence
- Demonstrates increased autonomy and reliance on self
- Expresses positive feelings about self
- Exhibits ability to control impulsivity and take turns with others
- Describes possible consequences of behavior
- Participates in planning and implementation of behavior improvement program
- Tolerates overnight separation periods from attachment figure
- Verbalizes decreased anxiety during separation from parent or love figure
- Exhibits decreased complaints of somatic symptoms.
- Identifies precipitating factors for anxiety
- Applies improved alternative coping strategies

Parents:

- Identify strengths and weakness of the child
- Participate in planning and implementation of behavior improvement program
- Establish and maintain consistency in boundaries for acceptable behavior
- Provide reinforcement of child's positive behaviors
- Describe appropriate ways to express feelings of frustration regarding child's inappropriate behaviors
- Develop appropriate ways to cope with anger and feelings toward the child

Nursing Interventions

Implications for nursing care of the child with a mental illness will vary based on the individual needs of the child and the disorder being addressed. Interventions may overlap in the child with more than one diagnosis. General nursing approaches may include:

- Maintain a safe physical environment.
- Identify any suicide risk, ideation, or actions.
- Keep sharp or hazardous items out of reach or in a locked area.
- Intervene to prevent injury from aggression or acting-out behaviors.
- Redirect and channel aggressive behavior into a controlled activity.
- Maintain consistency of caregivers and approach to behavior issues.
- Identify capabilities of the child related to self-care.
- Provide encouragement for the child toward independent self-care.
- Provide simple explanations for behavior boundaries.
- Establish a consistent pattern of reward for positive behavior and aversive stimuli response for negative behaviors.
- Identify association between nonverbal communication patterns and the child's individual needs.
- Use headgear such as a helmet or hand coverings to prevent self-inflicted injury during behaviors such as head-banging, scratching, or hair-pulling.
- Attempt to determine precipitating factors that lead to agitated and self-injurious behavior.
- Establish a trusting relationship by first using eye-contact reinforced with a smile.
- Use a slow approach when introducing tactile stimuli such as touch or hugs.
- Use positive reinforcement for child's attempts at interaction with others.
- Provide familiar security objects such as a favorite toy, pillow, or blanket.
- Provide adequate supervision and limits for the child's activity.
- Use a matter-of-fact approach in explanation of consequences for negative behaviors.
- Plan activities that provide a chance for the child to succeed.
- Provide a distraction-free environment for task-oriented activity.
- Help the child or adolescent to recognize and accept anger as a feeling.
- Teach the child or adolescent ways to channel anger into socially appropriate physical outlets.
- Include parents in discussions regarding events that trigger overwhelming fears and somatic symptoms in the child.

Evaluation

Criteria for evaluating the desired outcomes in the child will depend on the problematic behavior being addressed. It is anticipated that children with developmental disorders will increase their ability to interact and communicate with others. This can be measured by progress in their ability to trust others and initiate social contact with another person. Progress is also evaluated in the child's ability to control negative and self-harming behaviors.

Evaluation of the child with attention deficit or hyperactivity will include a consistent decrease in disruptive and dangerous behaviors along with the ability to function in a social or structured learning environment. Goals for the child with a conduct disorder are centered on the development of self-control and a decrease in impulsive behaviors. The outcome is measured by improvement in the ability to have satisfying relationships with both peer and family groups. Positive steps in developing self-esteem and feelings of self-worth should also be noted.

It is vital in each type of child or adolescent disorder that careful evaluation is given to the participation of parents and other family members in the treatment program. Take note of interactions between the child and family with emphasis on whether they are coping effectively with the child's behavioral symptoms. Evaluate the support given to the child and whether there is positive reinforcement of positive behaviors. A positive outcome is demonstrated in the child's ability to function and adapt appropriately to the environment around them.

Summary

There are many factors that may contribute to the incidence of a mental disorder in the child or adolescent. By far the most prevalent is the genetic component with a familial history of mental disorders. This risk is compounded when environmental issues such as poverty, violence, substance abuse, and poor family relationships provide a dysfunctional system in which the child lives.

Disorders may exist in various developmental areas including intelligence level, interactive and communicative skills, and coordination. Deficits may range from mild to profound, and they interfere with the child's ability to adjust and interact with the world around them. Because of their limited social skills and a lack of enthusiasm involving their environment, these children do not develop mentally or socially to a level consistent with their chronologic age.

Learning disorders and language impairment interfere with the child's performance both socially and academically. The frustration experienced by these children often leads to decreased motivation and premature exit from the school system. Because both society and academic advancement require basic skills in reading, mathematics, writing, and communicative language, it is difficult for these children to adjust and function as they grow older. Early intervention and treatment can help the child with one of these disorders to adapt and accommodate for the deficit.

Perhaps the most difficult situation for both clients and parents is the child with a behavior disorder. Because of the disruptive and destructive nature of the behaviors, these children often become entangled with law enforcement officials early in their lives. The child is unable to understand or control the erratic episodes of behavior, which leads to frustration and ambivalent feelings in parents, teachers, and others who come in contact with the child. Family maladjustment and poor parent–child interaction is common. If the child's conduct is aggressive or hostile in nature, the likelihood increases that the behavior will lead to arrest and disciplinary action by the judicial system. There is often a familial pattern of psychiatric problems in children who are diagnosed with conduct or defiant disorders of this level.

Other disorders in children are often the result of stress-related symptoms that manifest themselves in the form of anxiety, repetitive tic movements, or inappropriate elimination. The child often has a poorly developed self-concept that is further eroded by the embarrassment and lack of understanding about the disorder. Therapeutic intervention includes helping the child to understand the relationship between the psychologic symptoms and the condition.

Many of the mental disorders seen in children continue to manifest symptoms into the adult years. Some are not diagnosed until adulthood but may have been present since childhood. Others are not symptomatic until adolescence and beyond. Early intervention is necessary to assist both the child and those associated with him or her to develop the adaptive skills to encourage a functional level of existence.

Bibliography

American Psychiatric Association (2000). *Diagnostic and statistical manual of mental disorders* *text revision* (4th ed.). Washington, DC: American Psychiatric Association.

Biederman, J., Faraone, S. V., & Monteaux, M. C. (2002). ADHD risk factors independent of gender. *American Journal of Psychiatry, 159,* 1556–1562.

Costello, E. J., Mustillo, S. L., Erkanli, A., Keeler, G., & Angold, A. (2003). High risk of psychiatric disorders at 16 years. *General Psychiatry, 2003 (60),* 837–844.

Greene, R., Biederman, J., Zerwas, S., Monuteaux, M. C., Goring, J. C., & Faraone, S. V. (2002). Clinical significance of oppositional defiant disorder. *American Journal of Psychiatry, 159,* 1214–1224.

Kirk, S. A, & Hsieh, D. K. (2004). Diagnostic consistency in assessing conduct disorder: an experiment on the effect of social context, *American Journal of Orthopsychiatry,* 74(1), 43–55. Available at http://web4.epnet.com/citation. asp. Accessed on July 14, 2004.

Loeber, R., Burke, J D, Lahey, B B, Winters, A., & Zera, M. (2000). Oppositional defiant and conduct disorder: a review of the past 10 years, part I. *Journal of American Academy of Child Adolescent Psychiatry, 39,* 1468–1484.

Ruchkin, V., et al. (2003). Psychopathology and early conduct disorder explain persistent delinquency, *Journal of Clinical Psychiatry, 64,* 913–920.

FILL IN THE BLANK

Fill in the blank with the correct answer.

1. The _____ is the most common underlying contributor to the probability of a mental disorder in children.

2. _____ is the most common type of learning disorder.

3. One of the most common problems that develops from the learning disorders is that of _____ and _____ with others.

4. Individuals with mild mental retardation can be educated to approximately the _____ in addition to learning skills for adaptive living.

5. In the child with autism, the nonverbal behaviors such as _____, _____, and _____ used to communicate are profoundly deficient.

6. Speech that is characterized by repetitive or prolonged sounds or syllables that include pauses and monosyllable broken words is _____.

7. The filtering of sensory input to allow a select few to pass through into conscious awareness is termed _____.

8. Repetitive movements that occur in tic disorders are referred to as _____.

9. _____ describes the repeated passage of feces into inappropriate places such as clothing, trashcans, or the floor.

10. The disruptive or inappropriate behaviors and decreased self-esteem seen in most children and adolescents with mental disorders hinder their interpersonal relationships and support a nursing diagnosis of _____.

MATCHING

Match the following terms to the most appropriate phrase.

a. Repetitive and continuous behavior that infringes on the rights of others or defies rules of society appropriate for age level

b. Intellectual functioning with IQ of 70 or below

c. Failure to utilize sounds or articulate syllables intelligibly during speech

d. Repeated episodes of urine incontinence during day or night

e. Clumsiness in motor activities with significant delays in developmental milestones

f. Persistent patterns of inattention, hyperactivity, or impulsive behaviors, more frequent than those seen in the average child

g. Repetitive pattern of negative, defiant, disobedient, and hostile behavior toward authority figures

h. Marked abnormality in the development of ability to socially interact and communicate with the outside world

i. Limited speech and vocabulary with difficulty learning new words or applying concepts of grammar

1. _____ ADHD

2. _____ Developmental coordination disorder

3. _____ Enuresis

4. _____ Conduct disorder

5. _____ Mental retardation

6. _____ Oppositional defiant disorder

7. _____ Expressive language disorder

8. _____ Autism

9. _____ Phonologic disorder

MULTIPLE CHOICE

Select the best answer from the multiple-choice items.

1. Miguel is a 6-year-old who has been diagnosed with enuresis after tests show no physical reason for the symptoms. Miguel's mother is visibly upset and says, "It is his father's fault. He had the same problem." Which of the following would be the nurse's best response?

   a. "Why would you blame his father?"

   b. "This problem is not usually someone's fault."

   c. "You seem quite upset about your son's problem."

   d. "What is it in his father's background that makes you say that?"

2. Justin is a 7-year-old child who is having difficulty with reading and writing assignments in school. His teacher has suggested he be tested for a learning disorder. Which of the following categories would apply to Justin's problem?

   a. Stuttering

   b. Dyslexia

   c. Attention deficit

   d. Vocal tic

3. Amanda, a 6-year-old whose parents divorced 6 months ago, begins to cry and vomits each time her mother brings her to school. Her mother is asked to take her home each day. Which of the following is most descriptive of Amanda's behavior?

   a. Conduct disorder

   b. Separation anxiety disorder

   c. Oppositional defiant disorder

   d. Pervasive developmental disorder

4. School officials have contacted the parents of John, a 14-year-old who has been truant from school four times in the past month. John set fire to his grandmother's garage when he was 10, assaulted his father for telling him to clean his room at age 11, and was suspended from school for writing graphic language on the school sidewalk with spray paint. When John is admitted to the psychiatric center for adolescents, which of the following nursing diagnoses should receive priority?

   a. Risk for violence, directed at others

   b. Self-esteem, disturbance

   c. Dysfunctional family processes

   d. Social interaction, impaired

5. Monica is a 16-year-old who has been admitted to the psychiatric unit with severe depression. Monica is placed on suicide precautions. Which of the following signs might be suggestive of suicidal behavior?

   a. Limits her visitors to four people

   b. Asks the nurse for shampoo so she can wash her hair

   c. Sleeps during the day in between therapy sessions

   d. Gives her charm bracelet to her best friend

6. The child with expressive language disorder would most likely have a problem with which of the following tasks?

   a. Following rules for a game

   b. Being touched or held by another person

   c. Staying overnight with a relative

   d. Compromising during an argument

7. Beth is a 5-year-old who has difficulty articulating syllables in a way that her speech can be understood. She often has repetitive or prolonged sounds separated by pauses that make her anxious and upset. Which of the following describes the speech problem that Beth is experiencing?

   a. Syntax

   b. Copropraxia

   c. Stuttering

   d. Echopraxia

8. Richard is a 7-year-old who exhibits characteristic signs of delayed mental development. Upon testing, Richard is found to have an IQ level of 54. Which of the following situations would be a realistic outcome for Richard?

   a. Institutional care to provide adequate supervision

   b. Independent living with ability to provide own income

   c. Simple job with supervised independent living

   d. Self-care needs of feeding and toileting only

9. Bobby is a 7-year-old who is being evaluated for a learning disorder. While talking to his mother, the nurse receives the following information. Which of the following factors is most likely a contributing factor to the child's performance?

   a. Turns up the TV to volume that is uncomfortable for others

   b. Likes to play on swings and gym equipment at school

   c. Tends to pick on his little brother and sister

   d. Is afraid of the neighbor's dog

10. A 15-year-old is verbally aggressive toward the principal of his school after being reprimanded for breaking a school rule. He tells him, "You don't own me. Nobody owns me. I don't have to keep your silly rules." This type of behavior is characteristic in which of the following disorders?

    a. Mental retardation

    b. Oppositional-defiant disorder

    c. Separation anxiety disorder

    d. Tourette's disorder

SEEK AND FIND

Find the incorrect information in the following statements.

1. Tic movements are usually more obvious during sleep or during concentrated activity such as reading or playing the piano.

2. Encopresis is the repeated passage of urine into inappropriate places such as clothing and trashcans or onto the floor.

3. Separation anxiety disorder in the child or adolescent does not usually involve behavior that demands attention.

4. The child or adolescent with ADHD is usually aware of the potential consequences of his or her actions.

5. The symptoms of autism are most often detectable before the age of 6 months.

SCENARIO: "TOO MUCH FOR ANTHONY"

Anthony is a 14-year-old client who has been admitted to the adolescent psychiatric center after repeated incidents of suspension from school for disruptive and defiant behaviors toward his teachers and peers. He is an only child from a single parent family. His father died when he was 3 years old, leaving his mother with minimal employment skills to support her young son. Anthony was born with the congenital anomaly of imperforate anus, in which there is no anal opening for elimination of feces from the bowel. Surgery was performed to make an opening; however, without sphincter control, Anthony has had to endure the incontinence and embarrassment that accompanies this condition.

His mother relates that Anthony was always a hyperactive child. When he started school, the teachers were calling several times a week to tell her that they could not manage him in their classroom. He was given time-out suspensions from class in addition to receiving many failing grades in his academic learning. Anthony was placed in an alternate class situation for children with learning disabilities. In addition to being easily distracted, Anthony cannot sit still nor concentrate on any one task long enough for its completion.

Anthony's mother says that she is afraid he is going to end up in jail if something isn't done. She says, "He has been a hassle for me ever since he was born. Sometimes I really wish he had never been born. Maybe he would be better off in jail—then I wouldn't have to deal with him."

He is given a diagnosis of ADHD with oppositional-defiant disorder. It is also determined that Anthony has an intelligence level in the gifted range.

What psychologic factors may be underlying his disruptive behavior?

_____

_____

What may have contributed to his performance in the school setting?

_____

_____

What feelings may Anthony be having related to his mother's attitude toward him?

_____

_____

What approach might be used to help Anthony's mother to deal with her son's illness?

_____

_____

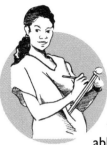

LEARNING OBJECTIVES

After learning the content in this chapter, the student will be able to:

1. Describe characteristics of those persons who are known as older adults.
2. Describe psychosocial issues relating to the mental health of the older adult.
3. Identify interventions that promote good mental health in the older adult.
4. Assess and differentiate between delirium, dementia, and depression in the older adult.
5. Describe the symptoms and stages in the progression of Alzheimer's disease.
6. Identify appropriate nursing diagnoses for delirium and dementia.
7. List expected outcomes for persons with delirium and dementia.
8. Identify nursing interventions for persons who demonstrate cognitive impairment.
9. Evaluate the effectiveness of implemented planned nursing care.

Disorders and Issues of the Older Adult

KEY TERMS

Ageism
Aging
Agnosia
Alzheimer's disease (AD)
Amnestic disorders
Anomia
Aphasia
Apraxia
Catastrophic event
Confabulation
Delirium
Dementia
Disorientation
Primary aging
Secondary aging
Sundowning syndrome
Vascular dementia

Issues of the Older Population

Definition of Aging

Aging is defined as a manifestation of changes that advance in a continuous and progressive manner during the adult years. The older adult population typically exhibits physical symptoms of aging such as graying of hair, a decrease in subcutaneous supportive tissue with wrinkling of the skin, and presbyopia (decline in the ability to focus on close-up objects). It is important to recognize the flexible nature of health and functioning among those older than 65 years. There are effects of **primary aging,** or those changes that occur as a result of genetics or natural factors, and those of **secondary aging,** which are influenced by the environment. A pattern of coping with environmental stressors is often established as a result of social learning early in life. Successful adaptation to the process of aging is encouraged by the ability to give meaning and perspective to life experiences. This is reflected in findings that most older adults, despite coexisting chronic medical conditions or disabilities, rate their physical or mental health as good or excellent. Although the changes that accompany aging are inevitable, it is recognized that older adults who can adapt to these changes with relative acceptance experience the highest level of satisfaction with their lives.

Mind Jogger

What implication do these demographics have for nursing?

Mind Jogger

How might childhood experiences influence how a person adapts to the aging process?

At a Glance 18-1 Chronic Medical Conditions Most Common in People 65 Years and Older

- Arthritis
- Visual disturbances
- Hypertension
- Peripheral vascular disease
- Congestive heart failure
- Urinary dysfunction
- Parkinson's disease
- Hearing loss
- Stroke
- Chronic obstructive pulmonary disease (COPD)
- Thyroid disease
- Diabetes mellitus

Psychosocial Issues Related to Aging

Chronic disease, memory impairment, and depressive symptoms affect large numbers of older adults, and the risk of these problems occurring often increases with age. Social and behavioral aspects of life and the link of loss to age can have much influence on the mental status and the prevalence of mental health disorders in late life. Losses that occur more frequently among the older population include loss of:

- Health
- Retirement and work
- Spouse or loved ones
- Income
- Status
- Friends
- Cognitive decline
- Home
- Independence
- Roles

Care of the older adult with mental illness has received some federal government attention with legislative regulation of both psychiatric treatment facilities and nursing homes. A high percentage of mental disorders are found among the residents of long-term care facilities. Specialized units and programs to address the needs of the mentally ill in these institutions have seen tremendous growth and are related to an increased focus on escalating inpatient hospital costs. Cost containment by Medicare, Medicaid, Health Maintenance Organizations (HMOs), and with mandates imposed by OBRA (Omnibus Budget Reconciliation Act of 1987) to regulate both pharmacologic and physical restraints have brought about the emergence of supportive community care. Nurses continue to have increasing roles of responsibility for the identification and assessment of needs, along with the care of older people experiencing mental disorders.

Obstacles to Mental Health Care for the Older Adult

Ageism is a commonly held belief that stereotypes and minimizes the worth of the aging person by indicating that senescence and mental health conditions are a part of the normal aging process. This promotes an assumption that older people are incompetent or senile and somehow an inferior segment of society. Discrimination in the form of limited access to the funds and services of mental health resources is shown by a reluctance to separate these disorders as abnormal and treatable in all age-groups. Unfortunately, many elderly people themselves accept as normal the coexistence of mental disorders and later life decline. Many symptoms are unreported by those who may see mental issues as a sign of weakness or loss of control, and there is also added fear of institutionalization. The person may be reluctant or unable to discuss

feelings or emotions, preventing recognition of the problem. The cost of mental health care is in itself a factor that often decreases the chances that the older adult will seek treatment. Limited income and existing medical and pharmacologic health care costs may also decrease the likelihood that mental health issues will be addressed.

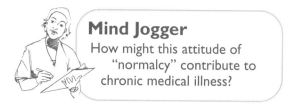

Cognitive Impairment

Impaired cognitive functioning implies that there is some measure of deterioration in a person's ability to perform the activities of daily living. The subtle mental decline attributed to the normal aging process is seldom evident in the day-to-day functioning of the older adult. Normal memory lapses such as misplacing an item, forgetting someone's name, or forgetting an appointment are considered typical as one ages. Changes may become more evident when there is an increase in anxiety produced by the need to perform under pressure. There is much variance among older adults and many continue to function at a very high level by compensating for their impairment with written reminders and lists. The greatest mental decreases with aging are seen in the areas of learning and retaining information. It is suggested that there is also some decline in abstract reasoning and complex problem-solving ability.

In contrast, cognitive impairment is a more defined problem centered on memory loss. There may be a significant loss in the ability to remember the content of what is read or descriptive details of what is seen or heard. Important events may be repeatedly forgotten. This degree of impairment is quite different from that seen in normal aging. Memory is the basis for our thinking processes. The loss of memory leaves the affected person unable to remember past experiences, which are used to make current decisions and judgments. The person is left in a state of confusion, unable to understand present experiences.

Cognitive Disorders

The term *cognitive disorders* has replaced the previously used terms of *organic brain* or *mental disorders.* In these disorders there is a noticeable change in cognition from the former level of functioning. This category of conditions includes delirium, dementia, and amnestic disorders. Underlying these disorders is a medical condition, a substance that may be a medication or toxin, or a combination of the two. In other words, there is an underlying cause for the altered cognitive state.

Delirium

Delirium is characterized by a disturbance of consciousness and a change in cognition that develop over a short time. The disorders in this category all present with a disturbance in level of awareness and cognitive functioning, but they may have different etiologies such as a medical condition, trauma, infections, medications, or a combination of factors. The most common underlying causes in older people are listed in At a Glance 18-2. Once the cause is determined and treated, the condition is usually reversed and improvement in the mental state is seen.

Common Signs and Symptoms. The pattern of delirium is progressive. The deterioration in the level of consciousness and cognitive functioning is evident in the client's behavior and inability to carry out previously routine activities of daily living. Delir-

At a Glance 18-2 Common Causes of Delirium in Older People	
Medical conditions	Systemic infections
	Metabolic disturbance
	Fluid and electrolyte imbalance
	Hepatic or renal disease
	Pathologic conditions of the brain
	Trauma
Substance induced	Medication toxicity
	Multiple drug interactions
Substance intoxication	High doses of narcotic drugs
	Alcohol
	Sedatives, hypnotics, or anxiolytics
Substance withdrawal	Abrupt discontinuation of any of the above drugs (any combination of pharmacologic or physical causes)

ium develops rapidly with symptoms that may fluctuate depending on the time of day. There is a decreased level of consciousness with impaired thinking, concentration, and awareness of the surrounding environment. Speech becomes incoherent and motor coordination or activity rapidly deteriorates. The person may experience hallucinations and

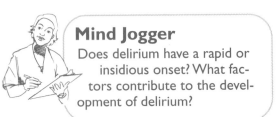

Mind Jogger
Does delirium have a rapid or insidious onset? What factors contribute to the development of delirium?

delusional thought processes. Appetite and sleep are disturbed as the mental decline continues.

Just the Facts

Perceptual disturbance may include hallucinations (e.g., seeing and talking to a dead parent), illusions (e.g., seeing intravenous tubing as a rope), or delusions (e.g., may see injection as a threat of harm).

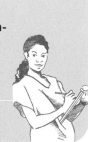

Just the Facts

Delirium is a disturbance in consciousness and cognition and occurs over a short period.

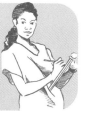

Incidence and Etiology. The symptoms may be caused by medical conditions, medications, substance toxicity or withdrawal, toxin exposure, or a combination of factors. Older adults are more at risk for delirium because of their higher incidence of chronic illness and their use of multiple medications to manage those disorders. The increased chance of hospitalization for acute infections, sepsis, and exacerbations of chronic illnesses such as congestive heart failure and chronic pulmonary disease adds to the risk. The combined use of both prescription and over-the-counter medications can contribute to the development of delirium. Significant risk factors for delirium are the body's decreased ability to metabolize and excrete drugs as the body ages, the smaller doses of some medications given to older people, and additional adverse drug reactions. In addition, other factors such as sensory deprivation, an altered sleep-wake cycle, and nutritional or fluid deficiencies can contribute to the onset of a delirious state.

Dementia

Because memory impairment is common to both delirium and dementia, it is necessary to recognize that a person with delirium can also have a preexisting dementia. One assessment that may help distinguish between them is that except in late dementia, most people with dementia alone are usually alert to the environment, whereas a person with delirium also has a disturbance in consciousness. This means that a person who is alert but disoriented and confused because of dementia may develop a deteriorating level of consciousness as a result of an acute state of delirium.

Dementia is characterized by irreversible, progressive declines in cognitive functioning, including a loss of memory, awareness, judgment, and reasoning ability. This decline in intellectual functioning is severe enough to interfere with a person's normal daily activities

Case Study: Bertha's Behavior Speaks

Bertha is an 86-year-old resident of the dementia unit in a nursing home facility. Her speech consists of irrational sentence fragments unrelated to any conversation directed to her. Her usual activity is ambulating down the corridor with her walker, going in and out of rooms at random. For the past 2 days, Bertha has resisted getting out of bed. She has been less responsive with few verbal utterances. Today the nurse finds her crying and restless. She has developed a fever and is shaking. The nurse notes a strong odor to the urine in the brief Bertha has been wearing. The nurse realizes that Bertha is unable to describe pain or the location of any discomfort.

What do the changes in Bertha's behavior indicate?

_____

_____

Describe how her behavior may be related to a problem.

_____

_____

_____

and ability to communicate or interact with others. There are different causes of dementia; Alzheimer's disease is the most common.

Just the Facts
Characteristics of Dementia
- Irreversible
- Progressive
- Loss of memory
- Loss of awareness
- Loss of judgment
- Loss of reasoning

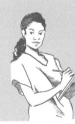

At a Glance 18-4 Other Conditions Associated with Dementia

- Pick's disease
- Trauma
- HIV disease
- Chronic drug/alcohol/nutritional abuse
- Brain tumors
- Huntington's disease
- Creutzfeldt-Jakob disease
- Parkinson's disease
- Multiple sclerosis
- Amyotrophic lateral sclerosis

Mind Jogger
How is dementia different from delirium?

Alzheimer's Type of Dementia

Alois Alzheimer, a German physician, first identified **Alzheimer's disease** in the early twentieth century. A female client in her fifties was described as having the signs of what appeared to be a mental illness. Following her death, an autopsy revealed this woman had dense deposits, or neuritic plaques, outside and around the nerve cells in her brain. Inside the cells were twisted strands of fiber, or neurofibrillary tangles. Today, a definite diagnosis of Alzheimer's disease is still only possible when an autopsy shows these classic signs of the disease.

Alzheimer's disease primarily affects the cerebral cortex, which is involved in conscious thought and language, the production of acetylcholine (a neurotransmitter involved in memory and learning), and the hippocampus, essential to memory storage. In the regions attacked by this disease, the neurons degenerate and lose their synaptic connections to other neurons.

Common Signs and Symptoms. As the neurons of the hippocampus degenerate, short-term memory fails. The ability to perform routine tasks begins to diminish. Once the disease progresses to the cerebral cortex, it begins to take away language and impairs judgment, leading to impulsive emotional outbursts and disturbing behaviors such as the wandering and agitation that are commonly seen in this disorder. The progression to remote memory loss leaves the person with the inability to recognize even close family members or to communicate in any meaningful way. In addition, there is a progressive, irreversible loss of memory that affects temporal and spatial orientation, abstract thinking, ability to carry out mathematical calculations, and capacity to learn new things or concepts. Personality changes lead to a diminished and lost sense of self as memory fades and with it the mental pictures that give meaning to one's life. Memories erode into small pieces that gradually disappear and are lost beyond recall.

Initially, the person may write down what they want to remember, and then forget to check the written reminder. There is difficulty encoding material to be recalled or an inability to make a connection between the meaning of the spoken word and words to be re-

membered. Early in the course of the disease, clients are usually aware of their memory deficit and try to compensate for their losses by using **confabulation** (filling in the gaps with fictitious statements), but increasingly they become frightened and anxious about the memory deficits and get discouraged. As the disease progresses, they lose insight into their memory loss and are no longer aware of it.

> ## Just the Facts
> Short-term (recent) memory: Remembering for a few minutes or hours
> Long-term (remote) memory: Remembering for a few years; memory is preserved

There is an inability to acquire and process new information—for example, a new house or address may not be recognized and the person shows up at a previous address. Language difficulties become more marked as the disease progresses. The problems related to language include:

Anomia—inability to find the right word (e.g., when shown a watch, the client may refer to it as a "timepiece," or referring to someone who has died, may say that the person is at the "resting place" or "sleeping place" instead of the cemetery).

Agnosia—inability to identify an object (e.g., the client may try to eat soup with a knife, eat the paper wrapper on a piece of candy, or attempt to shave with a toothbrush and toothpaste). This can also be sensory (e.g., unable to identify hot temperature [i.e., bath water], recognize the meaning of traffic lights, or recognize themselves in the mirror, thinking there is an intruder in the room).

Aphasia—impairment in the significance or meaning of language that prevents the person from understanding what is heard, following instructions, and communicating needs (e.g., the need to go to the bathroom or to communicate pain).

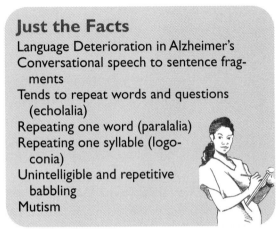

Just the Facts
Language Deterioration in Alzheimer's
Conversational speech to sentence fragments
Tends to repeat words and questions (echolalia)
Repeating one word (paralalia)
Repeating one syllable (logoconia)
Unintelligible and repetitive babbling
Mutism

Visual and special skills deteriorate, and the person may get lost while driving a car or walking. The person develops **apraxia,** or an inability to carry out purposeful movements and actions despite intact motor and sensory functioning. The person may try to water plants with a hose but is unable to connect the hose to the water faucet or is unable to transfer food from plate to mouth with silverware when trying to eat. The ability to use correct judgment or to make logical decisions is lost. Usually the first noticeable sign of this is a difficulty in managing finances and is often the deficit that leads families to seek medical attention. The person may pay bills twice or not pay bills, buy unnecessary items, make large charitable donations, or be unable to balance a checkbook.

In addition, there is evidence of self-neglect as the person shows carelessness and a lack of attention to appearance and dress. Layering of clothing and an unkempt appearance in one who was previously neat and well-groomed is typical. Personality and mood changes are noticeable as the person loses interest and energy for doing previously enjoyed activities. Depression is common, with decreasing interaction and social withdrawal. As the disease progresses, agitation and responses of fear and panic (both verbal and physical) may occur with a potential of harm to self and others, referred to as catastrophic events. These occurrences are often precipitated by frustration and a perceived threat or fear, often trivial in nature such as a change in routine or environment.

Behavior problems such as stubbornness, resistance to care, abusive language, acting out in response to hallucinations or delusions, or urinating in inappropriate places may occur. They tend to hide articles and develop a suspicion of others, thinking misplaced things have been stolen when the items cannot be found. There may also be increased restlessness that leads to rummaging, wandering, aimless walking (pacing), and interruption of the sleep-wake cycle. This behavior puts the person at risk for injury. Some persons exhibit a peak period of agitation and acting out behavior during the evening hours, which is sometimes referred to as **sundowning syndrome.**

In advanced dementia, the person may be totally unaware of his or her surroundings and require total and constant supervision and care. The people with this degree of impairment are at risk for accidents and infectious diseases that often lead to death. The three most common causes of death in the person with Alzheimer's are pneumonia, urinary tract infections, and infected decubitus ulcers. Clients live an average of 4 to 10 years,

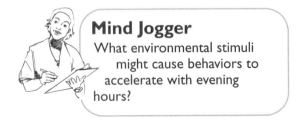

Mind Jogger
What environmental stimuli might cause behaviors to accelerate with evening hours?

At a Glance 18-5 Clinical Stages of Alzheimer's Disease

Stage	Duration	Characteristics
I. Mild	1–4 years	Poor short-term memory Unable to acquire new information (may have difficulty balancing a checkbook, preparing a complex meal, or remembering medication schedules) Mild anomia Personality changes Disorientation—may get lost Some decrease in judgment
II. Moderate	2–10 years	Significant memory loss Impaired judgment (difficulty with simple food preparation, housework or yard work, may require assistance with ADLs) Increased cognitive loss Anxiety, suspiciousness Agitation, depression Problems with sleeping Wandering or pacing Difficulty recognizing family or friends
III. Severe	8–12 years	Severe cognitive impairment Physical unsteadiness and loss of mobility (requires considerable assistance with personal care and ADLs; often chair or bed bound and dependent on others for care; may be mute) Total loss of speech Loss of appetite, weight loss Incontinence

although in some people, the duration from time of diagnosis to death may be as many as 20 years or more.

Incidence and Etiology. There is clearly a familial pattern with some forms of Alzheimer's disease. Some families exhibit an inherited pattern that suggests possible genetic transmission. There are studies that indicate that early-onset cases (those diagnosed before the age of 65 years) are more likely to be familial than late-onset cases. Estimates of the prevalence of dementia depends on how it is defined, but the incidence increases dramatically after the age of 75, with the risk doubling approximately every 5 years after age 65. More than half of the diagnosed cases of dementia can be attributed to Alzheimer's disease.

There is no cure for Alzheimer's disease. There are currently two medications that can sometimes delay the progression of the disease and symptoms (see At a Glance 18-6). Much research is being done to determine other approaches to the treatment of Alzheimer's disease. Support groups may be of help to spouses and family members who take care of the victims of this disease.

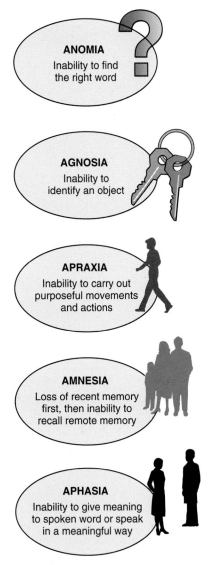

FIGURE 18-1. The five As of Alzheimer's disease.

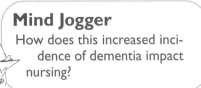

Mind Jogger

How does this increased incidence of dementia impact nursing?

At a Glance 18-6 Associated Signs and Symptoms of Alzheimer's Dementia

Confabulation
Short-term memory loss first—then remote
Decreasing ability to perform routine tasks
Hiding articles with inability to relocate them
Suspiciousness
Restlessness, rummaging, wandering, and pacing
Interruption of sleep-wake cycle
Language deterioration (anomia, aphasia)
Impaired judgment
Impulsive emotional outbursts (catastrophic events)
Inability to recognize family or friends
Inability to recognize familiar objects (agnosia)
Loss of spatial and temporal orientation
Loss of abstract thinking and mathematical concepts
Inability to learn anything new or encode incoming information
Personality changes
Inability to carry out purposeful movements (apraxia)
Stubbornness
Abusive language
Hallucinations and delusions
Eliminating in inappropriate places
Sundowning

Vascular Dementia

Vascular dementia is a condition caused by the effects of one or more strokes (cerebrovascular accident [CVA]) on cognitive functioning that is characterized by an abrupt onset and follows a steplike pattern of cerebrovascular disease and symptoms. The pattern of deficit is related to the portion of the brain that has been destroyed by the stroke. Some functions are affected while others may remain intact. Each step is accompanied by a decrease in cognitive functioning.

At a Glance 18-7 Medications Used in the Treatment of Alzheimer's Disease

- Tacrin hydrochloride (Cognex)
- Donepezil hydrochloride (Aricept)
  Both drugs inhibit the enzyme acetylcholinesterase in the CNS, increasing the level of acetylcholine. The drug may temporarily improve cognitive function in clients with Alzheimer's disease.
  Most common side effects:
  - Headache
  - Blurred vision
  - Insomnia
  - Nausea
  - Diarrhea
  - Urinary frequency
  - Muscle cramps
  - Urticaria
  - Dizziness
- Antipsychotic medications such as risperidone (Risperdal) and haloperidol (Haldol) may be used to decrease verbal and physical aggressiveness.
- Other alternative therapy methods are currently being studied to determine their effectiveness.

At a Glance 18-8 Associated Signs and Symptoms in Vascular Dementia

- Series of strokes (CVAs)
- History of hypertension or cerebrovascular disease
- Hemiplegia or weakness of extremities
- Gait disturbances
- Steplike cognitive decline
- Exaggerated reflexes
- Foot drop
- Inability to control emotions
- Aphasia
- Apraxia
- Agnosia
- Decreased thought processing
- Hallucinations and delusions

Common Signs and Symptoms. In the early stages, personality and insight tend to be better preserved than in the client with Alzheimer's disease. Depression is common as the condition advances. Neurologic symptoms such as hemiplegia, abnormal reflexes, gait disturbances, and uncontrollable emotional responses may develop as a result of the cerebral infarcts. The person may laugh or cry without a stimulus that would cause the response. There are multiple cognitive deficits such as aphasia, apraxia, agnosia, and the inability to organize thought processes.

Incidence and Etiology. The onset of vascular dementia may occur any time in the older adult but is less common after age 75. The initial onset is typically earlier than the onset of Alzheimer's disease. The two types of dementia can coexist in the same person. Vascular dementia tends to be more common in men than in women. The incidence of this form of dementia is much lower than that of the Alzheimer's type.

Depression and Dementia

Although not categorized as a cognitive disorder, studies show that depression is the most common mental disorder in the older population. Depression is categorized as a mood disorder (see Chapter 10) that can occur in any age-group. In the older adult, the cognitive deficits of depression tend to be nonprogressive and inconsistent with the degree of those found in dementia. Depression often accompanies the early stages of dementia, particularly in Alzheimer's disease. The person still has the mental ability to understand that something is happening, that memory lapses are occurring, and that they are unable to do things that previously were easily accomplished. These disturbing changes naturally lead the person to feelings of loss, decreased self-worth, hopelessness, and depression. These feelings can lead the person to thoughts that life is not worth living. The depression can actually intensify the effects of the disease. It is important to recognize these feelings in the early stages of dementia when the person still may have the ability to carry out a plan for suicide.

As many of the symptoms found in depression are also characteristic of dementia, it may easily go unrecognized. Changes in appetite, changes in sleep patterns, and loss of energy and initiative are common to both disorders. The person may demonstrate other symptoms such as withdrawal from others, self-neglect, and feelings of failure, inadequacy, helplessness, and powerlessness. The diagnostic work-up for all dementia of the AD type includes testing for depression. Usually when asked questions, the depressed person will answer with, "I don't know," indicating a lack of energy to formulate an answer, whereas the demented person will attempt to answer, demonstrating the existing mental deficits.

Risk factors for the development of depression in the early stages of dementia include a previous depressive episode or a very achievement-oriented lifestyle. Difficult family situations or financial strain may also precipitate depressive symptoms such as sadness and emptiness, which may be reinforced by a coexisting dementia. If the existence of depression is determined, it is important that treatment be initiated, because this can lead to improvement in the person's overall functioning. The most effective treatment in the older adult is a combination of antidepressant medication and various psychotherapeutic approaches. Nursing observations related to antidepressant therapy should take into consideration the age-related physiologic changes that slow the body's response and the elimination of drugs in older people. It is also important to monitor for the many side effects caused by these agents and to report and document any adverse effects. Elderly persons may experience negative effects that may worsen other existing conditions.

In addition, it is common for caregivers to experience signs of depression. The constant demands of the unpredictable behaviors in the demented person take their toll on the caregiver. The burden increases as an attempt is made to balance this schedule with other family responsibilities. Communication with family and friends may become strained or minimal as the caregiver becomes increasingly protective and isolated. Programs such as support groups can allow the caregiver to express feelings that are shared by others in the group. These groups can also provide information and suggestions for dealing with the problem behaviors and the frustration or fear that may accompany them.

At a Glance 18-9 Resources for More Information

- Alzheimer's Association: (800) 272-3900 or http://www.alz.org
- National Institute on Aging—Alzheimer's Disease Education and Referral Center: (800) 438-4380 or http://www.nih.gov/nia

---

Amnestic Disorders

According to the *DSM-IV-TR,* the **amnestic disorders** are characterized by a disturbance in memory that is due to either the direct physiologic effects of a general medical condition or trauma, the persisting effects of a substance, or effects not otherwise specified.

Common Signs and Symptoms. In amnestic disorders, the person has difficulty learning new information (short-term or recent memory) and is unable to recall previously learned information or past events (long-term or remote memory). The memory impairment must be severe enough to cause a distinct decline from a previous level of functioning in social or occupational situations. Confabulation, or filling in the gaps with imaginary events, is common early in the disease process.

These disorders differ from dementia in that there is no impairment in abstract thinking or judgment. The person may be disoriented to place and time, but rarely to person. There are usually no personality changes, although there may be apathy and emotional dullness.

The onset of symptoms may be acute or insidious, depending on the underlying pathology. The course of the illness may be unpredictable, and treatment will be determined by the cause of the manifesting symptoms.

At a Glance 18-10 **Associated Signs and Symptoms of Amnestic Disorders**

- Impaired ability to learn new information
- Unable to recall previously learned information
- Impaired social or occupational functioning
- Confabulation
- Disorientation to place and time, but rarely to person
- Apathy and emotional dullness

Incidence and Etiology. The amnestic disorders typically occur as a result of trauma, surgery, hypoxia, or other pathologic conditions affecting the brain. Age of onset and incidence are variable, depending on the cause.

Application of the Nursing Process for Delirium

Nursing Assessment

It is crucial to determine the cause of **disorientation** and mental decline. Sometimes it is a combination of sensory loss (e.g., hearing loss) and an unfamiliar environment such as hospitalization for an elderly person, sometimes there is a related mental disorder (such

as dementia), and other times there is an underlying physical or medical condition. When sensory factors are assessed as an issue, a simple adjustment of lighting or checking the battery in a hearing aid may be all that is needed to resolve the problem. In the case of physical causes, prompt detection and treatment is imperative to restoring mental function.

Assessment will include a complete history and physical examination. Nurses play a major role in obtaining information. If the client is unable to provide information, it may be acquired from family members or others who may be aware of the person's health history and circumstances leading up to the current disorder. A list of current medications should be obtained so that the possibility of medication toxicity or interaction can be determined. Treatment and nursing intervention will depend on the precipitating factors. When considering the assessment data, the nurse should also consider the person's baseline physical condition or previous level of functioning.

Nursing Diagnosis

Although each situation of delirium may differ, some commonalities exist in caring for the client with an acute deteriorating mental state. Nursing diagnoses to address the problems may include:

- Risk for injury or potential for violence
- Altered thought processes or acute confusion
- Self-care deficit
- Sensory-perceptual alterations
- Fear
- Sleep pattern disturbance
- Nutrition: altered, risk for less than body requirements
- Knowledge deficit

Expected Outcomes

Once problems are identified, the planning of realistic outcomes will depend on the individual problems. Outcomes for the client may include:

- Remains safe from harm or injury
- Accurately states time, place, person, situation
- Meets basic needs and independently performs ADL
- Responds appropriately to incoming stimuli
- Identifies the fear and focuses on eliminating or reducing the source
- Is free of signs of sleep deprivation
- Regains or maintains ideal body weight for height and age
- Demonstrates understanding of current health problems

Nursing Interventions

Most clients with delirium will be cared for in the acute care setting. In providing nursing care for the client, the nurse must carry out all interventions to ensure that permanent brain damage or death is avoided. Because the course of delirium is short and critical, plans of care and goals are short term, and the focus of the medical and nursing teams should be directed toward correcting the underlying problem. Nursing interventions will be directed toward the acute phase of the illness. Those specific for the delirious state may include:

- Monitor level of consciousness for further deterioration or improvement.
- Reduce environmental noise.
- Provide regular verbal, visual, or tactile stimulation.
- Provide glasses or hearing aids to facilitate orientation.
- Place family photographs or favorite objects within view.
- Provide a nightlight.
- Reorient client to date, time, and place.
- Explain all procedures and what is happening to the client.
- Initiate safety precautions.

Evaluation

Evaluation of the effectiveness of the care plan will be based on the degree to which successful reversal of the underlying problem is accomplished. Although most people with delirium will have a full recovery, this likelihood decreases in older people. Many older clients will develop delirium during a hospital stay because of existing medical conditions that increase their risk of complications. There is an increase in the morbidity rate associated with this risk.

Application of the Nursing Process for Dementia

Nursing Assessment

Assessment data for the client with dementia should include a past health and medication history. Asking the client questions or reviewing the current level of functioning with family members may help the nurse to obtain data concerning recent and remote memory loss. Other assessment information to obtain includes:

- Disorientation
- Mood changes, feelings of hopelessness
- Fear and frustration level—develops as the person is unable to give meaning to incoming sensory messages and leads to agitation and catastrophic reactions
- Inability to concentrate—leads to pacing behaviors
- Suspiciousness, agitation, or aggressive behaviors
- Self-care deficit
- Inappropriate social behavior—public disrobing or sexual behaviors such as masturbation
- Level of mobility, wandering or pacing behaviors
- Judgment ability—safety becomes a major concern

- Sleep disturbance—sleep more often for shorter periods of time
- Speech or language impairment
- Hallucinations, illusions, or delusions
- Bowel and bladder incontinence
- Apathy (flatness of gestures, tone of voice, facial expression)
- Recognition of family members, child, or spouse (may have difficulty deciding to whom feelings should be directed)
- Any decline in nutritional status
- Sensory needs and limitations

Identify the primary caregiver, support systems, and the knowledge base of the family members. The role of caregiver to the demented person is a difficult, stressful, and time-consuming task. A spouse or adult children most often assume this role. It is important for the nurse to actively listen to the feelings and concerns of the family members. The demented person is dependent on the caregiver and often will be reassured and calmed by his or her presence. However, caregivers often feel overwhelmed by the responsibility imposed by the disease as it progresses and may be increasingly isolated as the demented person continues to decline. Words cannot describe the emotional devastation of this disease on the caregiver and family as the one they love vanishes one day at a time. The nurse can assist in locating support groups and respite care (programs to temporarily relieve the burden of primary care giving) alternatives for the family.

Nursing Diagnosis

The problems of caring for the client with dementia are many. Each person must be viewed from the perspective of his or her own particular situation and the losses that are evident and continuous in the person's decline. Nursing diagnoses that may be applicable to the situation may include:

- Anxiety, related to accumulative losses
- Coping ineffective, individual, related to frustration and fear

- Risk for injury, related to wandering behaviors and disorientation
- Risk for violence, self-directed or directed at others, related to agitation
- Altered thought processes, related to hallucinations or delusions
- Self-care deficit, related to cognitive loss
- Sensory-perceptual alterations, related to agnosia
- Self-esteem disturbance, related to hopelessness and losses
- Nutrition altered: less than body requirements, related to decreased appetite
- Confusion, acute or chronic, related to cognitive losses
- Social isolation, related to anomia and agnosia
- Communication impaired, verbal, related to anomia and aphasia
- Sleep pattern disturbance, related to loss of time orientation
- Caregiver role strain, related to dependent state of the victim
- Family processes, altered, related to caregiving roles

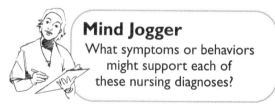

Mind Jogger
What symptoms or behaviors might support each of these nursing diagnoses?

Expected Outcomes

Once problems are identified, the planning of realistic outcomes will depend on the individual problems. Outcomes for the client may include:

- Demonstrates decreased anxiety levels
- Remains safe and free from injury
- Does not harm self or others
- Experiences minimal catastrophic reactions
- Maintains participation in self-care activities
- Remains oriented at level of ability

- Follows scheduled routine of activity and rest
- Feels valued and accepted

A final outcome is that the caregiver and family will identify and utilize community support systems.

Nursing Interventions

Perhaps one of the most important aspects of caring for the person with dementia is communication. Both verbal and nonverbal approaches must be adapted to the limited ability the demented person has to understand what is being said or the intended meaning.

- Use touch, eye contact, nonhurried movements, a smile, or a pleasant affect.
- Speak clearly, softly, and slowly using short simple words and sentences—a raised voice will trigger agitation.
- Identify yourself and call the person by name at each meeting.
- Avoid questions that challenge memory—instead of asking the person who a relative is, tell them the relative's name.
- Focus on one piece of information at a time.
- Use gestures or cues to accompany speech or commands.
- Use face-to-face contact.
- Repeat questions or commands exactly as they were first stated—saying them another way adds another challenge.
- Validate at the client's level of functioning—this helps the client to cope with feelings of loss.
- Ask questions and comments that allow the client to remember or reminisce on subjects that have emotional meaning for the client. Do not argue or disagree with what the client is saying. When the client is delusional, acknowledge his or her feelings and reinforce reality or divert attention to another issue.
- Recognize the client's feelings and redirect attention to another subject that is pleasant if a client becomes verbally aggressive.

- Keep clocks, pictures, calendars in view to help the client identify with reality.
- Play soft music, which has a soothing effect, or the television can be turned on without sound. Misleading stimuli such as excess noise or television can produce agitation—programs are often too confusing or move too fast.
- Cover mirrors to minimize the illusion that an intruder is in the room, because the client may no longer recognize self in a mirror.

As dementia advances, the ability to independently carry out the steps of self-care is diminished. Nursing interventions that may support the client's self-care deficit include:

- Allow client time to perform those tasks he or she is able to do.
- Assist with dressing—minimize the choices by selecting items of clothing. Different color items help the client to separate socks from pants, for example. Avoid tight clothing or complicated zippers and fasteners—Velcro fasteners decrease frustration with laces and buttons.
- Use step-by-step instructions, cueing as necessary.
- Try again later if client resists care—he or she may forget the issue in a few minutes.
- Maintain a consistent routine or schedule with the same caregivers as much as possible. This will promote calmness and decrease agitation.
- Use tub baths—many clients with dementia are frightened by the falling water of a shower on their skin.
- Use a same-sex person to bathe the client, which is sometimes accepted better by the client.
- Bathe the client at the time the client is accustomed to bathing (day vs. evening).
- Provide rest periods between activities—fatigue produces negative behaviors.
- Use a bed closer to the floor to prevent serious injury when ataxia is present.

Most clients with dementia will have weight loss. Nursing interventions related to maintaining adequate nutritional intake may include:

- Monitor intake of food and fluids.
- Provide finger foods that can be eaten while pacing—make sandwiches out of meat, vegetables, or fruit.
- Set one item or bowl of food in front of the client at a time—too many choices may be overwhelming and result in refusal to eat.
- Face the person if feeding—Alzheimer's tends to decrease peripheral vision and a side approach may frighten the client.
- Prevent the client from eating nonfood items such as napkins, food wrappers, or plants.
- Offer between-meal snacks.
- Consider a mechanical alteration in food consistency as the disease progresses, because swallowing may be impaired.

As dementia progresses, the ability to locate the bathroom and follow through with the steps of toileting is lost. The person may become incontinent with little recognition that urination or defecation has occurred. The nurse can best assist the demented client by doing the following:

- Label the bathroom door with a picture or large-print wording.
- Assist with clothing fasteners—simplify clothing (e.g., using pants with an elastic waist).
- Use toileting schedules.
- Watch the client for nonverbal messages such as fidgeting with pants, increased pacing, or going in and out of doors.

When a catastrophic reaction is occurring, distraction and redirection are the most useful interventions. It is important for the nurse not to overreact, as this may increase the intensity of the situation. Remember, the demented person is unable to control the behavior but will quickly forget the incident if allowed time to do so. It is important to intervene to prevent injury to the person or others. Nursing observations should be made as to *who* is involved in the incident (do certain persons tend to trigger the behavior), *what* is going on in the environment at the time of the

Case Study: Confusion in Motion

Patty is a 74-year-old woman who worked as a hotel custodian. She is constantly pacing the hallway with a broom, sweeping the floor as she goes. Patty has lost 14 pounds in the 3 months since her admission to the nursing home. She is unable to sit at the table long enough to eat her meals and resumes her constant walking after eating only a few bites.

Perform a nursing assessment of Patty's nutritional problem.

_____

_____

_____

What approaches could be used to address the problem and achieve the anticipated outcome?

_____

_____

incident, *where* the incidents tend to occur (does one location precipitate the behavior more than others), *when* the person tends to become more agitated (is there a particular time of day when the incidents reoccur), and *why* the person might be responding with agitation (e.g., pain, infection, uncomfortable clothing, incontinence).

Mind Jogger

What type of situation might cause a catastrophic response?

Just the Facts

Key areas of concern in the care of the person with dementia include communication, self-care deficit, nutrition, safety, fatigue, and confusion.

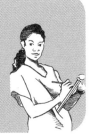

Evaluation

Outcomes for persons with dementia must be considered on a day-to-day and moment-to-moment basis, because their behavior is a response to the immediate world around them. The most important thing that caregivers can do is provide a safe environment and protection from injury. The nursing interventions suggested here allow clients to participate in self-care to the extent of their ability. With the assistance of caregivers and nursing personnel in controlling the environment, the person is helped to control the impulsive aggressive actions precipitated by frustration and confusion. Reassurance and calm is encouraged by consistency and simple, routine day-to-day activities. The nurse's reflection and evaluation of what works and what does not work with each client will promote a more

positive outcome to a very devastating situation. In addition, it is anticipated that the caregiver will understand the disease process and demonstrate adaptive coping strategies in dealing with the stress of the caregiver role.

Summary

Aging is an inevitable part of life in which changes occur that may have natural causes or be imposed by environmental and societal factors. Many senior adults continue to live active and viable lives beyond the retirement age, whereas others are restricted by decreased income and limitations imposed by chronic illness. With age comes the reality of loss in ways that may present the elderly person with emotional hurdles that are difficult to confront. Although some older persons may have conditioned coping adaptability, others may encounter difficulty in meeting these mental challenges. The aging person is often unaware of the signs that indicate a need for professional help in dealing with the psychologic issues. The lack of resources available to allow treatment of mental disorders in this segment of the population further discourages older adult from seeking help.

Although some cognitive decline is probable as one ages, it is subtle and causes few complications for the person. In contrast, cognitive impairment leads to a significant memory loss and a decline in the ability to perform activities of daily living. The three most common causes of cognitive impairment are delirium, dementia, and amnestic disorders. Delirium is marked by a sudden onset of a disturbance of consciousness and follows a short and critical course. In most cases, with treatment of the underlying cause, this disorder is reversible. Treatment is dependent on the cause, with the goal being to restore a previous level of functioning. Many elderly people develop delirium as a complication of an existing medical problem, which leads to a decrease in the likelihood of a full recovery.

In contrast, dementia is characterized by a deterioration in cognitive functioning that is irreversible and progressive, leaving the person with only a shadow of past experiences. Alzheimer's disease is the most common form of dementia. This is a condition that develops slowly; its destructive process leaves the person with an inability to recognize what once were familiar objects, functions, and people. Personality and mood changes accompany a loss of interest and energy in previously enjoyed activities. Behavior problems arise out of the fear and confusion the person is faced with as he or she attempts to cope with stimuli that are not understood. In advanced dementia, the person may be totally unaware of the environment and require constant care.

Nursing interventions should be directed at providing for the safety and basic needs of the person. Use of simple one-step commands in a stable and consistent environment provides a milieu that offers security and comfort to the demented person and promotes an optimal response. Excessive or misunderstood stimuli lead to fear, which in turn may result in outbursts or catastrophic events. These are best managed by a calm approach, using redirection and refocusing of the person's attention.

The symptoms of depression are often seen in the person with dementia. However, it is important to recognize the existence of depression in many older adults who are not demented. Because these two disorders have similar symptoms, a diagnostic work-up is essential to distinguish between the two conditions. Treatment usually leads to improvement in the cognitive level and overall functioning of the person.

It is important for the nurse to make assessments that provide a database from which applicable nursing diagnoses can be formulated. Plans of care should focus on providing a reasonable and measurable outcome. Nursing interventions are directed at maximizing the functional ability of the person with cognitive impairment. Whether the impairment be delirium or dementia, it is the responsibility of the nurse to initiate actions that, to whatever degree possible, improve the quality of the person's life and that of family members.

Bibliography

American Psychiatric Association (2000). *Diagnostic and statistical manual of mental disorders text revision* (4th ed.). Washington, DC: American Psychiatric Association.

Alzheimer's Disease (Revised 1997). Medical Library, American Psychiatric Association, Washington, D.C. (2:1:1997). Available at http://www.psych.org/public_info/alzheim.pdf. Accessed on July 12, 2004.

Federal Interagency Forum on Aging-Related Statistics (2000). *Older Americans 2000.* Washington, DC: National Institute of Health.

Fowles, D. G., & Greenberg, S. (2001). *A profile of older Americans:2001.* Administration on Aging, U.S. Department of Health and Human Services. Available at http://aoa.gov/prof/statistics/profile/2003.asp. Accessed on July 12, 2004.

Glass, R. M. (2001). JAMA patient page: Alzheimer's disease, *JAMA, 286,* 2194.

Greutzner, H. (1992). *Alzheimer's—A caregiver's guide and sourcebook.* New York, NY: John Wiley & Sons.

McNeil, C. (1995). Alzheimer's disease: Unraveling the mystery, National Institute on Aging/National Institute of Health. Available at http://www.alzheimers.org/unraveling/index.htm. Accessed on July 12, 2004.

National Council on Aging, Facts about older Americans (2002). Available at http://206.112.84.147/content.cfm?sectionID=106. Accessed on July 12, 2004.

Smyer, M. A., & Qualls, S. H. (1999). *Aging and mental health.* London: Blackwell Publishers, Inc.

FILL IN THE BLANK

Fill in the blank with the correct answer.

1. Changes that occur in the aging person as a result of genetics or natural factors are referred to as _____ aging.

2. Those changes that occur as a result of environmental influences are called _____ aging.

3. The most common causes of cognitive impairment are _____, _____, and _____.

4. Delirium is characterized by a change in _____ and a change in cognition that occur in a _____ period of time.

5. An altered response to the effects of medication is seen in older people because of the decreased ability of the body to _____.

6. Dementia is characterized by mental decline that is _____ and _____.

7. The three most common causes of death in the person with Alzheimer's dementia are _____, _____, and _____.

8. Periods of agitation in the client with Alzheimer's disease are referred to as _____.

MATCHING

Match the following terms to the most appropriate phrase.

a. Inability to carry out purposeful movement

b. Repetitive verbalization of one word

c. Inability to understand what is heard

d. Filling in the gaps with fictitious statements

e. Inability to find the right word

f. Repeating words or questions

g. Inability to identify an object

h. Repeating one syllable

1. _____ Confabulation

2. _____ Paralalia

3. _____ Anomia

4. _____ Echolalia

5. _____ Apraxia

6. _____ Logoconia

7. _____ Agnosia

8. _____ Aphasia

MULTIPLE CHOICE

Select the best answer from the multiple-choice items.

1. Hosea, a client diagnosed with Alzheimer's dementia, goes into the bathroom. As he glances in the mirror, he pulls up his pants and wanders back into the dayroom where he urinates in the trash can. This is an example of:
   a. Amnesia
   b. Anomia
   c. Agnosia
   d. Apraxia

2. Hosea's behavior is most likely related to:

   a. Anxiety created by an illusion that someone else is in the bathroom.

   b. Inability to remember why he is in the bathroom.

   c. Failure to recognize the purpose of the commode.

   d. Difficulty in managing his clothing to facilitate using the bathroom.

3. The nurse is caring for a client who is diagnosed with delirium related to urosepsis. Which of the following would correctly describe the course of this cognitive disorder?

   a. Progressive

   b. Insidious onset

   c. Reversible

   d. Long-term

4. Lilly is telling her family about her trip to the doctor yesterday afternoon. Although she is ill, she is unable to recall the reason for the visit and states she just needed some papers filled out. Which of the following describes Lilly's behavior?

   a. Anomia

   b. Confabulation

   c. Sundowning

   d. Logoconia

5. The nurse is feeding a nursing home resident who is diagnosed with Alzheimer's dementia. As the nurse attempts to place a spoonful of food in the resident's mouth, the resident says, "I don't want it, I don't want it, I don't want it." The term referring to this level of spoken language is:

   a. Babbling

   b. Paralalia

   c. Logoconia

   d. Echolalia

6. The nurse prepares to administer oral medication to Max, an elderly client with Alzheimer's disease. As the nurse attempts to put the tablets in his mouth, Max curses and strikes the nurse's hand. The nurse's best choice of action at this time would be to:

   a. Explain to Max that the medications are to help him get better.

   b. Leave Max alone and give the medication at a later time.

   c. Omit the dose and document the medication as refused.

   d. Call the physician and report the incident.

7. The nurse asks Mary, a client with dementia, to sit down so her shoestrings can be retied. Mary looks blankly at the nurse and continues to pace. How can the nurse best help Mary to understand this command?

   a. Repeat the command using different words to explain what is meant.

   b. Explain why it is important to keep her shoestrings tied.

   c. Guide her to a chair and point to the chair seat while telling her to sit.

   d. Allow her to pace and retie the shoestring when she sits down on her own.

8. Daisy has sustained several lacerations and bruises from falling as she gets out of bed and attempts to ambulate to the bathroom. With a memory deficit, Daisy does not remember verbal reminders to call for help when she needs to go to the bathroom. Which of the following nursing interventions would be the best approach to provide for her safety?

   a. Provide a bed closer to the floor.

   b. Provide a bedside commode.

   c. Place full side rails on the bed.

   d. Ask the doctor for a sedative at bedtime.

SEEK AND FIND

Find the incorrect information in the following statements.

1. Vascular dementia is characterized by a progressive decline in cognitive functioning.

2. In the patient with delirium, the symptoms develop with an insidious onset.

3. The depressed client will usually respond to questions asked by attempting to answer the question demonstrating the existing mental deficits.

4. The client with an amnesic disorder has difficulty learning new informaton and recalling previously learned information, along with an impairment in abstract thinking and judgment.

SCENARIO I: ANNIE'S DECLINE

Lately, Annie has been coming to the senior citizen center with unmatched earrings and shoes without hose. The supervisor of the center has been concerned about the obvious change in Annie's appearance. One day when Annie is delivering her assigned meals, she walks into the school where she taught and tells the secretary, "I don't know where I need to go with this food." When the center is advised of the situation, the supervisor remembers that several people on Annie's route have reported that they have not been receiving their meals. However, when she asks Annie about this, Annie states she must "have left them at another house by mistake." Realizing that there is a problem, the supervisor notifies Annie's daughter, Katy, of the situation. She arranges a visit to her mother's house the next day. She finds piles of unopened mail and bills with notices of nonpayment. There are spoiled food items in the refrigerator and soiled laundry is piled in a corner of the bathroom. Katy realizes something is very wrong with her mother and brings her to

the clinic for evaluation. After a diagnostic work-up, Annie is given a diagnosis of probable dementia, Alzheimer's type.

What assessment data would the nurse use to support a nursing diagnosis of risk for injury?

_____

_____

Katy feels that her mother can no longer continue to live independently and chooses to admit Annie to a nursing home. Annie does not understand why she has to be there, crying and saying she needs to go—"I have to feed the hungry children."

What would be the best nursing approach to Annie at this time?

_____

_____

Annie begins to take food items from the plates of other clients, stating they have stolen "her food." She becomes physically aggressive if they are taken away from her.

The nurse's best approach to Annie when she is removing the food is

_____

_____

How can distraction and redirection be used when Annie becomes agitated?

_____

_____

SCENARIO 2: HIDDEN MESSAGES

Frank is a 67-year-old resident of a special dementia unit of a long-term care facility. His family admitted him following an incident in which he drove a neighbor's car to the interstate and proceeded to enter an exit access going the wrong direction. Several vehicles were forced into the median to avoid an accident. He was eventually stopped by police officers who informed his wife, Ruth, that arrangements would have to be made for his safety.

Frank owns a construction business and told the police officers he was "going to work," although he had been unable to work for the past 3 years because of diagnosed early-onset Alzheimer's dementia. Since admission to the nursing home facility, Frank paces the halls, pulling on hand rails, doorknobs, and window casings. He repeatedly runs his hands over all door hinges and latches, kicks the wall and doors, and moves furniture around in the rooms. Frank wears a sock on his left foot, but refuses to wear shoes. He becomes agitated and strikes out with a fisted hand if any attempt is made to put a sock or shoe on the right foot. Frank will only take a bath if Ruth is present. He becomes physically aggressive when nursing personnel try to attend to his hygiene needs unless she is talking to him. The staff has placed pictures of Ruth on several doors in his room and in the shower room hoping to give him a feeling of security with her perceived presence. Ruth comes to the facility several times each day to help with her husband's care.

What may be the precipitating factor in Frank's aggressive behavior?

_____

_____

What methods can the nurse use to deal with the behavior?

_____

_____

What purpose do the pictures serve for Frank?

_____

_____

It is noted that Frank is limping with limited weight bearing on his right foot. An order is received for an x-ray that reveals a comminuted fracture of the third metatarsal. Calcification surrounding the fracture indicates the injury occurred several weeks ago, and it is decided to allow calcification to continue and not to intervene surgically at this point.

How is this injury affecting Frank's behavior?

_____

What approach can the nurse use to help Frank with the pain he does not understand?

_____

What nursing approaches may be used to relieve some of the caregiver strain for Ruth?

_____

_____

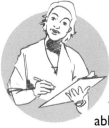

LEARNING OBJECTIVES

After learning the content in this chapter, the student will be able to:

1. Identify the function of psychopharmacology in the psychotherapeutic treatment regimen.
2. Name five classes of psychotropic drug agents.
3. Associate drug actions with uses in treating psychiatric disorders.
4. Identify side effects, therapeutic dosages, and contraindications of psychotropic medications.
5. Discuss effects of psychotropic agents in older people.
6. Describe nursing interventions and responsibilities in the administration of psychotropic agents.
7. Identify criteria for evaluating a therapeutic outcome for anti-anxiety, antidepressant, and antipsychotic drugs.
8. Describe guidelines for monitoring psychotropic drug therapy.
9. Develop a client teaching plan for psychopharmacologic agents.

CHAPTER

19

Psycho-pharmacology

KEY TERMS

Acetylcholine
Akathisia
Antidepressant
Antimanic
Antipsychotic
Anxiolytic
Dystonia
Extrapyramidal
Monoamine oxidase inhibitor (MAOI)
Neuroleptic malignant syndrome
Neurotransmitter
Postsynaptic receptors
Presynaptic compartment
Psychotropic
Reuptake
Serotonin
SSRIs
Synaptic cleft
Tardive dyskinesia

Pharmacologic Agents and Mental Illness

Psychiatric disorders that result in changes of cognition, mood, and behavior are historic and common among all societies of the globe. Throughout history, there are documented efforts at treating these disorders using drugs and various approaches in psychotherapy. Early pharmacotherapy used plants, mineral salts, and herbs. Today, the major approach to the treatment of psychiatric disorders is the use of psychotherapeutic drugs used in conjunction with psychotherapy. In most disorders a combination of the two is required to maintain stability of the client. The actual causes of most disorders have not been identified. However, regardless of the etiology, the psychiatric disorders are considered medical illnesses. Research studies of people with psychiatric symptoms demonstrate a pattern of both genetic and environmental factors that predispose a person to the development of the illness.

Medically, the disorders tend to present in an aggregate of symptoms often referred to as a *syndrome*. Much as a group of symptoms characterize the illnesses such as diabetes or gastroesophageal reflux, the symptoms of the psychiatric disorders are recognizable and linked to the particular disorders as described by the *DSM-IV-TR*. The most common symptoms fall into the following categories:

- Mood alterations
- Irritability and anxiety
- Altered thought processes
- Misperceptions of the environment
- Impaired and illogical communication or interaction patterns
- Disorientation and confusion

Since the 1950s, the development of psychopharmaceuticals has provided symptomatic relief for many people. These drug agents have provided a sense of normalcy for many clients with altered feelings, perceptions, and thinking. The use of psychotropic medications has also expanded our understanding of how the brain and mind are affected by the psychiatric disorders. **Psychotropic** agents are drugs that affect psychic function, behavior, or experience. These drugs do not cure or resolve the underlying problem. Rather, they are used in combination with counseling and other therapeutic modalities to reduce the disabling symptoms and promote restoration of a manageable and functional level of existence.

Psychotropic drug agents have their primary effect on neurotransmitter systems of the body. **Neurotransmitters** are the chemical messenger proteins stored in the **presynaptic compartment** located before the nerve synapse. There are many types of neurotransmitters that combine with individual receptors of the body. Once the neurotransmitter is mobilized into the **synaptic cleft**—the space between two neurons—it will continue to activate a response in the postsynaptic receptor until it is inactivated. Neurotransmitters can be inactivated either by enzymatic action or by **reuptake.** In the case of reuptake, the neurotransmitters are absorbed back into the presynaptic compartment of the previous neuron. Some drugs, such as the antiparkinson agents, cause the release of neurotransmitters **(acetylcholine)**, whereas others, such as the antipsychotic agent clozapine, interfere with the binding of chemical messengers to the intended receptors in the brain. Lithium carbonate, a drug used in the treatment of bipolar disorders, accelerates the destruction of monoamine neurotransmitters (dopamine, norepinephrine, and serotonin), inhibits their release, and decreases the sensitivity of **postsynaptic receptors.** These receptors, which bind with the drug, are located in the neuron distal to the synapse. The understanding of these processes has contributed to the development of psychotropic agents. The drugs are effective because they either enhance or decrease the brain's ability to use a specific neurotransmitter, a deficiency or excess of which is linked to the mental disorder. (See At a Glance 19-1.)

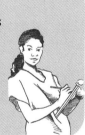

All drugs do not penetrate the brain cells equally. The chemical property known as *lipid-solubility* is a major determinant of a drug's molecular infusion into the brain tissue. The selectivity of the barrier between the blood and the brain further protects the brain by regulating the extent to which the drug penetration can occur. Drugs such as alcohol, heroin, and diazepam have high lipid solubility and are readily absorbed into the cerebral cells through the blood-brain barrier, increasing their potential for abuse. By the same token, the rate at which a medicinal agent is absorbed affects its efficacy. Scientists continue to study the specific effects of individual psy-chotropic drugs on psychologic processes and the use of these drugs in treating psychiatric disorders.

Classification of Psychotropic Drug Agent

Most drugs used to treat psychiatric disorders fall into the following categories:

- Antianxiety agents
- Antidepressants
- Antimanic agents
- Antipsychotic agents
- Antiparkinson (anticholinergic) agents

Each class of drugs is discussed according to their desired effect, side effects, adverse effects, normal dosage ranges, and related nursing responsibilities or interventions.

Antianxiety Agents

Current antianxiety medications **(anxiolytics)** were preceded by studies involving the calming effects of alcohol on the level of discomfort caused by anxiety. The effects of alcohol are limited by its rapid metabolism by the body, the tendency for tolerance to develop, and the tendency for rebound anxiety to occur. Researchers have attempted to find chemical agents that will produce the calming effects without the toxic and addictive qualities of alcohol. In the 1950s, drugs chemically related to the barbiturates were developed and remain in existence. Their use, however, has been replaced by a more popular group of drugs known as the benzodiazepines. The earliest were Librium (chlordiazepoxide) and Valium (diazepam); they were felt to be much safer and less addicting than the barbiturate drugs. Today, many long- and short-acting benzodiazepines are available that are used effectively in treating all levels of anxiety and anxiety disorders. (See At a Glance 19-2.) It must be recognized, however, that tolerance is common and addictive tendencies are possible. Used continuously and without adjunctive psychotherapy, their anxiety-reducing effects tend to diminish and tolerance develops. Their usefulness lies in the rapid onset of symptom relief because they enhance the binding of γ-aminobutyric acid (GABA) receptors, which causes an inhibitory or calming effect on the excited response in the brain. Higher doses can create a more profound effect, inducing sleep or perhaps even coma, indicating their depressive action on the subcortical levels of the central nervous system (CNS). The benzodiazepines and other commonly used anti-anxiety agents are listed in At a Glance 19-3.

At a Glance 19-2 Half Life of Benzodiazepine Drug Agents

Alprazolam (Xanax)	Short (7 to 15 hours)
Chlordiazepoxide (Librium)	Long (5 to 30 hours)
Clonazepam (Klonopin)	Long (20 to 40 hours)
Clorazepate (Tranxene)	Long (30 to 100 hours)
Diazepam (Valium)	Long (20 to 50 hours)
Lorazepam (Ativan)	Short (8 to 15 hours)
Oxazepam (Serax)	Short (5 to 15 hours)
Prazepam (Centrax)	Long (30 to 100 hours)

Indications for Use. Anxiolytics or antianxiety drugs are used in the treatment of anxiety disorders, anxiety symptoms, acute alcohol withdrawal, skeletal-muscle spasms, convulsive and seizure disorders, status epilepticus, and preoperative sedation.

Contraindications. The main contraindications are hypersensitivity, narrow-angle glaucoma, pregnancy and lactation, pre-existing CNS depression or psychosis, children under 12 years, and shock or coma. Anxiolytics should not be taken in combination with other CNS depressants. They should be used with caution in older people and in those with hepatic or renal dysfunction, a history of drug dependence or abuse, and depression. Physical dependence is indicated by withdrawal symptoms if discontinued abruptly. Severe symptoms are most likely in clients who have taken higher doses for a period of more than 4 months. The symptoms are caused by the acute separation of the drug molecules at the receptor site and the acute decrease in GABA neurotransmitters. These symptoms most commonly include increased anxiety, psychomotor agitation, insomnia, irritability, headache, tremors, and palpitations. In severe cases, psychotic manifestations and seizures may occur.

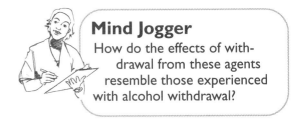

Mind Jogger
How do the effects of withdrawal from these agents resemble those experienced with alcohol withdrawal?

Nursing Diagnoses. Nursing diagnoses applicable to the client who is taking antianxiety medication may include:

- Risk for injury, related to effects of the drug, seizures, increased anxiety, effects of medication toxicity or overdose
- Risk for activity intolerance, related to side effects of sedation, confusion, or lethargy
- Confusion, related to effects of drug on CNS
- Knowledge deficit, related to medication regimen and drug effects

Nursing Interventions. Implementation of nursing actions to accompany the administration of antianxiety medications may include:

- Instruct the client to avoid driving or operating dangerous machinery while taking the drug.

At a Glance 19-3 Antianxiety or Anxiolytic Drug Agents

Chemical Group	Generic Name (Brand Name)	Usual Dosage (Daily)	Adverse Reactions and Side Effects
Antihistamines	Hydroxyzine (Atarax, Vistaril)	100–400 mg*	Dry mouth, drowsiness, pain at site of intra-muscular injection
Benzodiazepines	Alprazolam (Xanax)	0.75–4 mg*	Drowsiness, dizziness, ataxia, lethargy, hypo-tension, blurred vision, nausea, vomiting, anorexia, sleep distur-bance, tolerance, physi-cal and/or psychologic dependence
	Chlordiazepoxide (Librium)	15–100 mg*	
	Chlonazepam (Klonopin)	1.5–20 mg*	
	Clorazepate (Tranxene)	15–60 mg*	
	Diazepam (Valium)	8–40 mg*	
	Lorazepam (Ativan)	2–6 mg*	
	Oxazepam (Serax)	30–120 mg*	
	Prazepam (Centrax)	20–40 mg*	
Propanediols	Meprobamate (Equanil, Miltown)	400–2400 mg (not recom-mended for older people)	Drowsiness, dizziness, ataxia, reduced seizure threshold, tolerance, dependence
Miscellaneous	Buspirone (BuSpar)	15–60 mg	Drowsiness, dizziness, ex-citement, fatigue, head-ache, insomnia, nervous-ness, weakness, blurred vision, nasal congestion, palpitations, tachycardia, nausea, rashes, myalgia, incoordination

*Reduced dosages recommended for older people.

- Advise the client not to discontinue taking drug abruptly. Abrupt withdrawal can be life-threatening. (Symptoms may include depression, anxiety, abdominal and muscle cramps, tremors, insomnia, vomiting, diaphoresis, convulsions, and delirium.)
- Instruct the client not to drink alcohol or take other CNS depressants while taking these drugs.
- Assess client mood and orientation daily.
- Instruct the client to rise slowly from reclining position.
- Monitor lying and standing blood pressure daily.
- Assess for paradoxical excitement—notify the physician if it occurs.
- Offer ice chips, hard candy, frequent sips of water, or sugarless gum to relieve dry mouth.
- Give medication with food or milk to prevent nausea and vomiting.
- Report any indications of blood dyscrasias (sore throat, fever, malaise, easy bruising, or unusual bleeding).
- Instruct clients taking buspirone (BuSpar) that a lag time of 10 days to 2 weeks should be anticipated between onset of therapy and reduction in anxiety symptoms. (Client

should continue taking medication during this time.)

Client Teaching—Client and Family. In addition to the points listed under Nursing Interventions above, the following points should be included in client teaching:

- Do not take over-the-counter (OTC) or non-prescription drugs without the permission of the physician.
- Report any symptoms of fever, sore throat, malaise, easy bruising, bleeding, or increased motor restlessness to the physician.
- Be aware of side effects and potential adverse effects.

Outcome Evaluation. The following criteria may be used to evaluate the effectiveness of the antianxiety agents in the client:

- Experiences no physical injury or seizure activity
- Demonstrates decreased anxiety and associated symptoms
- Is able to tolerate usual activity without excessive sedation
- Maintains cognition pattern free of confusion

In addition, both the client and family will verbalize an understanding of the:

- Need for the medication and its potential side effects
- Dosage regimen
- Importance of not discontinuing the drug abruptly

Antidepressants

Antidepressants are used in the treatment of depression to elevate mood, increase physical activity and mental alertness, improve appetite and sleep, and restore interest or pleasure in usual activities and things previously enjoyed. Because the neurotransmitters involved in depression also affect these other body functions, they can be used to treat other types of disorders such as eating disorders and sleep dysfunction. Most medications that are used to treat depression increase the amount of chemicals in the brain that help to balance the moods. Depression results from a decrease in monoamine neurotransmitter (norepinephrine, **serotonin,** and dopamine) concentration to a level insufficient to stimulate the receptors. The effects of these neurotransmitters last longer than those of GABA chemicals. Research has demonstrated that by inhibiting the breakdown of the monoamines or promoting their reuptake, thus increasing their presence in the brain, mood can be effectively elevated.

Antidepressants generally fall into three types: monoamine oxidase inhibitors, tricyclic antidepressants, and serotonin-specific reuptake inhibitors. Early pharmacologic studies led to a group of drugs called the monoamine oxidase inhibitors (MAOIs). Monoamine oxidase is an enzyme that metabolizes or inactivates the monoamine neurotransmitters. Specifically, MAOIs work by releasing monoamine neurotransmitters in the brain, blocking their reuptake into the presynaptic compartments, or mimicking the effects of the monoamines at the receptors.

The tricyclic antidepressants (TCA), named for their three-ring chemical structure, were developed in the 1950s. These drugs work to correct the chemical imbalance of neurotransmitter concentrations in the synaptic cleft of CNS nerve cells. They effectively inhibit the reuptake of the neurotransmitters back into the cells, promoting a higher concentration of the neurotransmitters within the brain. TCAs also affect other body chemicals and characteristically produce a number of adverse and potentially dangerous side effects, including cardiac arrhythmias. This factor requires that all clients taking these agents be monitored closely.

The 1980s brought a new class of antidepressants that were designed to block the reuptake of serotonin, rather than norepinephrine. The serotonin-specific reuptake inhibitors (SSRIs) are all chemically related and have relatively fewer side effects than the TCAs, making them a safer and more desirable alternative. **SSRIs** selectively block the reuptake of serotonin into the presynaptic compartment of the nerve cell. (See Figure 19-1.) This causes increased concentration of serotonin at nerve endings in the CNS. These drugs have little or no effect on the cardiovascular system and fewer anticholinergic side effects. Since the advent of the SSRIs, physicians have readily prescribed them, and more people are being treated and benefiting from treatment.

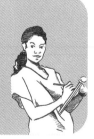

Just the Facts

Antidepressant drugs fall into three categories: monoamine oxidase inhibitors, tricyclic antidepressants, and serotonin-specific reuptake inhibitors.

The effect of antidepressant drugs on the state of depression is not immediate. They must be taken continuously for several weeks before therapeutic effects are evident and the client begins to feel better. This is because a continuous presence of the drug is needed in the brain for the level of the neurotransmitters to balance the deficit causing the depression. It is important that the client continues taking the medication, even if it does not seem to be helping. All of these drugs are effective, but some drugs work better for certain types of depression. A withdrawn client, for example, may benefit from a drug with stimulating effects, whereas another client may benefit from a drug that has a calming effect. Dosage and type of drug used will depend on the type and severity of the condition and the age of the client. It must be remembered that these drugs are not curative and cannot solve the problems underlying the client's mental state. Clients with suicidal tendencies must be closely observed, because therapeutic levels of these drugs can energize their ability to

carry out a suicide plan. Antidepressant medication combined with therapy and counseling is usually the preferred approach.

Mind Jogger

How might antidepressant therapy impose a greater risk for self-harm in the suicidal client?

Indications for Use. Antidepressant drugs are used in the treatment of major depression, dysthymic and bipolar disorders, depression accompanied by anxiety, childhood enuresis, depression associated with organic disease (alcoholism, schizophrenia, mental retardation), obsessive-compulsive disorder, ADHD in children, panic disorder, chronic pain, and bulimia. Bupropion (Zyban) is indicated for use with smoking cessation.

Contraindications. The main contraindications are hypersensitivity to the drug class and pregnancy and lactation. Tricyclic antidepressants are also contraindicated in the acute recovery period following a myocardial infarction. They should be used with caution in clients with a history of urinary retention or benign prostatic hypertrophy, glaucoma, asthma, or hepatic or renal disease. Concomitant use with MAOIs is contraindicated for all classes of antidepressants. MAOIs are further contraindicated in hepatic or renal insufficiency, a history of or existing cardiovascular disease, hypertension, severe headaches, or children under the age of 16 years. They should be used cautiously in clients with a history of seizures, diabetes mellitus, suicidal tendencies, angina pectoris, or hyperthyroidism. There are many drug-drug interactions that may occur with antidepressant medications. A physician or pharmacist should be consulted before combining these drugs with any other prescription or nonprescription (OTC) drugs.

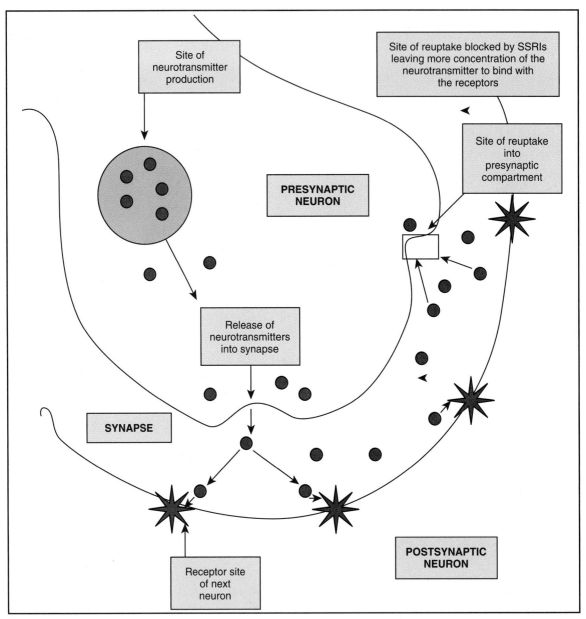

FIGURE 19-1. The release of serotonin from the presynaptic nerve ending into the synaptic cleft, where the neurotransmitter is free to connect with the receptors of the next neuron. The neurotransmitter may be deactivated by chemical processes or be taken back into the presynaptic compartment (reuptake). Serotonin-specific reuptake inhibitors (SSRIs) block the site of reuptake so that more of the neurotransmitter is available at the receptor sites.

Nursing Diagnoses. Nursing diagnoses that may be indicated in the client receiving anti-depressant therapy include:

- Risk for injury, related to side effects of sedation, orthostatic hypotension, photosensitivity, lowered seizure threshold, priapism, arrhythmias, or hypertensive crisis
- Risk for self-directed violence, related to mood dysphoria
- Social isolation, related to depression
- Constipation or urinary retention, related to side effects of the medication
- Self-care deficit, related to fatigue and low self-esteem
- Coping, individual, ineffective related to depressed mood
- Anxiety, related to situational crisis
- Sleep pattern disturbance, related to psychologic factors
- Sexual dysfunction, related to effects of medication or decreased libido
- Self-esteem, low related to mood disturbance
- Knowledge deficit, related to prescribed drug and side effects

Nursing Interventions. Nursing actions that should be implemented when caring for the client on antidepressant drug therapy include:

- Provide explanations of drug action and side effects.
- Monitor vital signs and observe for orthostatic hypotension.
- Advise to change positions slowly.
- Administer with food or milk to avoid gastrointestinal upset.
- Assist with ambulation or activity requiring mental alertness.
- Encourage increase in fluid intake.
- Offer hard candy or sugarless gum for dry mouth.
- Assess for suicidal ideation.
- Monitor mood at frequent intervals.
- Monitor for hoarding of drugs and other overdosing cues.
- Ensure use of protective sunscreen when outdoors (tricyclic antidepressants).
- Discourage caffeinated beverages.

Client Teaching—Client and Family. The client for whom an antidepressant drug is prescribed should be taught to:

- Take medication exactly as directed by the physician.
- Not use more of the drug, use it more often, or for a longer period than the physician ordered.
- Take the drug as directed consistently for several weeks to see a therapeutic effect.
- Take the medication with food or milk to avoid stomach upset.
- Keep regular doctor appointments.
- Use caution when driving, operating dangerous equipment, or engaging in activities that require mental alertness and coordination.
- Not mix with alcohol or other CNS depressants.
- Report any side effects to your physician.
- Not suddenly stop taking the medication—it must be withdrawn gradually.
- Take a missed dose as soon as possible—if several hours have lapsed or it is nearing the time for the next dose, the dose should not be doubled to catch up.
- Avoid smoking when taking tricyclic drugs—smoking enhances the metabolism and increased dosage may be required.
- Wear protective sunscreen when outdoors (tricyclic antidepressants).
- Rise slowly from a reclining position.

Outcome Evaluation. The following criteria may be used to evaluate the effectiveness of antidepressant drug therapy in the client:

- Is free of injury or adverse effects of drug
- Has not harmed self
- Interacts and communicates with staff and others
- Demonstrates more positive view of self
- Performs activities of daily living
- Communicates feelings about present situation
- Experiences normal sleep patterns and appetite
- Reports decreased feelings of anxiety
- Participates in unit activities

The client and the family will:

- Acknowledge need for ongoing therapy
- Demonstrate knowledge of medication and side effects

The antidepressant classes of drugs with side effects common to each group are listed in At a Glance 19-4.

Mood-Stabilizing Agents

Lithium carbonate is a naturally occurring metallic salt, much like sodium carbonate. It is used in the management of bipolar illness (severe mood swings), both to treat manic episodes and to prevent the recurrence of these episodes. Lithium is more effective in treating the "high" than in preventing the

At a Glance 19-4 Antidepressant Drug Agents

Chemical Group	Generic Name (Brand Name)	Usual Dosage (Daily)	Adverse Reactions and Side Effects
Tricyclic antide-pressants	Amitriptyline (Elavil, Endep)	50–100 mg	Lethargy, sedation, blurred vision, dry eyes, dry mouth, cardiac arrhythmias, hypotension, electrocardiogram changes, constipation, urinary retention, photosensitivity, blood dyscrasias, nausea and vomiting, increased appetite and weight gain, changes in blood glucose
	Amoxapine (Asendin)	50–100 mg	
	Desipramine (Nor-pramin, Pertofrane)	75–300 mg in divided doses	
	Doxepin (Sinequan, Adapin)	75–300 mg	
	Imipramine (Tofranil)	75–150 mg	
	Nortriptyline (Aventyl, Pamelor)	40–150 mg	
	Protriptyline (Vivactil)	15–60 mg	
	Trimipramine (Surmontil)	75–300 mg	
Heterocyclics	Bupropion (Wellbutrin, Zyban)	100 mg (1–3 times)	Agitation, headache, dry mouth, nausea, vomiting, change in appetite, weight gain or loss, photosensitivity, tremors, changes in blood sugar, possible seizures, priapism, hypotension, tachycardia
	Maprotiline (Ludiomil)	75–300 mg	
	Mirtazapine (Remeron)	15 mg	
	Trazodone (Desyrel)	100–600 mg	
Serotonin-specific reuptake inhibitors (SSRIs)	Citalopram (Celexa)	20–40 mg	Apathy, confusion, drowsiness, insomnia, weakness, agitation, anxiety, increased depression, cough, orthostatic hypotension, tachycardia, dry mouth, nausea, altered taste, ejaculatory delay, impotence, amenorrhea, photosensitivity, rash, pruritus, weight changes, tremors
	Fluoxetine (Prozac)	20–80 mg	
	Fluvoxamine (Luvox)	50–300 mg	
	Paroxetine (Paxil)	20–50 mg	
	Sertraline (Zoloft)	50–200 mg	

continues

At a Glance 19-4 Antidepressant Drug Agents *(Continued)*

Chemical Group	Generic Name (Brand Name)	Usual Dosage (Daily)	Adverse Reactions and Side Effects
Nonselective re-uptake inhibitors (serotonin and norepinephrine)	Nafazodone (Serzone) Venlafaxine (Effexor)	200–600 mg 75–225 mg	Abnormal dreams, anxiety, dizziness, headache, insomnia, nervousness, weakness, dry mouth, parasthenia, rhinitis, visual disturbances, altered taste, abdominal pain, nausea, vomiting, constipation, diarrhea, tachycardia, palpitations
Monoamine oxidase inhibitors	Isocarboxazid (Marplan) Pheneizine (Nardil) Tranylcypromine (Parnate)	20–40 mg 60–90 mg 20–30 mg	Dizziness, headache, orthostatic hypotension, constipation, nausea, arrhythmias, tachycardia *May interact with numerous foods and drugs to produce hypertensive crisis (severe hypertension, severe headache, fever, possible myocardial infarction or intracranial hemorrhage). See At a Glance 19-5.*

*Decreased dosages recommended for older people.

At a Glance 19-5 Foods and Drugs to Avoid When Taking an MAOI Drug Agent

Foods to avoid contain tyramine, a monoamine precursor of norepinephrine. The metabolism of tyramine is blocked by the MAOIs and a surge of norepinephrine is available at the adrenergic nerve receptors.

Foods. Aged cheese (cheddar, swiss, blue cheese, parmesan, provolone, romano), alcoholic beverages (beer, red wines), avocados, bananas, caffeine-containing beverages, smoked and processed meats (salami, pepperoni, bologna, summer sausage), caviar, corned beef, chicken livers, chocolate, fava bean pods, figs, meat tenderizers, pickled herring, raisins, sour cream, soy sauce, yogurt.

Drugs. Amphetamines, antihistamines containing ephedrine derivatives, antidepressants (tricyclic and SSRIs), antiallergy or antiasthmatic agents containing ephedrine derivatives, antihypertensive drugs, levodopa, meperidine.

Just the Facts

MAOIs can interact with numerous foods and drugs to produce a hypertensive crisis. Foods to avoid contain tyramine, a precursor of norepinephrine.

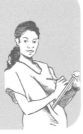

lows or depressive periods. Lithium is well absorbed from the gastrointestinal tract and may be given by capsule or concentrate. It has a peak blood level of 1 to 3 hours. The half-life of this drug is about 24 hours. Lithium is not metabolized by the body and is entirely excreted by the kidneys unchanged, so adequate renal functioning is necessary for its use. Most of a lithium dose is reabsorbed in the proximal renal tubules. The reabsorption of sodium and lithium are closely related, with any increase or decrease in dietary sodium intake affecting the levels of lithium in the blood plasma. A decrease in dietary sodium or loss through perspiration, vomiting, or diarrhea causes more lithium to be re-

absorbed and increases the risk of lithium toxicity. Excessive intake of sodium causes an increase in the excretion of lithium and may lower the serum level to a nontherapeutic level. Therapeutic serum levels are 0.6 to 1.2 milliequivalents per liter (mEq/L), with adverse effects occurring at levels in excess of 1.5 mEq/L and severe toxic reactions possible when levels reach 2 to 2.5 mEq/L. It is important to note that the therapeutic serum level of lithium is not much lower than a toxic serum level. Lithium dosage is determined based on both the clinical response and serum levels of the drug. In recent years, more drug agents have become available for the treatment of bipolar illness. Information on the mood-stabilizing drugs is found in At a Glance 19-6.

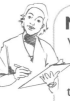

Mind Jogger

What information about the sodium content of food should be included when teaching a client about lithium carbonate?

At a Glance 19-6 Mood-Stabilizing Drug Agents

Chemical Group	Generic Name (Brand Name)	Usual Dosage (Daily*)	Adverse Reactions and Side Effects
Antimanic	Lithium carbonate (Eskalith, Lithane)	900–1200 mg (Maintenance) 1800–2400 mg (Acute mania)	Lethargy, drowsiness, headache, fatigue, dry mouth, metallic taste, nausea, vomiting, diarrhea, thirst, polyuria, leukocytosis, muscle weakness, fine tremors **Life-threatening:** Arrhythmias, bradycardia, renal toxicity, epileptiform seizures, coma

continues

At a Glance 19-6 Mood-Stabilizing Drug Agents *(Continued)*

Chemical Group	Generic Name (Brand Name)	Usual Dosage (Daily*)	Adverse Reactions and Side Effects
Anticonvulsants	Carbamazepine (Tegretol)	800–1200 mg	Sedation, headache, nausea, vomiting, indigestion, diarrhea, diplopia, elevated liver enzymes, drowsiness, sore gums, changes in appetite, vertigo, ataxia, dry mouth, confusion, hallucinations, prolonged bleeding
	Clonazepam (Klonopin)	3–20 mg	
	Divalproex (Depakote, Depakene, Epiva)	500–1500 mg	
			Life-threatening: Heart failure, arrhythmias, worsening of seizures, blood dyscrasias, toxic hepatitis, respiratory depression
Calcium-channel blocker	Verapamil (Calan, Isoptin)	240–320 mg	Dizziness, headache, transient hypotension, constipation, nausea, elevated liver enzymes, prolonged bleeding time
			Life-threatening: Heart failure, bradycardia, ventricular arrhythmias, AV block

*Decreased dosages recommended for older people.

Indications for Use. Antimanic agents are indicated for manic episodes associated with bipolar disorder and maintenance therapy to prevent or diminish future episodes. Lithium is also used in the treatment of migraine headaches and schizoaffective disorders.

Contraindications. The main contraindications are hypersensitivity to the drug, cardiac or renal disease, sodium imbalance, and pregnancy and lactation. It should be used cautiously in older people and those with metabolic disorders, urinary retention, or seizure disorders.

The action of anticonvulsants and calcium channel blockers in the treatment of bipolar disorders is not clear. However, they have been used effectively to stabilize the manic episodes in bipolar disorders.

Contraindications. Anticonvulsants and calcium channel blockers should not be used in those who are hypersensitive to these drugs, have a history of bone marrow suppression, or have taken an MAOI within 14 days of therapy. They should be used with caution in older people, pregnant and lactating women, and those with hepatic or cardiac disease.

Nursing Diagnoses. Nursing diagnoses applicable to the client receiving a mood-stabilizing agent may include:

- Risk for injury, related to side effects of drowsiness and dizziness
- Risk for poisoning, related to lithium toxicity (narrow therapeutic range of drug)
- Risk for injury, related to sodium imbalance
- Risk for violence, related to manic excitement, impulsive behaviors
- Risk for fluid volume deficit, related to side effects of medication (nausea, vomiting, diarrhea)
- Sensory/perceptual alterations, related to chemical alterations
- Self-esteem, chronic low, related to perceived lack of control

Nursing Interventions. Nursing actions that should be included in planning care for the client receiving mood-stabilizing drugs include:

- Educate the client to look for expected side effects of the drug without creating anxiety.
- Teach the client that side effects such as nausea, dry mouth, flatulence, dizziness, mild tremors, and insomnia should subside with continued treatment.
- Administer medication with food to avoid nausea and dyspepsia.
- Increase fluid intake to 2000 to 3000 mL daily.
- Maintain consistent dietary intake of sodium, and increase sodium if activity results in heavy perspiration.
- Assess for signs of toxicity in the client taking lithium carbonate therapy (muscle weakness, diplopia or blurred vision, severe diarrhea, persistent nausea and vomiting, tinnitus, and vertigo).
- Notify the physician of any indication of lithium toxicity.
- Monitor for changes in mood.

Client Teaching—Client and Family. When teaching the client and his/her family about mood-stabilizing drug therapy, it is important to include the following:

- Use caution when operating a motor vehicle or dangerous machinery.
- Do not stop taking the drug abruptly—serious withdrawal symptoms can occur.
- Take medication regularly, even when feeling well.
- Report any symptoms of drug side effects to the physician.
- Emphasize the importance of keeping physician appointments and having regular blood samples drawn (usually drawn 8 to 12 hours after the last dose was taken).
- Take medication at the same time each day. If a dose is missed, do not double the dose the next time (could result in toxicity).
- Consult with physician or pharmacist before taking any prescription or nonprescription medication with lithium.
- Report any mood swings or extreme changes in mood to the physician.
- For client taking lithium: Instruct to increase fluid intake to eight to ten 8-oz glasses of water each day. Instruct to include consistent intake of dietary sodium each day and to increase this amount if activity results in heavy perspiration.
- For clients taking calcium-channel blocker: Rise slowly from a sitting or reclining position.

Outcome Evaluation. Criteria that may be used to evaluate the effectiveness of mood-stabilizing agents in the client include:

- Experiences no physical injury while on medication therapy
- Maintains consistent therapeutic levels of lithium
- Is able to participate in normal day-to-day activities
- Maintains consistent dietary intake of sodium and fluid intake
- Does not experience extreme mood swings
- Has not harmed self or others

The client and family will verbalize:

- Importance of continuing drug therapy even if feeling well
- Importance of keeping appointments with physician and having drug blood levels drawn regularly
- Understanding of medication side effects and which symptoms to report to the physician

Antipsychotic Agents

Common to the psychotic disorders are the symptoms of delusions, hallucinations, disorganized speech, and disorganized or catatonic behaviors. People with psychosis rarely have insight into the pathologic complexity of these symptoms, often not realizing they are ill. This unusual lack of insight in many with psychosis during both periods of wellness and acute exacerbations of the symptoms is another dimension of the disabling and bizarre nature of these disorders. There is often the mistaken belief that because they are "feeling better" when taking medications that control the symptoms, they can stop taking them. This leads to acute exacerbations and hospitalization to restabilize the client.

Because the symptoms of the psychoses are extremely uncomfortable for most people, the effects of antipsychotic drugs are one of the most dramatic in modern medicine. Today, these drugs can reverse most or all symptoms in many with psychotic illness. Early agents, such as Thorazine (chlorpromazine), produced remarkable reversal in symptoms and resulted in a dramatic decrease in the number of clients confined to institutions and hospitals for the mentally ill. This trend continues today, with shortened hospital stays and longer periods of functional community living for many whose symptoms are controlled with antipsychotic medication. Compliance with drug therapy is inconsistent. Clients who lack insight into the necessity for continued treatment may abruptly discontinue taking their medication thinking that because

they feel well, they no longer need medication. This revolving scenario of "on and off" compliance often results in hospitalization for restabilization of drug regimens.

Antipsychotics are classified in several ways. Because of their varied chemical structures, the strength of the agent delineates its grouping into high, moderate, and low potency classes that are also referred to as *traditional antipsychotic groups*. (See At a Glance 19-7.)

At a Glance 19-7 Grouping of Antipsychotic Drugs by Chemical Potency

High-Potency

- Haloperidol (Haldol)
- Thiothixene (Navane)
- Trifluoperazine (Stelazine)
- Fluphenazine (Prolixin)

Moderate Potency

- Loxapine (Loxitane)
- Molindone (Moban)
- Perphenazine (Trilafon)

Low Potency

- Thioridazine (Mellaril)
- Mesoridazine (Serentil)
- Chlorprothixene (Taractan)
- Chlorpromazine (Thorazine)

The potency of the drug will influence the level and frequency of side effects experienced by the client. This also accounts for the need for some persons to receive higher dosages to achieve optimum clinical results. For example, a much larger dose of a low-potency drug such as Mellaril may be needed to produce the same level of symptom control that a lower dose of Haldol, a high-potency drug, offers. There is, however, a significant difference in the side effects they produce. Low-potency agents cause more anticholinergic effects, whereas high-potency drugs cause more extrapyramidal effects. These effects are discussed later in the chapter. Knowledge of the side effects enables the nurse to prepare the client for both the therapeutic benefits and potential adverse effects of the drug.

Later generation antipsychotic drugs are classified as atypical, not falling into any particular chemical class. The newer agents have had a major impact on the reduction of negative symptoms of psychoses (those developed over a prolonged period of time such as flattened affect, verbal deficits, and diminished drive) with a reduced risk of extrapyramidal side effects. The reduction of negative symptoms is ultimately the desired outcome of antipsychotic therapy and is a tool to measure progress of treatment. As a rule, the typical or positive psychotic symptoms (hallucinations and delusions) are those that lead to the most bizarre behavior. These symptoms are quite responsive to the typical antipsychotic agents. Along with reduced symptoms, these agents improve reasoning and decrease the ambivalent feelings and delusional thought processes that are both frustrating and frightening to the person experiencing them. By reducing the inner turmoil the person is feeling, these agents allow the person to devote more energy to external activity and interpersonal relationships.

Antipsychotic drug agents are listed in At a Glance 19-8, including categories, usual dosages, and side effects and adverse effects. In addition to inhibition of postsynaptic receptors of the neurotransmitters, these drugs also have properties that affect the cholinergic, α-1-adrenergic, and histamine receptors. This allows them to be used as antiemetics and in treating neurologic conditions such as intractable hiccups and tics (Tourette's disorder).

Side Effects of Antipsychotic Agents. The drugs in this group of agents are capable of producing numerous side effects. The lower potency drugs tend to produce the anticholinergic (dry mouth, urine retention, constipation, blurred vision) and antiadrenergic (hypotension) actions, whereas the higher potency drugs can produce severe **extrapyramidal** side effects (EPSEs). These reactions are much more devastating and contribute to the noncompliance exhibited in many clients for whom these

At a Glance 19-8 Antipsychotic Drug Agents

Chemical Group	Generic Name (Brand Name)	Usual Dosage (Daily*)	Adverse Reactions and Side Effects
Phenothiazines	Chlorpromazine (Thorazine)	40–800 mg	Extrapyramidal reactions, tardive dyskinesia, sedation, pseudoparkinsonism, EEG changes, drowsiness, dizziness, blurred vision, dry mouth, constipation, increased appetite, urine retention, weight gain, mild photosensitivity
	Fluphenazine (Prolixin)	1–40 mg	
	Mesoridazine (Serentil)	30–400 mg	
	Perphenazine (Trilafon)	12–64 mg	
	Prochlorperazine (Compazine)	15–150 mg	
	Promazine (Sparine)	40–1200 mg	
	Thioridazine (Mellaril)	150–800 mg	
	Trifluoperazine (Stelazine)	4–40 mg	
	Triflupromazine (Vesprin)	60–150 mg	**Life threatening:** seizures, neuroleptic malignant syndrome, blood dyscrasias

continues

At a Glance 19-8 Antipsychotic Drug Agents (Continued)

Chemical Group	Generic Name (Brand Name)	Usual Dosage (Daily*)	Adverse Reactions and Side Effects
Benzisoxazole	Risperidone (Risperdal)	2–6 mg	Somnolence, extrapyramidal symptoms, headache, insomnia, agitation, anxiety, tardive dyskinesia, aggressiveness, tachycardia, rhinitis, constipation, nausea, vomiting, dyspepsia, arthralgia, cough, rash, dry skin, photosensitivity **Life-threatening:** neuroleptic malignant syndrome, prolonged QT interval
Butyrophenone	Haloperidol (Haldol)	1–15 mg (maximum 100 mg)	Severe extrapyramidal reactions, tardive dyskinesia, sedation, drowsiness, lethargy, headache, insomnia, confusion, vertigo, tachycardia, hypotension, blurred vision, dry mouth, anorexia, constipation, diarrhea, nausea, dyspepsia, urine retention, rash **Life-threatening:** seizures, neuroleptic malignant syndrome, leucopenia
Dibenzoxazepine	Loxipane (Loxitane)	60–100 mg	Extrapyramidal reactions, sedation, drowsiness, numbness, tardive dyskinesia, pseudoparkinsonism, dizziness, tachycardia, orthostatic hypotension, blurred vision, dry mouth, constipation, urine retention, weight gain, rash **Life-threatening:** neuroleptic malignant syndrome, blood dyscrasias
Dibenzodiazepine	Clozapine (Clozaril)	25–450 mg	
Dibenzothiazepine	Quetiapine (Seroquel)	25–50 mg	
Dihydroindolone	Molindone (Moban)	15–225 mg	
Thienobenzodiazepine	Olanzapine (Zyprexa)	10–15 mg	
Thioxanthene	Thiothixene (Navane)	20–60 mg	

*Decreased dosages recommended for older people.

drugs are prescribed. The resistance to treatment leads to relapse and the return of symptoms and readmission to acute hospitalization. EPSEs can be grouped as:

- **Akathisia** (motor restlessness, inability to sit still)
- **Dystonias** (rigidity in muscles that control posture, gait, or eye movement)
- **Tardive dyskinesia** (late-appearing and irreversible movements of the mouth and face that include lip-smacking and grinding of teeth, protruding tongue movements, as well as pill-rolling of the fingers)
- **Drug-induced parkinsonism** (symptoms that mimic parkinsonism such as tremors, rigidity, akinesia, or absence of movement with diminished mental state) and neuroleptic malignant syndrome
- **Neuroleptic malignant syndrome** (A potentially fatal reaction most often seen with the high-potency antipsychotic agents. This response typically has an onset from 3 to 9 days after treatment is initiated. Symptoms include muscular rigidity, tremors, inability to speak, altered level of consciousness, hy-

perthermia, autonomic dysfunction (hypertension, tachycardia, tachypnea, diaphoresis), and elevated white blood cell count. Although it occurs in a very low percentage of clients taking these medications, the need for early recognition and immediate medical intervention is imperative.)

Indications for Use. All antipsychotic drugs are used in the treatment of acute and chronic psychoses, mania, and dementia-induced psychosis. The phenothiazines and haloperidol are also indicated in the treatment of intractable hiccups and control of tics and vocal disturbances. In addition, the phenothiazines may be used as antiemetics.

Contraindications. Important contraindications are hypersensitivity; coma or severe depression; liver, renal, or cardiac insufficiency; blood dyscrasias; and Parkinson's disease. They are used with caution in older clients; those with diabetes mellitus, chronic pulmonary disease, or prostatic hypertrophy; and during pregnancy and lactation.

Nursing Diagnoses: Nursing diagnoses that may accompany the administration of antipsychotic agents include:

- Risk for violence, directed at others, related to psychotic symptoms
- Risk for injury, related to medication side effects
- Potential for activity intolerance, related to medication side effects
- Noncompliance with medication regimen, related to suspiciousness and lack of trust in health care workers
- Thought process alteration, related to psychotic symptoms

Just the Facts

Extrapyramidal Side Effects

Akathisia: Motor restlessness, inability to sit still

Dystonias: Rigidity in muscles that control posture, gait, eye movement

Tardive dyskinesia: Late-appearing and irreversible movements of the mouth and face that include lip-smacking, grinding of teeth, protruding tongue movements, as well as pill-rolling of fingers

Drug-induced parkinsonism: Tremors, rigidity, akinesia, diminished mental state

Neuroleptic malignant syndrome: Potentially fatal reaction with muscle rigidity, tremors, inability to speak, altered level of consciousness, hyperthermia, autonomic dysfunction, and leukocytosis

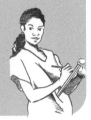

Mind Jogger

How might the altered processes of psychosis contribute to noncompliance with drug therapy?

- Coping, ineffective, individual, related to medication compliance and medication side effects

Nursing Interventions. When planning care for the client taking an antipsychotic agent, it is important to include the following nursing interventions:

- Reassure the client that interventions to help him or her with behavior control will be initiated.

At a Glance 19-9 **National Institute of Mental Health AIMS Scale**

Abnormal Involuntary Movement Scale

Facial and oral movements

1. Muscles of facial expression (frowning, blinking, smiling, grimacing)
2. Lips and periorbital area (puckering, pouting, smacking)
3. Jaw (biting, clenching, chewing, mouth opening)
4. Tongue (thrusting, tremors, athetoid movements)

Extremity movements

5. Upper (include choreic or rapid objectively purposeless, irregular, spontaneous movements; athetoid or slow irregular, complex, serpentine movements); does NOT include tremors (repetitive regular and rhythmic)
6. Lower (lateral knee movement, foot tapping, heel dropping, foot squirming, inversion and eversion of foot)

Trunk movements

7. Neck, shoulders, hips (rocking, twisting, squirming, pelvic gyrations)

Global judgment

8. Severity of abnormal movements
9. Incapacitation due to abnormal movements
10. Client's awareness of abnormal movements

Dental status

11. Current problems with teeth and/or dentures?
12. Does the client usually wear dentures?
13. Level of cooperation

Monitoring scale

0—Abnormal movements are not observed
1—Minimal or infrequent movements difficult to detect
2—Mild infrequent, but easy to detect lateral movements)
3—Moderate, frequent, easy to detect
4—Severe, almost continuously

0—No awareness
1—Aware, no distress
2—Aware, mild distress
3—Aware, moderate distress
4—Aware, severe distress

0—None
1—Partial
2—Full

continues

At a Glance 19-9 National Institute of Mental Health AIMS Scale *(Continued)*

AIMS Examination Procedure

Observe the client unobtrusively at rest. The chair used in the examination should be hard, firm, and without arms.

1. Ask client whether there is anything in mouth (e.g., gum, candy), and if there is, to remove it.
2. Ask client about current condition of his/her teeth. Ask if client wears dentures. Do teeth or dentures bother client now?
3. Ask whether client notices any movement in mouth, face, hands, or feet. If yes, ask to describe and to what extent they currently bother client or interfere with activities.
4. Have client sit in chair with hands on knees, legs slightly apart, and feet flat on floor. (Look at entire body for movement while in this position.)
5. Ask client to sit with hand hanging unsupported. If client is a man, between legs, if client is a woman and wearing a dress, hanging over knees. (Observe hands and other body areas.)
6. Ask client to open mouth. (Observe tongue at rest within mouth.) Do this twice.
7. Ask client to protrude tongue. (Observe abnormalities of tongue movement.) Do this twice.
8. Ask client to tap thumb, with each finger, as rapidly as possible for 10 to 15 seconds, separately with right hand, then with left hand. (Observe facial and leg movements.)
9. Flex and extend client's left and right arms (one at a time). Note any rigidity separately.
10. Ask client to stand up. (Observe in profile. Observe all body areas again, hips included.)
11. Ask client to extend both arms outstretched in front with palms down. (Observe trunk, legs, and mouth.)
12. Have client walk a few paces, turn, and walk back to chair. (Observe hands and gait.) Do this twice.

- Set limits with expectations for nonaggressive behavior.
- Encourage the client to discuss feelings of anxiety or frustration.
- Monitor the client for decreased symptoms of psychosis.
- Monitor the client for EPSEs of antipsychotic drug agents. (See AIMS assessment screening tool—At a Glance 19-9.)
- Maintain a calm attitude with matter-of-fact responses to reinforce reality.
- Maintain a low level of stimuli.
- Provide the client with sugarless candy, gum, or frequent sips of liquid to combat dry mouth.
- Encourage frequent oral hygiene.
- Observe elimination pattern for difficulty urinating or constipation.
- Monitor intake and output.

Client Teaching—Client and Family. Both the client and his or her family should be included in client teaching. It is important to integrate the following into the teaching plan:

- The medication regimen and the importance of taking medication as directed
- Side effects and interventions to help relieve them
- Signs and symptoms of tardive dyskinesia, and instructions to report any incidence to the physician
- Effects of noncompliance and the return of symptoms when medications are discontinued
- Importance of taking medication with food or milk to decrease stomach irritation
- Avoiding taking antipsychotic medications

within 1 hour of taking antacids or antidiarrheals (may decrease effectiveness of antipsychotic drug)

- That several days to several weeks of drug therapy may be needed before full effects of treatment are achieved
- Importance of keeping appointments with physician and for laboratory testing
- Use of caution when operating motor vehicle or machines that require coordination and mental alertness Because of drowsiness that may occur with this medication
- Importance of avoiding direct exposure to sunlight or using a sunscreen when in the sun
- Avoidance of vigorous exercise and overheating while taking this medication
- Possibility of phenothiazines turning urine pinkish red to red to reddish brown (this is harmless and may be expected)
- Importance of not stopping medication abruptly without checking with the physician
- Avoiding alcoholic beverages while taking these drugs (potentiate CNS action)
- Avoiding orthostatic hypotension by rising slowly from a sitting or reclining position

Outcome Evaluation. Once planned interventions have been implemented, the following criteria may be used to evaluate the effectiveness of drug therapy in the client:

- Experiences reduced incidence of psychotic symptoms and behaviors
- Seeks help when beginning to feel behavior is out of control
- Experiences minimal drug side effects
- Complies with therapeutic drug regimen
- Participates in planning care and long-term drug compliance
- Expresses understanding of relationship between psychotic symptoms, medication compliance, and behavior

Finally, it is important that the client and the client's family verbalize an understanding of the prescribed medication regimen and potential side effects.

Antiparkinson Drug Agents

Antiparkinson drug agents are used to relieve the drug-induced extrapyramidal symptoms associated with the antipsychotic drug agents. The two most commonly used are benztropine (Cogentin) and trihexyphenidyl (Artane), synthetic anticholinergic agents that resemble both atropine and diphenhydramine in their chemical structure. They are available only with a prescription, and the dosage is determined by the severity of symptoms.

Contraindications. The main contraindications are hypersensitivity reaction to the drug, narrow-angle glaucoma, myasthenia gravis, urinary retention, peptic ulcer disease, prostatic hypertrophy, and children under 3 years of age. These drugs must be used with caution in older people because of significant side effects, including urinary retention, visual disturbances, palpitations, and increased intraocular pressure.

Psychotropic Drug Agents and Older People

For older clients who have dementia-related aggression, distressing repetitive behaviors, catastrophic reactions, delusions, hallucinations, or agitation, the use of antipsychotic drugs has become a common approach to reducing and managing the incidence of these symptoms. The Omnibus Budget Reconciliation Act (OBRA) of 1987 limited the use of psychotropic medications for residents in long-term care facilities. These guidelines have been modified but with specific diagnostic and monitoring specifications. Antipsychotic medications can cause serious side effects such as extrapyramidal symptoms and tardive dyskinesia. The newer generation of psychotropic drugs is associated with fewer side effects, and they have thus become the drugs of choice for older people. Guidelines set by OBRA specify that these drugs can only be used for specific diagnoses and when behavioral and environmental measures are unsuccessful in managing symptoms.

The impact of age-related physiologic changes on antipsychotic drug therapy accounts for many of the serious side effects that occur in older people. Many of the drugs by themselves or in interaction with other drugs can cause the very symptoms they are prescribed to treat, such as agitation or delusions. Because many older clients commonly take medications for other illnesses, this situation is all too familiar. Because older adults have a higher body fat-to-lean ratio, less serum albumin, less total body water, fewer brain cells, and slower liver metabolism and renal clearance than young adults, they need far less of these drugs to produce a therapeutic effect. Effects and side effects persist longer, sometimes even after the drug is discontinued. Because there is less protein to bind with the drug, more of the drug is free to circulate. The drug remains in the body longer because of slower liver metabolism and slower renal excretion.

It is extremely important that all alternative approaches be considered before the use of these drugs in the older client. If used, their effects should be monitored closely and treatment discontinued if the person is adversely affected by the drug.

Just the Facts

Age-Related Physiologic Changes in Older People

  Higher body fat-to-lean ratio
    Less serum albumin
    Less total body water
    Fewer brain cells
    Slower liver metabolism and renal clearance

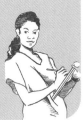

Mind Jogger

What are the potential implications of these age-related changes for the older client living at home who takes combinations of drugs to treat multiple conditions?

Summary

Psychopharmacology has provided symptomatic relief from the devastating effects of psychotic illnesses, providing some retrieval of normalcy for many clients with altered thinking, feeling, and perception. Psychotropic medications do not provide a cure or resolve the underlying problem; they must be used in combination with counseling and other therapeutic modalities to achieve the most desirable results of treatment.

Psychotropic drug agents have their primary effect on neurotransmitter systems. The drugs are effective because they either enhance or decrease the brain's ability to use a specific neurotransmitter, a deficiency or excess of which is linked to the mental disorder. Anxiolytics or antianxiety drugs are used in the treatment of conditions such as anxiety disorders, anxiety symptoms, acute alcohol withdrawal, and convulsive and seizure disorders. Antidepressant therapy assists the client with depression to elevate mood, increase physical activity and mental alertness, improve appetite and sleep, and restore interest in previously enjoyed activities.

Antidepressant drugs must be taken continuously for several weeks before therapeutic effects of treatment are evident. Time is needed for the continuous presence of the low levels of neurotransmitters to be restored and to balance the deficit causing the depression. Clients with suicidal tendencies must be closely observed because therapeutic levels of antidepressant drugs can give them the energy to carry out a suicide plan.

Lithium carbonate is a metallic salt used in the treatment of bipolar illness, both to treat acute episodes and to prevent their reoccurrence. Antipsychotic drug agents have also revolutionized the care of those with psychotic symptoms by reducing or reversing the discomfort of the delusions, hallucinations, and disorganized behaviors common to these disorders. The incidence of adverse side effects and the lack of insight into the need for continued treatment contribute to the noncompliance seen in many with psychosis who require antipsychotic medications to stabilize their illness.

The potency of the antipsychotic drug will influence the level and frequency of side effects experienced by the client. Low-potency agents tend to cause more anticholinergic side effects, whereas high-potency drugs cause more extrapyramidal effects. The AIMS assessment tool is used to monitor the extrapyramidal and irreversible group of movements that appear late in the use of these drugs. Antiparkinson (anticholinergic) drug agents are used to decrease the extrapyramidal effects exhibited in those taking the antipsychotic drug agents.

Antipsychotic drug agents are used with caution to control psychotic manifestations in the older client because of age-related physiologic changes. The drug effects persist longer and the drugs remain in the body longer, many times causing the very symptoms they are prescribed to treat. Careful monitoring is mandated to avoid the adverse consequences of using these agents in the older client.

It is important to reiterate that a combination of psychotropic drug therapy and psychotherapeutic intervention is required to maintain a consistent balance in the control of symptoms. Noncompliance with the treatment plan may compromise the outcome and lead to a reoccurrence of the symptoms. These drugs in and of themselves do not impose a cure, but they can allow the person with mental illness to function in an adaptive role within society.

Bibliography

Sherese, A., Roumen, M. (2003). Switch to mania upon discontinuation of antidepressants in patients with mood disorders: a review of the literature, *Canadian Journal of Psychiatry, 4(48),* 258–264. Available at http://www.cpa-apc.org/Publications/Archives?CJP/2003/may/ali.asp. Accessed on July 12, 2004.

American Psychiatric Association (2000). *Diagnostic and statistical manual of mental disorders text revision* (4th ed.). Washington, DC: American Psychiatric Association.

Chernin, T. (2001). New studies target side effects of psychotropic drugs, *Drug Topics,* 145(4):16.

Cohen, B. M. (2001). Mind and medicine drug treatments for psychiatric illnesses, *Social Research,* September 22.

Guiterrez, M. A., Roper, J. M., & Hahn, P. (2001) Paradoxical reactions to benzodiazepines, *American Journal of Nursing, 7*(101), 34–39.

Karch, A. M. (2003). *Lippincott's nursing drug guide 2004,* Springhouse Publishing Co.

Mancama, D., & Kerwin, R. W. (2003). Pharmacogenomics; mental illness—treatment, *CNS Drugs, 3 (17),* 143.

Martin, A., Scahell, L., Klin, A., & Volkmar, F. R. (1999). Higher-functioning pervasive developmental disorders; rates and patterns of psychotropic drug use. *Journal of American Academy of Child and Adolescent Psychiatry,* 38(7):923–931.

Nursing drug handbook 2004, 24th ed., Springhouse Publishers.

Viguera, A., & Baldessarini, R. (1998). Focus on lithium, *Atlantic Psychopharmacology Quarterly, 1[Autumn (1)].*

Weitzel, C. A. (2000).Could you spot this psychiatric emergency? *RN, 9(63),* 35–38.

FILL IN THE BLANK

Fill in the blank with the correct answer.

1. Psychotropic drug agents have their primary effect on _____ of the body.

2. The effects of the neurotransmitter dopamine are seen in _____ and _____.

3. The usefulness of the anxiolytic (antianxiety) drugs lies in their _____ that causes an inhibitory or calming effect on the excited response in the brain.

4. A continuous presence of an antidepressant drug is needed in the brain for the level of _____ to _____ causing the depression.

5. The client taking antidepressant medications is at risk for injury related to _____.

6. The effectiveness of antidepressant medication can be evaluated by observations of the client _____.

7. Foods to avoid when taking an MAOI drug include _____.

8. Side effects of lithium carbonate that contribute to noncompliance include _____.

9. Low-potency antipsychotic drugs cause more _____ side effects, whereas high-potency antipsychotic drugs cause more _____ side effects.

10. Extrapyramidal reactions are monitored by the _____.

MATCHING

Match the following terms to the most appropriate phrase.

a. Antianxiety drug

b. Antidepressant drug

c. Mood-stabilizing drug

d. Antipsychotic drug

e. Antiparkinson agent

1. _____ Effexor

2. _____ BuSpar

3. _____ Tegretol

4. _____ Mellaril

5. _____ Klonopin

6. _____ Ativan

7. _____ Wellbutrin

8. _____ Risperdal

9. _____ Celexa

10. _____ Centrax

11. _____ Clozaril

12. _____ Cogentin

MULTIPLE CHOICE

Select the best answer from the multiple-choice items.

1. A client admitted to the psychiatric unit with agitation and anxiety is pacing up and down the corridor. The nurse approaches the client and asks if he would like to talk about what is bothering him. He states he doesn't need to talk, he just needs a larger dose of medication. The best approach for the nurse at this time is to:

   a. Explain that medication will help the anxious feelings, but will not resolve the problem.

   b. Suggest he get involved in activities to divert his attention from his anxiety.

   c. Check to see if a sedative is ordered as needed for increased agitation.

   d. Notify the physician of the client's request.

2. A 58-year-old client with psychotic symptoms of hallucinations and delusional thinking is admitted for stabilization. The physician orders haloperidol 1 mg two times a day. When assessing the client's behavior, which of the following observations should the nurse report?

   a. Is often seen in dayroom asleep.

   b. Repeatedly licking lips with a swiping movement.

   c. Makes frequent trips to the water fountain during waking hours.

   d. Talks to self and laughs inappropriately at least 4 to 6 times daily.

3. The nurse is caring for a client whose serum lithium carbonate level is 1.5 mEq/L. The nurse would expect the physician to:

   a. Order an additional dose to be given one time only.

   b. Increase the daily dosage of the medication.

   c. Order the next dose of the drug to be held.

   d. Stop the medication.

4. The nurse is preparing to administer a dose of fluphenazine (Prolixin) to a client who has been diagnosed with schizophrenia. Which of the following side effects is more common with this medication?

   a. Motor restlessness

   b. Arthralgia

   c. Anorexia

   d. Abnormal dreams

5. It is important for the nurse to include which of the following instructions when doing client teaching for the client taking a tricyclic antidepressant medication:

   a. Take the medication with coffee or tea to enhance its effect.

   b. The medication can be discontinued after a few weeks of therapy.

   c. You can omit the morning dose of your medication if it makes you too sleepy.

   d. Wear a hat and long-sleeve shirt when you are outdoors in the sun.

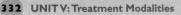

6. The client for whom an MAOI is pre-scribed should be taught to avoid which of the following dietary items?

a. Milk or milk products

b. Smoked or processed meat

c. Foods high in sodium

d. Legumes and nuts

7. The physician has ordered the drug benz-tropine (Cogentin) for a client who has been taking the antipsychotic medication haloperidol (Haldol). Which of the following would the nurse expect to assess in this client?

a. Increased delusional thinking

b. Intractable hiccups

c. Diminished drive and apathy

d. Protruding tongue movements

SEEK AND FIND

Find the incorrect information in the following statements.

1. Lithium carbonate is more effective in treating the "lows" than the "highs" of bipolar illness.

2. Drugs such as alcohol, heroin, and diaze-pam have a low lipid solubility and are absorbed slowly into the cerebral cells of the brain.

3. Clients taking lithium carbonate should decrease fluid intake to no more than 1000 mL in 24 hours.

4. The effect of antidepressant drugs is usu-ally noted within several days after the initial dose is taken.

5. Smoking tends to diminish the body's metabolism of tricyclic drugs and a decreased dosage may be required.

6. Low-potency antipsychotic agents cause more extrapyramidal side effects, whereas high-potency agents cause more anticholinergic effects.

7. Because of their ability to increase the effectiveness of antipsychotic drugs, antacids or antidiarrheal drug agents should not be administered within 1 hour of an antipsychotic agent.

SCENARIO: LIFE ON THE EDGE

Bianca is a 32-year-old who has been managing a local department store for the past 4 years. She has been divorced for 2 years and has two daughters, 6 and 9 years of age. She is admitted to the psychiatric unit after being brought to emergency room by her grandmother who states that her 9-year-old granddaughter called and said, "My mom won't wake up!" The grandmother hands the nurse an empty bottle containing a label for alprazolam (Xanax). She tells the nurse that her daughter was also drinking alcohol. She states, "Bianca has been drinking more since her divorce. She just doesn't seem to care about herself anymore."

What is the nursing priority for Bianca at this time?

_____

_____

Why is it dangerous to mix a psychotropic drug with alcohol?

_____

_____

The physician prescribes the antidepressant citalopram (Celexa) for Bianca. What teaching should the nurse do concerning this drug?

_____

_____

_____

What side effects may occur with an SSRI drug?

_____

_____

How will the nurse evaluate the effectiveness of the drug?

_____

_____

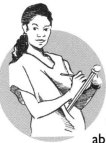

LEARNING OBJECTIVES

After learning the content in this chapter, the student will be able to:

1. Describe the goals of treatment in the mental health setting.
2. Define what is meant by a therapeutic milieu.
3. Differentiate between mental health professionals who are integral in the treatment process.
4. Identify the basic principles of psychotherapeutic treatment methods.
5. Discuss the role of the nurse in the psychotherapeutic process.

The Therapeutic Process in Mental Health Settings

KEY TERMS

Behavioral therapy

Biofeedback

Biomedical therapy

Clinical psychologist

Cognitive therapy

Contracting

Electroconvulsive therapy (ECT)

Group therapy

Humanistic therapy

Psychiatrist

Psychodynamic therapy

Psychotherapy

Therapeutic milieu

Overview of the Mental Health Care Environment

Mental health care is a multifaceted integration of varied approaches that have developed in an attempt to meet the treatment needs of those with mental disorders and their families. In the past, those with psychiatric problems were shunned and locked away from society in institutional settings; the present trend is to recognize mental disorders as treatable illnesses with more optimistic outcomes. Those in need of mental health care have the right to humane and individualized treatment plans. Treatment includes the preservation of personal and patient rights in both outpatient and inpatient settings. Our society is moving in the direction of promoting resources for more research and for application of these studies to preventive treatment, education, and community-oriented support as a common goal. Those who spearhead these efforts advocate availability and funding to ensure quality and equal access for those who need mental health services. Recent studies have shown that mental illness accounts for more than one-fourth of all cases of disability in the United States, Canada, and Western Europe. Although treatment may be available, a large percentage of people with mental illness do not receive treatment. There continues to be a need to improve public understanding, attitudes, and actions regarding mental health and illness.

Mind Jogger
What factors may contribute to the public attitude toward those with mental illness?

The goals of treatment are designed to reduce the symptoms of mental disorders and to allow those who suffer from these disorders to live and function in society with improved personal and interpersonal skills. There are many specific types of therapies that may be used, either as a single treatment method or in various combinations. The more common therapeutic treatment modalities are discussed in this chapter along with the various mental health professionals of the treatment team who provide these interventions.

Therapeutic Milieu

Within the mental health care environment, the concept of a **therapeutic milieu** emerges as a combination of the social and therapeutic environment. This type of structured community provides a setting conducive to providing therapeutic interaction between clients and members of the professional team. The objective of this milieu is to provide a supportive network in which there is a sense of common goals within safe and secure surroundings. Group activities are scheduled that maximize the functional ability of each client. The nurse is often in a position to maintain the milieu as a place where dignity and acceptance allow the client to practice skills without reprisal. Because of time spent with the client, the nurse is also a role model for social behaviors and communication skills, which reinforces the trusting relationship needed for successful treatment.

Just the Facts
During the process of treatment, clients are encouraged to be as independent as possible.

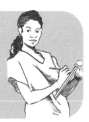

Mind Jogger
What benefit would a group home milieu provide over a return to the general social climate when the client is discharged from inpatient status

Treatment Team

Within the various mental health care settings such as mental health centers, private practices and clinics, psychiatric hospitals, residential group homes, and social service agencies, helping professionals work together to provide a diversified approach toward a common outcome of improved access to treatment for those needing care.

Psychiatrist. A psychiatrist is a physician licensed to practice medicine and specializes in psychiatric or mental disorders. A board-certified physician has passed the examinations of the American Board of Psychiatry and Neurology. A psychiatrist can evaluate, diagnose, and treat all types of mental illness, including pharmacologic, biomedical, and psychotherapeutic interventions. Some psychiatrists subspecialize in the pediatric, adolescent, or geriatric sector of the population.

Clinical Psychologist. Most licensed clinical psychologists have received a master's or doctoral level degree specializing in psychology with advanced training and field requirements. These professionals administer and interpret psychologic testing that can be used in the diagnostic process. The clinical psychologist also provides individual, family, and group therapy to assist in the resolution of mental health issues. The licensed psychologist can work independently or as a member of the mental health team.

Psychiatric Nurse. Psychiatric nursing is a specialized area of nursing practice that focuses on the prevention and treatment of mental health related problems. Most psychiatric nurses are registered nurses with some advanced-practice nurses working in specialized areas such as geriatric-psychology, consultation, education, and administration.

- *Registered Nurse.* A registered nurse (RN) may have an associate degree, diploma, or bachelor's degree in nursing. In the psychi-
atric setting, the registered nurse is accountable for both the physical and mental health care of the client. They are responsible for developing the individualized care plan and ensuring that it is implemented within a safe and therapeutic environment.
- *Licensed Practical/Vocational Nurse (LPN/LVN).* The licensed practical/vocational nurse has received a certificate in vocational nursing from an approved college-based, technical, or hospital-based program. The practical/vocational nurse assists in all aspects of the nursing process. The LPN/LVN may be responsible for basic nursing care including: observation of behaviors and data collection, administering medications, monitoring for medication side effects, therapeutic communication with clients, and documentation on the client record. The nurse is often able to establish and maintain a therapeutic relationship with the client while doing basic nursing interventions such as vital signs, dressing changes, or assisting with hygiene needs. The nurse works closely with other members of the care team to facilitate the best possible rehabilitative efforts for the clients.

Mental Health Technician. A mental health technician usually receives on-the-job training and has a high school education. Some of them may have additional studies at the vocational, technical or college level. Some people with baccalaureate degrees in psychology or related fields may also be employed in this capacity. Technicians assist clients with physical and hygiene needs as needed, monitor unit activities, and assist with group or recreational activities.

Social Workers (LCSW). Clinical social workers usually have a master's or doctoral level degree in their discipline and are trained as client advocates. Their role includes counseling of all types, providing referrals, and acting as a client liaison with government and civil agencies. The social worker works with placement agencies, such as community group homes and nursing homes, to secure a continued support and care system for the client who is unable to live in an independent or home setting.

Licensed Professional Counselors (LPC). Most clinical mental health counselors have a master's level degree with specialized training and licensure in professional counseling. Counseling incorporates approaches that best meet the clients' needs and help them to resolve problem areas toward a more satisfying and rewarding lifestyle.

Case Managers and Outreach Workers. Agencies such as mental health centers, psychosocial rehabilitation programs, and government agencies employ these workers to monitor and ensure that a client's needs are met. Most persons with severe mental illness need medical care, social services, housing, and financial assistance. Case workers provide assistance in securing these services. They also provide follow-up support to ensure the client's ability to live in the community setting.

Therapeutic Recreation Specialist. A bachelor's or master's prepared therapist receives national certification and is licensed or certified by the state in which he or she works. Recreation therapy uses various approaches such as art, music, leisure education, and recreation participation to help people with limitations make the most of their lives physically, mentally, and socially. This type of therapy provides ways for people to help themselves and to feel good about themselves and their accomplishments by improvements in the areas of concentration, decision-making, and completion of task-oriented projects. This enhances the client's self-confidence and improves the ability to work in a team environment with improved social and communication skills.

Occupational Therapist. Occupational therapists have a bachelor's or master's level degree in occupational therapy. They work with clients to improve their level of functioning for everyday living. Activities such as cooking, money management, grocery shopping, and transportation are used to improve self-esteem and promote a realistic level of independent living. Occupational therapists work with other members of the treatment team toward rehabilitation and discharge planning.

Religious Advisor. Religious advisors have bachelor's or master's level degrees in theology and provide spiritual support for clients and their families. They participate in treatment team meetings and spiritual counseling as indicated.

Dietician. Dieticians usually have a master's level degree in nutrition. They serve as a resource person by providing nutrition information and counseling to clients with specific nutritional problems and needs.

At a Glance 20-1 The Mental Health Treatment Team

- Psychiatrist
- Clinical psychologist
- Registered nurse
- Licensed practical/vocational nurse
- Mental health technician
- Social worker
- Licensed professional counselor
- Case managers and outreach workers
- Therapeutic recreation specialist
- Occupational therapist
- Religious advisor

Mind Jogger
What is the therapeutic benefit of a collaborative team approach to mental health care?

Role of the Nurse in Mental Health Care

At the hub of the mental health team, the nurse functions in a variety of different roles. The nurse-client relationship provides multiple opportunities for the nurse to obtain information that is often a vital resource to other team members. Information may be communicated verbally or documented in the medical record. This may be helpful for intervention strategies developed by other professionals. The nurse also serves as a liaison between the client and therapist or physician. The nurse assesses, evaluates, and interacts with clients on a day-to-day basis. The nurse is a vital component of maintaining a therapeutic milieu that supports and encourages clients in appropriate behavioral responses. In addition, the nurse models and assists the client with communication skills and social interactions with others in the milieu.

The nurse is an important source of unbiased and nonjudgmental support for the client. The nurse is able to maintain an objective view of the client's situation by understanding his or her own feelings and emotional responses toward the client. Ongoing self-assessment, allows the nurse to separate reaction from therapeutic action and remain focused on ways to promote a positive outcome for the client and their family.

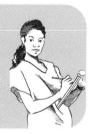

Just the Facts

The psychologic state of the nurse can influence the nurse's perception of the client and intended behavioral message.

Caregiver. The nursing process provides the foundation for the implementation of all nursing interventions. Basic to the nursing assessment is the observation of appropriate and inappropriate behaviors, noting both precipitating factors and situational reinforcers. This information is documented in the client record and provides feedback for other members of the mental health care team for evaluating effectiveness and progress of the treatment plan. A response to therapy is often observed by the nurse while performing other nursing interventions such as medication administration, physical assessment, or assisting with personal care. It is important for the nurse to positively reinforce appropriate behavior and encourage clients to participate in all aspects of the psychotherapeutic process.

Counselor. Nurses are often the person that is available and willing to provide an attitude of genuine concern for the client through active listening and therapeutic communication. The client should be encouraged to openly express feelings and thoughts without reprisal. Although not all behavior is acceptable, the nurse must separate inappropriate behavior from the client. Unconditional acceptance of the client as a person is imperative to a therapeutic outcome.

Educator. Nurses are often the link between clients and information about their illnesses and treatment. Compliance with treatment is more probable when clients are informed about the problem and how the treatment works. Education is provided at the client's level of understanding through verbal explanation, demonstration, and printed materials about the illness and treatment regime. It is important for the nurse to evaluate the client's understanding of the instructions by verbal response or return demonstration.

Advocate. As a client advocate, the nurse functions to protect the rights of the client through acceptance and support for decisions that are made. Compliance with treatment usually improves as the nurse demonstrates an empathetic positive regard for client needs. Empathy involves the nurse's willingness to understand the situation from the client's perspective. By being willing to listen, the nurse is able to view a problem through the client's eyes and assist in providing the resources necessary for the client to make a decision.

The Therapeutic Process (Inpatient Setting)

Members of the therapeutic treatment team work toward a common goal that is developed in collaboration with the client. The therapeutic process consists of those strategies that are used to achieve that objective. During the admission process, an initial intervention that helps to establish a sense of client trust is the provision of any unit rules or policies to the client and significant others. These rules may vary from facility to facility, but usually include things such as:

- Hours of visitation and client approval for certain persons to visit
- Types and times for therapy sessions
- Personal free time
- Mealtimes and bedtime
- Caffeine restrictions, available food or snack items
- Shaving or cosmetic items
- Sharp items, cords, and belts
- Violent or threatening behaviors
- Medication schedule
- Activities
- Telephone privileges

Close supervision is necessary to maintain compliance with all unit rules. It is important for each member of the mental health team to maintain consistency in enforcing these rules to establish limits and boundaries for behavior. Clients are encouraged to comply with all the rules and to attend all activity and therapy sessions.

Treatment team meetings are held daily or weekly in which each member contributes any new information regarding the client being discussed. The frequency of the meetings will depend on the individual needs or problems the client is experiencing. The exchange of ideas focuses on what will be the best approach to facilitate a positive outcome for each person. Discharge planning is also a topic during the meeting. From the time of admission, all strategies are aimed toward discharge as an outcome.

The Client's Place in the Process. Behaviors such as aggression and physical violence, foul language, or inappropriate confrontation are not tolerated in a therapeutic milieu. Clients are encouraged to express thoughts and feelings they experience during times when these actions occur. Interventions are used to help the client identify the unacceptable behavior and develop constructive approaches to deal with similar situations in the future. This provides the client with a way to effectively manage self-control toward behavior modification.

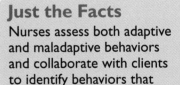
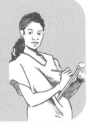

Just the Facts

Nurses assess both adaptive and maladaptive behaviors and collaborate with clients to identify behaviors that need to change.

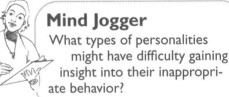

Mind Jogger

What types of personalities might have difficulty gaining insight into their inappropriate behavior?

Clients also attend therapeutic community groups with nurses functioning as leaders. Clients are given the opportunity to voice complaints, concerns, or feedback regarding the staff, other clients, or the environment in general. The security of a safe environment to express these feelings is essential. Guidelines for behavior are established and maintained in a consistent manner by the group leader. This structured milieu helps the client toward improved social skills and functioning as a member of a society. The client learns how to express concerns in a rational and acceptable manner as well as tolerance and acceptance of the views of others.

> **Just the Facts**
>
> Therapeutic intervention begins with the assumption that everyone can experience functional growth in interpersonal relationships and the demands of daily living.

Types of Psychotherapeutic Treatment

Psychotherapy is described as a dialogue between a mental health practitioner and the client with a goal of reducing the symptoms of the emotional disturbance or disorder and improving that individual's personal and social well-being. The aim of this dialogue is not to give advice, but to allow clients to learn about themselves, their life, and their feelings, and to make choices toward change. The intent is for clients to rediscover their own person, their priorities, and inner courage to act on them. Credible psychotherapy fosters insight into feelings, behavior, and interpersonal skills with success resting in the quality, not the type of therapy method used. Most clinical licensed mental health practitioners embrace an eclectic theoretical orientation, meaning their belief is in using components of many types of therapies, which they in turn utilize in their practice. People are complex beings with diverse and unique individual problems that are more successfully addressed by a flexible approach. Regardless of the method used, psychotherapy is successful when issues in the person's life are uncovered and energy and power are released to allow constructive change. An important variable in this success is the relationship between the client and therapist, and how the client views this relationship. Various types of approaches have proven to be comparably effective, although each may have its advantages and disadvantages in different client situations.

Individual Psychotherapy

There are five main approaches to individual therapy. **Psychodynamic therapy** is primarily based on psychoanalytic theory, or the assumption that when a client has insight into early relationships and experiences as the source of his or her problems they can be resolved. It is further assumed that these experiences can be analyzed to resolve current emotional problems. This Freudian-based therapy characteristically lasts several years with biweekly sessions.

Humanistic therapy centers on the client's view of the world and his or her problems. The goal is to help clients realize their full potential through the therapist's genuineness, unconditional positive regard, which fosters the client's sense of self-worth, and empathetic understanding of the client's point of view. This therapy is nondirective but focuses on helping the client to explore and clarify his or her own feelings and choices.

Behavioral therapy does not foster awareness but emphasizes the principles of learning with positive or negative reinforcement and observational modeling. The goal is to incur behavioral change within a relatively short time. In this therapy, the behavior or symptom is the problem. The underlying belief is that the original causes of maladaptive behavior may have little to do with present factors invoking the behavior. The plan of treatment is formulated and executed by the therapist, often with a variety of exercises to be done by the client between sessions. Gradual exposure to an anxiety-producing situation (such as in phobias) may be used along with relaxation exercises (examples are breathing, visualization, or meditation). Skills are modeled and taught for real-life situations with emphasis on what works best on specific symptom situations. It is important that reinforcement schedules, limits, and consequences be consistently followed.

Contracting is a behavioral technique in which the client and therapist draw up a contract to which both parties are obligated. The contract requires the client to demonstrate specific behaviors that are included in the therapy. In exchange, the therapist will give certain rewards the client has requested. The criteria for success are clearly outlined in the pact between the two parties engaged in the therapy.

Cognitive therapy focuses on identifying and correcting distorted thinking patterns that can lead to emotional distress and problem behaviors. Cognitive therapists believe that clients change their behaviors by changing their maladaptive thinking about themselves and their experiences. Clients are taught problem-solving skills and stress reducing methods. They learn that their psychologic difficulties or problems can be solved through cognitive processing.

Biomedical Therapy

A form of **biomedical therapy** using psychopharmacotherapy has benefited many clients with mental disturbances and disorders. The use of drugs is often combined with psychotherapy for a more successful outcome. The medication prescribed depends on the disorder being treated and the client's overall medical condition. (Specific psychotherapeutic drugs are discussed in Chapter 20.)

Electroconvulsive therapy (ECT) is another biomedical treatment that is generally reserved for clients with severe mental illness that are unresponsive to medications and other forms of therapeutic intervention. Some conditions where ECT may be used are major depression, psychosis, catatonia, and severe suicidal ide-

ation. Modern technology uses low-voltage electric shock waves to the brain along with general anesthesia and muscle relaxants to minimize the risk and negative impact on the client. The adjunctive use of medication helps to prevent severe muscle contractions that can inadvertently result in fractures or dislocated bones. Other adverse effects include temporary memory loss and confusion. Studies continue regarding the long-term effects of ECT.

Group Therapy

In **group therapy,** a trained and competent therapist leads a small group of people with similar problems who discuss individual and common issues. Remedial groups are concerned with ill persons who are not currently coping effectively with the stresses and strains of living. Groups often must work through negative content before positive results can surface. The success of the group interaction depends on the degree of trust, openness, and interpersonal risk-taking among the members. Interaction between members allows each to hear from others about their perceptions and behavior, either confirming or contradicting these self-views. Arguments and debates often indicate the attempt of each member to validate his or her own sense of reality.

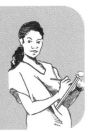

Just the Facts

Success in the group setting is dependent on the degree of trust, openness, and interpersonal risk taking of the individual group members.

Couples therapy is a highly effective group model used in helping couples resolve interpersonal conflict and initiate enhanced communication skills. In cases of marital conflict, the therapy tends to be most effective if the differences are of short-term duration. The therapist facilitates by listening to points of view and reality expressed by both partners.

Family therapy involves discussions and sessions designed to assist members with problem-solving skills within the family system. The problem may be troubled communication among family members or centered on the behavior of one particular person. The underlying belief is that individual problems originate from the family system. To treat the basic issue, the whole family must undergo therapy.

Other Types of Therapy

Biofeedback is used for specific types of anxiety and involves monitoring the client's heart rate, muscle tension, and other body functions. The feedback allows the person to learn to control these body functions under different emotional situations. This therapy method works best if used consistently. Neurobiofeedback is currently being used in the treatment of attention deficit disorder.

Agitation therapy may be used in problematic and aggressive people who do not respond positively to other therapies. The person is exposed to external agitation from other clients in a controlled atmosphere. This is designed to increase that person's self-awareness of maladaptive behavior and limitations. The goals of this therapy are to teach sublimation of aggression and anger impulses with insight and a willingness to change. The desired outcome is for the client to achieve control over his or her behavior and assume responsibility for emotional and social growth. It is often used in combination with other types of therapy.

Play therapy is often used with children and allows the therapist to treat the child during the dynamic process of play. The therapist is able to assess the child's internal affective state and psychologic response during the various stages of the treatment process.

Other adjunctive therapies may include occupational, recreational, and creative art therapies. These provide a relaxed atmosphere in which the client is often able to express emo-

tions and feelings that may be subdued during other forms of therapy. Recreational therapy provides an outlet for sublimating frustration and internal drives of emotion, along with encouraging social interactive skills. In the clinical setting, participation in all forms of therapy sessions is encouraged to provide the client with every opportunity for maximum benefit of treatment.

Summary

It is important to recognize that mental health care includes an umbrella of therapeutic approaches to the treatment of the client with mental illness. This multidisciplinary strategy enlists the skills of professionals such as psychiatrists, psychologists, psychiatric nurses, social workers, counselors, case managers, recreation therapists, and more. This team effort is directed at reducing the symptoms of mental disorders and improving the client's personal and interpersonal skills, and his or her functioning in society.

A therapeutic milieu provides a social and therapeutic community setting that supports the combined effort of treatment goals within a safe, secure, and encouraging environment. An attitude of acceptance within the group reduces the fear many clients have as they emerge from treatment into the boldness of societal living. Clients often feel a sense of unworthiness or inability to "fit in" as the phase of readjustment to these demands confronts them. A milieu can serve as a halfway mark to merge this gap between an inpatient setting and independent living. A case manager is usually assigned to each client, while social workers and counselors or therapists continue working with the client on an outpatient basis as long as needed to support the mental health treatment goals.

The nurse is a vital part of the treatment mental health care team. The nurse plays a daily interactive role with the client, providing a therapeutic atmosphere in which assessment and evaluation of behaviors and communication skills is facilitated. The nurse serves as a model for the client in appropriate social and interactive skills while reinforcing and rewarding this behavior in the client.

The therapeutic process focuses on interactive relationships between a mental health practitioner and the client with an expected outcome of reducing the effects of the emotional disturbance or disorder and improving both the personal and social well-being of the person. Licensed mental health practitioners work together toward optimizing the client's chance for a more fulfilling existence individually and in their daily interaction with others. Each person is a unique being that distinguishes his or her needs as a priority in the therapeutic methods utilized in treatment. Individual psychotherapy focuses on the problems or situations with which the client is having difficulty; it guides and assists the client to work toward resolution of the roadblocks in mental functioning. Other types of therapy, such as group, family, play, or recreational therapy, and biofeedback, may be used to address contributing issues.

A combination of these psychotherapeutic methods combined with the benefits of psychotherapeutic drug agents provides an effective model of treatment for the client with mental health disorders or dysfunction. The ultimate goal of all avenues of treatment remains an improvement in the personal and social functioning of each client to an optimal and satisfying level of existence.

Bibliography

Horne, A. M. & Passmore, J. L. (1991). *Family counseling & therapy* (2nd ed.). Itasca, Illinois: Peacock Pub., Inc.

Long, P. W. (2003). President's new freedom commission on mental health. Available at http://www.mentalhealth.com. Accessed on July 12, 2004.

Martens, W. H. (2003). Agitation therapy, *American Journal of Psychotherapy, 56(3),* 234–250.

Seligman, M. E. (1995). The effectiveness of psychotherapy, Consumer Reports Study. *American Psychologist, 50(12),* 965–974. Available at www.apa.org/journals/seligman.html. Accessed on July 12, 2004.

Spinelli, E. (2003). Client-therapist relationship, *American Journal of Psychotherapy, 56(3),* 357–363.

Sternberg, R. J. (1997). *In Search of the Human Mind.* Orlando, Florida: Harcourt, Brace.

Student Worksheet

FILL IN THE BLANK

Fill in the blank with the correct answer.

1. A therapeutic milieu combines a
_____ and _____ envi-
ronment.

2. The process of working toward a common
care goal that is mutually shared by the
client is referred to as the _____.

3. _____ in enforcing unit rules by
each member of the treatment team helps
to set limits and standards for client behavior.

4. _____ is described as a dialogue
between a mental health practitioner and
the client with a goal of reducing the emotional symptoms and improving the
client's personal and social well-being.

5. _____ is often used with children and allows the therapist to treat a
child during the dynamic process of play.

6. The role most closely associated with
nurses is that of _____.

MATCHING

Match the following terms to the most appropriate phrase.

a. Focuses on identifying and correcting
distorted thinking patterns.

b. Behavioral method with a mutually obligated agreement between therapist and
client.

c. Provides relaxed environment for developing social interactive skills and personal accomplishment.

d. Discussion among a small number of
people with common and individual issues led by a trained therapist.

e. Focuses on the client feelings, views, and
choices in resolution of the problem.

f. Person learns to control anxiety response
through instrumental monitoring of body
functions during exposure.

g. Psychopharmacologic and electroconvulsive methods of treating mental disorders.

h. Involves therapy sessions with other
members of client's family.

i. Fosters reinforcement and observational
modeling to resolve problems.

j. Uses insight into early experiences to resolve current problems.

1. _____ Psychodynamic therapy

2. _____ Humanistic therapy

3. _____ Behavioral therapy

4. _____ Cognitive therapy

5. _____ Biomedical therapy

6. _____ Group therapy

7. _____ Family therapy

8. _____ Biofeedback

9. _____ Recreation therapy

10. _____ Contracting

MULTIPLE CHOICE

Select the best answer from the multiple-choice items.

1. The role of the nurse working with the client who has a mental disorder includes:
   a. Conducting psychologic testing
   b. Daily individual psychotherapy sessions
   c. Monitoring behavioral responses to therapy
   d. Acting as a liaison with government and civil agencies

2. Which of the following demonstrates an expected client outcome of a therapeutic milieu environment in the mental health setting?
   a. Behavioral responses are monitored and documented
   b. Improved social and communication skills observed during activities
   c. Changes in cognitive thoughts will be demonstrated by testing
   d. Early life experiences will provide insight into present behavior

3. When caring for the client with outbursts of uncontrolled anger, which of the following nursing actions would most reinforce the desired outcome?
   a. Model an appropriate response to the situation
   b. Provide insight into the cause of the observed response
   c. Reprimand the client for the inappropriate actions
   d. Observe and document a detailed description of the incident

4. Which of the following best describes the function of a clinical psychologist as a member of the treatment team?
   a. Attend to the personal and emotional needs of the client
   b. Coordinate recreational and occupational therapy
   c. Function as coordinator of outpatient resources
   d. Administer and interpret results of psychologic testing

5. Which of the following mental health professionals assists clients to use energy more constructively?
   a. Licensed professional counselor
   b. Recreational therapist
   c. Mental health technician
   d. Clinical social worker

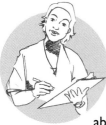

LEARNING OBJECTIVES

After learning the content in this chapter, the student will be able to:

1. Apply concepts of mental health care to clients in nonpsychiatric settings.

2. Identify types of client situations in which interventions may be needed to meet mental health needs.

3. Utilize principles of grief and loss to meet psychosocial needs of the person experiencing physical disease and loss.

4. Identify factors that can precipitate aggressive behaviors in clients who are confined in a controlled environment.

5. Describe the role of the nurse in the deliverance of mental health care within the correctional institution.

Mental Health Care in Nonpsychiatric Settings

KEY TERMS

Duo-diagnosis

Holistic

Manipulation

Powerlessness

Psychologic crisis

Nonpsychiatric Setting

The **holistic** concept of nursing care incorporates the entire scope of human needs, addressing the physical, psychosocial, cultural, and spiritual issues of the individual client. Nurses practice in a variety of nonpsychiatric settings, providing an array of situations in which the emotional and psychosocial needs of clients may emerge. Among these practice settings are emergency rooms, inpatient units, long-term care facilities, home health care, hospice care, physician clinics, and the criminal justice system. In some instances, mentally healthy individuals may experience temporary mental instability as a result of a situational crisis, such as rape, trauma, abuse, or environmental disaster. Crisis intervention and supportive nursing strategies can make a major difference in the ability of the client to access and mobilize coping resources at a time when life seems to be unraveling. In many situations, the nurse is the health care worker who observes and assesses these feelings or behaviors that may demonstrate symptoms of mental health dysfunction.

Among the most common emotional and psychologic responses to trauma, physical illness, or loss are depression, fear, anxiety, denial, withdrawal, anger, apathy, regression, and dependency. Levels of these emotions may accelerate as a person feels a loss of control over what is happening when pain, disability, hospitalization, or death may loom in the unknown. The stage of the illness and the possible treatment options will be a factor in this reaction. The economic impact of health care in any setting can also produce an overwhelming flood of emotions and fears. In addition, a projection of these fears is often demonstrated by the client in self-centered demanding behaviors such as unreasonable requests of health care providers. Regardless of the setting, the nurse should be prepared to initiate interventions to address the psychosocial needs, as well as the physical needs, of each client.

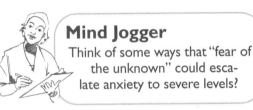

Mind Jogger
Think of some ways that "fear of the unknown" could escalate anxiety to severe levels?

Mental Health Nursing in Nonpsychiatric Health Care Systems

DSM-IV-TR addresses conditions or problems that pose a psychologic factor that affects a medical condition. These factors can influence the course of a general medical condition, resulting in an exacerbation of the illness or a delayed recovery. Sometimes the factors may interfere with treatment of the medical condition such as continued noncompliance with diet or medication therapy in the client with diabetes, or continued smoking by the client with chronic pulmonary disease. Each problem is addressed based on the individual psychologic factors that are present (see At a Glance 21-1).

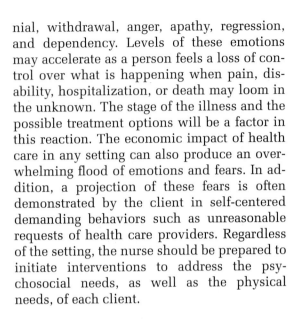

Just the Facts

Factors affecting one's ability to cope include:

Individual factors, such as age, personality, intelligence, values, cultural beliefs, and emotional state

Environmental factors, such as support system and financial stability

Illness-related factors, such as type of illness, rate of progression, functional impairment, and prognosis

At a Glance 21-1 Psychologic Factors That Affect Medical Conditions

- Mental Disorders: Psychiatric disorders such as bipolar, schizophrenia, or major depression in combination with myocardial infarction, renal disease, asthma, or surgery.
- Psychologic Symptoms: Significantly affect the course or treatment of the medical condition (e.g., apathy or depressed state may affect recovery from surgery).
- Personality Traits or Coping Styles: Personality trait or maladaptive coping strategy can adversely affect the course or treatment of the medical condition (e.g., controlling, hostile personality trait may interfere with post-treatment myocardial infarction progress, or continued denial of need for a diagnostic procedure or surgery).
- Maladaptive Health Behaviors: Behavior practices such as unsafe sexual practices, lack of exercise, or excessive use of food, drugs, or alcohol.
- Stress-Related Physiological Response: Stress-related physiologic responses might initiate increased incidence of hypertension, cardiac arrhythmias, angina, migraine headache, or respiratory crisis.

Just the Facts

Common coping strategies in physical illness include asking questions to obtain information and guidance for treatment, sharing concerns and finding support from others, a change in emotional climate with light-hearted humor, and suppression of fears and "what ifs."

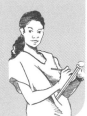

A physical illness that imposes a severe threat to a person's health status and a lifetime of chronic disease may elicit a grief response to this real or perceived loss. The disease process may restrict the person's lifestyle and socioeconomic status, which may threaten both the self-esteem and sense of security previously enjoyed. Future goals and family roles may be shattered by the imposition of the physical and psychologic effects of the symptoms. At a Glance 21-2 lists some physical illnesses or surgeries that have the potential to elicit major psychologic effects on the client and the client's family.

At a Glance 21-2 Physical Illnesses and Surgeries with Major Psychologic Effects

- Alzheimer's disease
- AIDS/HIV disease
- Diabetes mellitus
- Parkinson's disease
- Multiple sclerosis
- Lou Gehrig's disease
- Hemophilia
- Stroke (CVA)
- COPD, asthma
- Cancer/chemotherapy
- Myocardial infarction
- Hemodialysis
- Mastectomy
- Prostatectomy
- Colostomy, ileostomy, nephrostomy
- Amputation
- Quadriplegia or hemiplegia
- Radical facial and/or neck surgery

Role of the Caregivers

The lack of control over the devastating effects imposed by many of these conditions may be described as a state of helplessness or **powerlessness.** This may be true of both the person who has the illness and the family involved.

The nurse should assume an empathetic and supportive role as the emotional and psychologic defenses of those persons are attacked by the decision making and coping necessary to deal with the illness or surgery. The nurse should plan to include time for active listening, allowing and encouraging the release and expression of feelings and concerns. Explanations concerning diagnostic tests, procedures, permits, and consent forms are vital to allow the person to make informed decisions regarding their situation. A sense of empowerment is returned to the client when he or she is included in planning to meet care needs and has the opportunity to make choices about those needs. The nurse's sensitivity to the anxiety the client is experiencing will also be a major factor in client's ability to adapt to the situation.

caregivers in providing the needed help also provides a sense of security during a time when ego defenses are weakened and the client needs a sense of stability to allow and encourage trust in the environment. It is most important to teach the client problem-solving skills and provide support for self-care efforts. The increase in self-care responsibilities as appropriate helps to preserve self-esteem and provides a sense of control over a situation that may seem overwhelming.

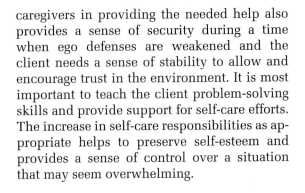

Just the Facts

Adaptive coping behaviors—Client demonstrates ability to mobilize internal and external resources to adapt to a situation.

Maladaptive coping behaviors—Client is unable to mobilize internal and external resources resulting in disorganized and destructive behaviors.

Crisis—Situation in which client's available coping mechanisms are inadequate.

Mind Jogger

How does informed decision making help to defuse the anxiety of the client?

Just the Facts

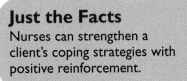

Nurses can strengthen a client's coping strategies with positive reinforcement.

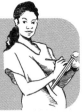

Mind Jogger

How can the nurse assist in strengthening the client's support system? What referrals could be utilized?

A **psychologic crisis,** in which the person is totally overwhelmed by the situation, can be averted through the support of the client's caregivers, friends, and family. Assessment of the client's emotional reaction to the diagnosis, past and current coping abilities, and available support resources provides the nurse with a baseline for intervention to facilitate adaptation as the outcome. Consistency of

Medical-Surgical Client with a Psychiatric Illness

The client with a diagnosed psychiatric illness who is hospitalized can present a nursing challenge. Whereas the nurse may prioritize the medical-surgical needs of the client, the secondary diagnosis must be considered in all aspects of care planning. Critical thinking leads the nurse to ask: How will the client mentally view this procedure? What environmental stimuli could be misinterpreted? What explanations will be needed to reinforce reality to the client with a psychotic disorder? How might this client misperceive pain? What approach could be used if the client exhibits delusional thinking or hallucinations? What psychologic signs and symptoms might be anticipated in a client with schizophrenia or major affective disorder who is diagnosed with a serious medical or surgical condition?

It is important for the nurse to consider the situation in the accompanying case study and answer the questions posed there.

Case Study: More Than One Problem

John, a 48-year-old unemployed mechanic, is admitted to the emergency room with the following symptoms: acute upper left abdominal pain, abdominal distention, febrile, elevated WBC, nausea, and vomiting. Initial medical assessment leads to a diagnosis of a perforated diverticuli of the splenic flexure with peritonitis. The client also has a diagnosis of chronic schizophrenia, undifferentiated type, and has lived in a group home milieu for the past 6 months. John is given sedation prior to the emergency abdominal surgery. When John returns to the medical-surgical unit, he has a nasogastric tube connected to intermittent suction, a left triple-lumen subclavian intravenous line, a right jugular intravenous line with total parental nutrition (TPN) infusion, and an open abdominal incision with wet-to-dry packing secured with 4 x 8 dressings and Montgomery straps.

Because John also has a diagnosis of schizophrenia, his behavior may be altered by the events of anesthesia and surgery. What response might the nurse expect as John emerges from sedation and anesthesia?

_____

How might he misinterpret the array of "tubes" connected to his body?

_____

_____

Do you think John will understand that the pain is related to his surgery? What approach might the nurse use to help John understand the reality of the pain?

_____

_____

The second postoperative day, John begins to question the invasive equipment lines entering his body. The nurse enters his room to find him drinking water, with his nasogastric tube lying on the floor beside the bed. He tells the nurse he was thirsty, and "that hose was siphoning all the water out of my body to water the plants neglected by my inability to turn the shower on, and I got some water so I can water the shower."

continues

Case Study: More Than One Problem (Continued)

What type of psychotic behavior is seen in John's actions?

_____

What physical assessments related to his surgical care would be important to report?

_____

How should the nurse respond to John's altered thinking?

_____

_____

_____

_____

The nurse assesses that bowel sounds are present and that no nausea or vomiting has occurred with the oral intake. The physician orders a liquid diet for John. While passing his room several hours later, the nurse hears John talking. When entering the room, no one is present except John. The water faucet in the sink and the shower are both turned on with hot water running. John tells the nurse, "It can't flow through me if it is not running. Don't turn it off or I will shrivel up." How could the nurse use the IV and TPN fluid to divert John's delusional thinking back to reality?

_____

The nurse proceeds to change the packing and dressing on John's abdominal incision. John tells the nurse, "If you take that off, the water will become contaminated and kill the plants." What misperception does John have concerning the open abdominal incision? How could the nurse use the wet-to-dry packs to reinforce reality?

_____

_____

_____

Application of the Nursing Process

Nurses facing the challenge of a duo-diagnosis situation such as this can use the nursing process to identify the problems related to both physiologic and psychologic issues. Communication techniques and nursing interventions for altered thought processes are critical to the outcome in John's situation. His psychologic state complicates his compliance with treatment and his recovery from surgery.

Both the physiologic and psychologic needs of the individual client must be assessed and met. Acute assessment skills and creative interventions are needed to avoid complications and promote the client's return to a state of wellness and discharge from the hospital.

Nursing Diagnosis. Nursing diagnoses that are commonly used in planning the care of clients with psychologic needs related to a medical illness or surgical condition include:

- Adjustment impaired, related to chronic illness
- Anxiety, related to situational crisis
- Alteration in self-image, related to functional changes imposed by illness
- Coping ineffective, family; related to inability to care for client
- Coping ineffective, individual; related to situational crisis
- Denial, ineffective; related to fear or anxiety
- Grieving, anticipatory; related to potential for loss
- Hopelessness, related to chronic illness
- Powerlessness, related to situational crisis
- Role performance alteration, related to change in health status
- Self-care deficit, related to effects of medical or surgical condition
- Self-esteem, situational low, related to increased dependence on caregivers
- Social isolation, related to factors imposed by illness

Evaluation. The anticipated outcome for the client with psychologic problems related to a medical illness is that optimal healthy physiologic functioning is preserved within the restrictions imposed by the disease process. An understanding of the disease process and any effects of the illness facilitates a productive interdependence of the client, caregivers, and support persons. Participation in treatment, progress toward rehabilitative efforts, and reduction in stress or anxiety-related symptoms will strengthen the ability of the person to cope effectively with the situational crisis confronting them.

Mental Health Nursing in the Criminal Justice System

There are many theories and assumptions as to why individuals commit acts against society that secure them time living behind the walls and locks of a prison. What happens? Is it related to environmental factors, or is it fostered by a predisposition to engage in behaviors that defy the legal boundaries that define right from wrong? In his book, *Inside the Criminal Mind,* Stanton Samenow describes the criminal's irresponsible pattern of behavior as predominant "throughout his life." School, work, family, and friends are all victims of deceit, devious thinking, and **manipulation** to meet criminal's self-serving coercive views of the world. Feeling no obligation to anyone, the criminal believes people, their property, and society in general exist for his or her benefit. Criminals will do virtually anything to acquire whatever they want. They have a voracious and ruthless need for power, caring very little about whom they injure or things they destroy as they manipulate others. Samenow states, "They have an inflated self-image in which they regard themselves as special and superior and assume that people will do their bidding."

Although there are some types of crimes that are viewed by psychiatric professionals as the result of mental instability, it must be considered that all criminals think differently. In a distorted form of logic, they think their behavior is acceptable as long as it benefits them. Correctional facilities have continuously sought ways to reform and rehabilitate those whose thinking is dominated by devising ways to be a better criminal. Prison is an environment where antisocial thoughts and behaviors are the norm, and the exchange of crime-related ideas is fostered by the commonality of narcissistic and self-serving personalities. The same behaviors demonstrated on the street are continued in prison. The incarcerated person usually uses the system to his or her favor, continuing manipulative and power-seeking behaviors. Fear, remorse, or regret may be temporarily displayed by the inmate new to the system. However, the hard-core truth of survival leads many to play the game of toughness in an atmosphere where stabbing, rape, gang warfare, and rioting are common. There is a constant struggle within the confines of the prison walls to maintain some sense of self. Security becomes a control issue with prison guards often waging power struggles to maintain their authority. The criminal often engages in psychologic warfare with security personnel, seeking favors or special treatment and playing con games to win "good-time" credits. Inmate complaints are common, along with selfish requests and expectations, and charges that their rights are being violated when their wishes are denied, all the time ignoring the fact that their present situation is the result of their own choices.

Theft, homosexuality, and rape are widespread within the prison system. The homosexual inmates fall prey to other prisoners who use fear and threats if sexual acts are not performed. The weak, both physically and mentally, are vulnerable to the aggravation of the strong. Cigarettes, commissary items, and tennis shoes become bargaining bait to ward off the avengers. For those who know aggression and crime as a way of life, it is understandable that incarceration with a living environment where privacy, dignity, and individuality are absent further contributes to the underlying hostility. The obvious sense of powerlessness stimulates the inmates to search for power and control within the system. This need, combined with time to devise their manipulative acts, breeds a potential for violence and disruption. Fighting and impulsive rebellious acts result in punishment that only adds to their psychologic stockpile of perceived injustices.

Prison Healthcare Issues and Practices

The medical division of a correctional facility is one of the bargaining bases for the inmates. Real or perceived ailments become a means to seek special privileges and excuses from assigned labor and regimental routines. Medications are coveted and requested for both actual and nonsensical reasons. The need for treatment must be separated from the exploitative methods devised by the criminal to assure that any legitimate condition receives the appropriate medical attention.

Many policies and guidelines of the criminal justice organization govern the boundaries of medical treatment available to the inmates. An introduction to these policies is included in the initial orientation of inmates on their arrival to the prison facility. In addition, an explanation of the risk factors precipitated by aggregate and confined living is provided. Most of the prison population are presently dealing with or have a history of some type of substance abuse. Risk behaviors related to drug use gives rise to the growing numbers of those who test positive for HIV. Hepatitis B and C are rampant within the system. A portion of the population has developed AIDS. Regardless of whether a person is a prison inmate, the psychologic impact and verdict imposed by hearing that one has tested positive for these diseases is the same. The result is devastating. Nurses within the prison system do the same counseling for these victims as for those in the outside world. For this victim, the nurse may be the sole support system. There are no families or friends from whom consolation and sympathy can be sought. Silence is absolute to avoid the harassment of fellow inmates. Although treatment is available, the cold reality of another sentence engulfs their being.

Nurse's Role in the Prison System

Nurses who work in a correctional facility must learn to separate what is real from what is a manipulative endeavor by the inmate. A calm, but firm and matter-of-fact approach is essential to command compliance with rules and policies of the institution. Security is always present in the medical department. The same standards of behavior are expected from the inmates regardless of where they are in the prison. The empathy and compassion that is so integral to other areas of nursing may quickly be seen by criminals as an opportunity for their con games. The nurse must be vigilant to avoid being victimized by these actions. It is also important, however, to accept the inmate as a person with human feelings and needs. If psychologic symptoms are voiced or observed, the nurse should refer the information through the appropriate channels so that counseling or treatment can be provided. A psychiatric evaluation process is required by the American Correctional Association, the national accrediting body for prisons and jails.

Data collected in this process may include:

- Previous counseling or psychiatric treatment
- Current or previous use of psychotropic medications
- Any history of inpatient psychiatric treatment, either court mandated or voluntary
- Family history of psychiatric problems
- History of seizures or head trauma
- History of suicide attempts
- Any hallucinations or delusional thinking
- Any objective psychotic symptoms
- History or current use of illicit drugs
- Any criminal history as a juvenile
- Convictions for sex offenses
- History of violence, assault, or destructive behaviors
- History of being the target of violence while incarcerated

Further diagnostic evaluation is recommended and referral is warranted if the inmate demonstrates symptoms or behaviors of psychiatric illness, has a history of previous mental health treatment, voices current suicidal ideation or prior suicidal gestures, indicates affective distress, or is at high risk for problems with adjustment to confinement, or the offense committed is of an unusual nature.

Summary

Mentally healthy individuals may at times experience periods of psychologic disarray and instability when confronted with crisis or situations that threaten physical or emotional well-being. Psychologic factors such as diagnosed psychotic mental illness, depression, personality disorders, maladaptive health behaviors, or stress-related responses can all affect the outcome and treatment process of a medical condition.

The person's ability to cope with chronic illness or the outcome of major surgery can also contribute to psychologic stress and potential crisis. The support of family, friends, and caregivers offers a sensitivity and balance that can avert a psychologic crisis. The client with a psychiatric illness who is hospitalized for a medical or surgical condition requires skilled intervention to address both physiologic and psychologic needs.

Nurses who practice within the criminal justice system must be alert to the manipulative tactics used by the criminal to gain favors or unprescribed medicinal drugs. Aggressive forces within the prison environment result in a psychologic warfare between inmates, as well as between security and inmates.

A growing proportion of the inmate population in correctional facilities has a history of risk behaviors and is testing positive for HIV and Hepatitis B and C. Criminal behavior is the result of distorted criminal thinking. Time in prison often feeds the criminal's search for ways to be a better criminal and avoid being caught, rather than ways to conform to the laws of society. A combination of these factors presents the need for the nurse to use a nontraditional approach to the client population. While seeing the medical needs of the client as the primary focus of providing healthcare to the inmates, their psychologic games and issues must always be considered.

Bibliography

American Psychiatric Association (2000). *Diagnostic and statistical manual of mental disorders text revision* (4th ed.). Washington, DC: American Psychiatric Association.

Samenow, S. E. (1984). *Inside the criminal mind*, New York, NY: Random House.

Texas Department of Criminal Justice Diagnostic and Evaluation Process Diagnostic Screening Interview. Revised 5/94.

FILL IN THE BLANK

Fill in the blank with the correct answer.

1. When the client is included in the planning of care needs and choices made, it returns a sense of _____ to the person.

2. The lack of control over the devastating effects imposed by serious physical illnesses and surgeries is referred to as a state of _____ .

3. Psychologic factors can affect a medical condition causing a(n) _____ of the illness or a(n) _____ recovery.

4. _____ in caregivers in providing care offers as sense of security when ego defenses are weakened.

5. Although some types of crimes are viewed by psychiatric professionals as related to mental instability, the common link between criminals is the difference in their _____ .

6. _____ are rampant within the prison system.

7. A calm, but _____ nursing approach is essential for compliance of prison inmates with rules and policies of the institution.

MATCHING

Match the following terms to the most appropriate phrase.

a. Concept that includes entire scope of human needs.

b. Purposeful self-serving behavior directed at getting needs met.

c. Temporary state of high anxiety in which usual coping mechanisms fail.

d. Combination of physical and mental illness.

e. Loss of ability to act or sense of control.

1. _____ Duo-diagnosis

2. _____ Psychologic crisis

3. _____ Holistic

4. _____ Powerlessness

5. _____ Manipulation

MULTIPLE CHOICE

Select the best answer from the multiple-choice items.

1. The nurse is doing interventions for a client who is experiencing a psychologic crisis. The most essential tool the nurse can teach the client at this time is:

    a. How to avoid similar situations in the future.

    b. Behavior modification to deal with current anxiety level.

    c. Steps in problem solving to confront the issue systematically.

    d. Anticipatory grieving to deal with the posttraumatic period.

2. Edward has had a radical perineal prosta-tectomy for metastasized cancer of the prostate gland. The nurse can best develop a sense of trust and cooperation with Edward by:

   a. Providing total care needs for the length of his hospital stay.

   b. Involving him in care planning necessary to meet his needs.

   c. Minimizing the choices he has to make during his recovery period.

   d. Teaching him adaptive coping mechanisms for dealing with loss.

3. The nurse is caring for a client who has recently been diagnosed with leukemia. Which of the following is important for the nurse to include in a psychologic assessment of this client?

   a. Adaptive and maladaptive coping behaviors

   b. Relaxation techniques

   c. Opportunities for spiritual counseling

   d. Explanation of diagnostic tests

4. The nurse is doing a psychiatric evaluation for an inmate of a correctional facility. Which of the following factors would indicate a need for referral and further evaluation?

   a. Has difficulty sleeping well

   b. Anger toward the judicial system

   c. Previous treatment for depression

   d. Ambivalent feelings about other inmates

SEEK AND FIND

Find the incorrect information in the following statements.

1. Prison inmate complaints that rights are being violated when their requests are not granted are usually based in reasonable expectations of the system.

2. A personality trait or maladaptive coping strategy does not usually interfere with the course or treatment of a medical condition.

3. Mentally healthy individuals usually are able to cope with crisis situations without a threat to their physical or emotional well-being.

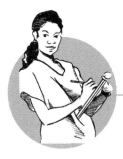

A

DSM-IV-TR
Classification

Disorders Usually First Diagnosed in Infancy, Childhood, or Adolescence

MENTAL RETARDATON	317	Mild Mental Retardation
	318.0	Moderate Mental Retardation
	318.1	Severe Mental Retardation
	318.2	Profound Mental Retardation
	319	Mental Retardation, Severity, Unspecified
LEARNING DISORDERS	315.00	Reading Disorder
	315.1	Mathematics Disorder
	315.2	Disorder of Written Expression
	315.9	Learning Disorder NOS
MOTOR SKILLS DISORDER	315.4	Developmental Coordination Disorder
COMMUNICATION DISORDERS	315.31	Expressive Language Disorder
	315.32	Mixed Receptive-Expressive Language Disorder
	315.39	Phonological Disorder
	307.0	Stuttering
	307.9	Communication Disorder
PERVASIVE DEVELOPMENTAL DISORDERS	299.00	Autistic Disorder
	299.80	Rett's Disorder
	299.10	Childhood Disintegrative Disorder
	299.80	Asperger's Disorder
	299.80	Pervasive Developmental Disorder NOS
ATTENTION DEFICIT AND DISRUPTIVE BEHAVIOR DISORDERS	314.xx	Attention Deficit/Hyperactivity Disorder
	.01	Combined Type
	.00	Predominantly Inattentive Type
	.01	Predominantly Hyperactive-Impulsive Type
	314.9	Attention Deficit/Hyperactivity Disorder NOS
	312.xx	Conduct Disorder
	.81	Childhood-Onset Type
	.82	Adolescent-Onset Type
	.89	Unspecified Onset
	313.81	Unoppositional Defiant Disorder
	312.9	Disruptive Behavior Disorder
FEEDING AND EATING DISORDERS OF INFANCY OR EARLY CHILDHOOD	307.52	Pica
	307.53	Rumination Disorder
	307.59	Feeding Disorder of Infancy or Early Childhood
TIC DISORDERS	307.23	Tourette's Disorder
	307.22	Chronic Motor or Vocal Tic Disorder
	307.21	Transient Tic Disorder
	307.20	Tic Disorder NOS

NOS = Not Otherwise Classified

continues

ELIMINATION DISORDERS	—.—	Encopresis
	787.6	With Constipation and Overflow Incontinence
	307.7	Without Constipation and Overflow Incontinence
	307.6	Enuresis (Not Due to a General Medical Condition)
OTHER DISORDERS OF INFANCY, CHILDHOOD, OR ADOLESCENCE	309.21	Separation Anxiety Disorder
	313.23	Selective Mutism
	313.89	Reactive Attachment Disorder of Infancy or Early Childhood
	307.3	Stereotypic Movement Disorder
	313.9	Disorder of Infancy, Childhood, or Adolescence

Delirium, Dementia, Amnestic, and Other Cognitive Disorders

DELIRIUM	293.0	Delirium Due to a *(General Medical Condition)*
		Substance Intoxication Delirium
		Substance Withdrawal Delirium
	780.09	Delirium Due to Multiple Etiologies
		Delirium NOS
DEMENTIA	294.xx	Dementia of the Alzheimer's Type, With Early Onset
	.10	Without Behavioral Disturbance
	.11	With Behavioral Disturbance
	294.xx	Dementia of the Alzheimer's Type, With Late Onset
	.10	Without Behavioral Disturbance
	.11	With Behavioral Disturbance
	290.xx	Vascular Dementia
	.40	Uncomplicated
	.41	With Delirium
	.42	With Delusions
	.43	With Depressed Mood
DEMENTIA DUE TO A GENERAL MEDICAL CONDITION	294.1x	Dementia Due to HIV Disease
	294.1x	Dementia Due to Head Trauma
	294.1x	Dementia Due to Parkinson's Disease
	294.1x	Dementia Due to Huntington's Disease
	294.1x	Dementia Due to Pick's Disease
	294.1x	Dementia Due to Creutzfeldt-Jakob Disease
	294.1x	Dementia Due to *(Other Medical Condition)*
	—.—	Substance-Induced Persisting Dementia
	—.—	Dementia Due to Multiple Etiologies
	294.8	Dementia NOS
AMNESTIC DISORDERS	294.0	Amnestic Disorder Due to *(General Medical Condition)*
	—.—	Substance-Induced Persisting Amnestic Disorder
	—.—	Amnestic Disorder NOS
OTHER COGNITIVE DISORDERS	294.9	Cognitive Disorder NOS

continues

Mental Disorders Due to a General Medical Condition Not Elsewhere Classified

MENTAL DISORDERS DUE TO A GENERAL MEDICAL CONDITION NOT ELSEWHERE CLASSIFIED	293.89	Catatonic Disorder Due to *(General Medical Condition)*
	310.1	Personality Change Due to *(General Medical Condition)*
	293.9	Mental Disorder NOS Due to *(General Medical Condition)*

Substance-Related Disorders

ALCOHOL-RELATED DISORDERS (Alcohol Use Disorders)	303.90	Alcohol Dependence
	305.00	Alcohol Abuse
	303.00	Alcohol Intoxication Delirium
	291.81	Alcohol Withdrawal
	291.0	Alcohol Intoxication Delirium
	291.0	Alcohol Withdrawal Delirium
	291.2	Alcohol-Induced Persisting Dementia
	291.1	Alcohol-Induced Persisting Amnestic Disorder
	291.x	Alcohol-Induced Psychotic Disorder
	.5	With Delusions
	.3	With Hallucinations
	291.89	Alcohol-Induced Mood Disorder
	291.89	Alcohol-Induced Anxiety Disorder
	291.89	Alcohol-Induced Sexual Dysfunction
	291.89	Alcohol-Induced Sleep Disorder
	291.9	Alcohol-Related Disorder NOS
CAFFEINE-RELATED DISORDERS (Induced Disorders)	305.90	Caffeine Intoxication
	292.89	Caffeine-Induced Anxiety Disorder
	292.89	Caffeine-Induced Sleep Disorder
	292.9	Caffeine-Related Disorder NOS
CANNABIS-RELATED DISORDERS (Cannabis Use Disorders)	304.30	Cannabis Dependence
	305.20	Cannabis Abuse
(Cannabis-Induced Disorders)	292.89	Cannabis Intoxication *(Specify if With Perceptual Disturbance)*
	292.81	Cannabis Intoxication Delirium
	292.xx	Cannabis-Induced Psychotic Disorder
	.11	With Delusions
	.12	With Hallucinations
	292.89	Cannabis-Induced Anxiety Disorder
	292.9	Cannabis-Related Disorder NOS
COCAINE-RELATED DISORDERS (Cocaine Use Disorders)	304.20	Cocaine Dependence
	305.60	Cocaine Abuse
(Cocaine-Induced Disorders)	292.89	Cocaine Intoxication *(Specify if With Perceptual Disturbance)*
	292.0	Cocaine Withdrawal

continues

292.81	Cocaine Intoxication Delirium
292.xx	Cocaine-Induced Psychotic Disorder
.11	With Delusions
.12	With Hallucinations
292.84	Cocaine-Induced Mood Disorder
292.89	Cocaine-Induced Anxiety Disorder
292.89	Cocaine-Induced Sexual Dysfunction
292.89	Cocaine-Induced Sleep Disorder
292.9	Cocaine-Related Disorder NOS

HALLUCINOGEN-RELATED DISORDERS

(Hallucinogen Use Disorders)

304.50	Hallucinogen Dependence
305.30	Hallucinogen Abuse

(Hallucinogen-Induced Disorders)

292.89	Hallucinogen Intoxication
292.89	Hallucinogen Persisting Perception Disorder (Flashbacks)
292.81	Hallucinogen Intoxication Delirium
292.xx	Hallucinogen-Induced Psychotic Disorder
.11	With Delusions
.12	With Hallucinations
292.84	Hallucinogen-Induced Mood Disorder
292.89	Hallucinogen-Induced Anxiety Disorder
292.9	Hallucinogen-Related Disorder NOS

INHALANT-RELATED DISORDERS

(Inhalant Use Disorders)

304.60	Inhalant Dependence
305.90	Inhalant Abuse

(Inhalant-Induced Disorders)

292.89	Inhalant Intoxication
292.81	Inhalant Intoxication Delirium
292.82	Inhalant-Induced Persisting Dementia
292.xx	Inhalant-Induced Psychotic Disorder
.11	With Delusions
.12	With Hallucinations
292.84	Inhalant-Induced Mood Disorder
292.89	Inhalant-Induced Anxiety Disorder
292.9	Inhalant-Related Disorder NOS

NICOTINE-RELATED DISORDERS

(Nicotine Use Disorder)

305.1	Nicotine Dependence

(Nicotine-Induced Disorder)

292.0	Nicotine Withdrawal
292.9	Nicotine-Related Disorder NOS

continues

OPIOID-RELATED DISORDERS

(Opioid Use	304.00	Opioid Dependence
Disorders)	305.50	Opioid Abuse
(Opioid-Induced	292.89	Opioid Intoxication *(Specify if With Perceptual Disturbances)*
Disorders)	292.0	Opioid Withdrawal
	292.81	Opioid Intoxication Delirium
	292.xx	Opioid-Induced Psychotic Disorder
	.11	With Delusions
	.12	With Hallucinations
	292.84	Opioid-Induced Mood Disorder
	292.89	Opioid-Induced Sexual Dysfunction
	292.89	Opioid-Induced Sleep Disorder
	292.9	Opioid-Related Disorder NOS

PHENCYCLIDINE (OR PHENCYCLIDINE-LIKE)-RELATED DISORDERS

(Phencyclidine Use	304.60	Phencyclidine Dependence
Disorders)	305.90	Phencyclidine Abuse
(Phencyclidine-Induced	292.89	Phencyclidine Intoxication *(Specify if With Perceptual Disturbance)*
Disorders)	292.81	Phencyclidine Intoxication Delirium
	292.xx	Phencyclidine-Induced Psychotic Disorder
	.11	With Delusions
	.12	With Hallucinations
	292.84	Phencyclidine-Induced Mood Disorder
	292.89	Phencyclidine-Induced Anxiety Disorder
	292.9	Phencyclidine-Related Disorder NOS

SEDATIVE, HYPNOTIC, OR ANXIOLYTIC-RELATED DISORDERS

(Sedative, Hypnotic,	304.10	Sedative, Hypnotic, or Anxiolytic Dependence
or Anxiolytic Use	305.40	Sedative, Hypnotic, or Anxiolytic Withdrawal *(Specify if With Perceptual Disturbances)*
Disorders)		
(Sedative, Hypnotic,	292.89	Sedative, Hypnotic, or Anxiolytic Intoxication
or Anxiolytic-Induced Disorders)	292.0	Sedative, Hypnotic, or Anxiolytic Withdrawal *(Specify if With Perceptual Disturbances)*
	292.81	Sedative, Hypnotic, or Anxiolytic Intoxication Delirium
	292.81	Sedative, Hypnotic, or Anxiolytic Withdrawal Delirium
	292.82	Sedative, Hypnotic, or Anxiolytic-Induced Persisting Dementia
	292.83	Sedative, Hypnotic, or Anxiolytic-Induced Persisting Amnestic Disorder

continues

	292.xx	Sedative, Hypnotic, or Anxiolytic-Induced Psychotic Disorder
	.11	With Delusions
	.12	With Hallucinations
	292.84	Sedative, Hypnotic, or Anxiolytic-Induced Mood Disorder
	292.89	Sedative, Hypnotic, or Anxiolytic-Induced Anxiety Disorder
	292.89	Sedative, Hypnotic, or Anxiolytic-Induced Sexual Dysfunction
	292.89	Sedative, Hypnotic, or Anxiolytic-Induced Sleep Disorder
	292.9	Sedative, Hypnotic, or Anxiolytic-Related Disorder NOS

POLYSUBSTANCE-RELATED DISORDER	304.80	Polysubstance Dependence

OTHER (OR UNKNOWN) SUBSTANCE-RELATED DISORDERS

Other (or Unknown) Substance Use Disorders	304.90	Other (or Unknown) Substance Dependence
	305.90	Other (or Unknown) Substance Abuse
Other (or Unknown) Substance-Induced Disorders	292.89	Other (or Unknown) Substance Intoxication *(Specify if With Perceptual Disturbances)*
	292.0	Other (or Unknown) Substance Withdrawal *(Specify if With Perceptual Disturbances)*
	292.81	Other (or Unknown) Substance-Induced Delirium
	292.82	Other (or Unknown) Substance-Induced Persisting Dementia
	292.83	Other (or Unknown) Substance-Induced Persisting Amnestic Disorder
	292.xx	Other (or Unknown) Substance-Induced Psychotic Disorder
	.11	With Delusions
	.12	With Hallucinations
	292.84	Other (or Unknown) Substance-Induced Mood Disorder
	292.89	Other (or Unknown) Substance-Induced Anxiety Disorder
	292.89	Other (or Unknown) Substance-Induced Sexual Dysfunction
	292.89	Other (or Unknown) Substance-Induced Sleep Disorder
	292.9	Other (or Unknown) Substance-Related Disorder NOS

Schizophrenia and Other Psychotic Disorders

	295.xx	Schizophrenia Residual Symptoms *[Episodic, Continuous, or Single Episode of Negative Symptoms],* Other, or Unspecified Pattern
	.30	Paranoid Type
	.10	Disorganized Type
	.20	Catatonic Type
	.90	Undifferentiated Type
	.60	Residual Type

continues

	295.40	Schizophreniform Disorder *(Specify With/Without Good Prognosis)*
	295.70	Schizoaffective Disorder *(Specify Bipolar/Depressive Type)*
	297.1	Delusional Disorder *(Erotomanic Type/Grandiose Type/Jealous Type/Persecutory Type/Somatic Type/Mixed Type/Unspecified Type)*
	298.8	Brief Psychotic Disorder *(With/Without Marked Stressors, With Postpartum Onset)*
	297.3	Shared Psychotic Disorder
	293.xx	Psychotic Disorder Due to *(General Medical Condition)*
	.81	With Delusions
	.82	With Hallucinations
	—.—	Substance-Induced Psychotic Disorder
	298.9	Psychotic Disorder NOS

Mood Disorders

DEPRESSIVE DISORDERS	296.xx	Major Depressive Disorder
	.2x	Single Episode
	.3x	Recurrent
	300.4	Dysthymic Disorder *(Early/Late Onset With/Without Atypical Features)*
	311	Depressive Disorder NOS
BIPOLAR DISORDERS	296.xx	Bipolar I Disorder
	.0x	Single Manic Episode *(Specify if Mixed)*
	.40	Most Recent Episode Hypomanic
	.4x	Most Recent Episode Manic
	.6x	Most Recent Episode Mixed
	.5x	Most Recent Episode Depressed
	.7	Most Recent Episode Unspecified
	296.89	Bipolar II Disorder *(Specify Hypomanic or Depressed)*
	301.13	Cyclothymic Disorder
	296.80	Bipolar Disorder NOS
	293.83	Mood Disorder Due to *(General Medical Condition)*
	—.—	Substance-Induced Mood Disorder
	296.90	Mood Disorder NOS

Anxiety Disorders

	300.1	Panic Disorder Without Agoraphobia
	300.21	Panic Disorder With Agoraphobia
	300.22	Agoraphobia Without History of Panic Disorder
	300.29	Specific Phobia
	300.23	Social Phobia
	300.3	Obsessive-Compulsive Disorder
	309.81	Posttraumatic Stress Disorder *(Specify if Acute/Chronic or With Delayed Onset)*
	308.3	Acute Stress Disorder

continues

	300.02	Generalized Anxiety disorder
	293.84	Anxiety Disorder Due to *(General Medical Condition)*
	—.—	Substance-Induced Anxiety Disorder
	300.00	Anxiety Disorder NOS

Somatoform Disorders

	300.81	Somatization Disorder
	300.82	Undifferentiated Somatoform Disorder
	300.11	Conversion Disorder *(With Motor Symptom or Deficit/With Sensory Symptom or Deficit/With Seizures or Convulsions/ Mixed Presentation)*
	307.xx	Pain Disorder
	.80	Associated With Psychological Factors
	.89	Associated With Both Psychological Factors and General Medical Condition *(Acute or Chronic)*
	300.7	Hypochondriasis *(Specify if With Poor Insight)*
	300.7	Body Dysmorphic Disorder
	300.82	Somatoform Disorder NOS

Factitious Disorders

	300.xx	Factitious Disorder
	.16	With Predominantly Psychological Signs/Symptoms
	.19	With Predominantly Physical Signs/Symptoms
	.19	With Combined Psychological and Physical Symptoms
	300.19	Factitious Disorder NOS

Dissociative Disorders

	300.12	Dissociative Amnesia
	300.13	Dissociative Fugue
	300.14	Dissociative Identity Disorder
	300.6	Depersonalization Disorder
	300.15	Dissociative Disorder NOS

Sexual and Gender Identity Disorders *(Applies to all primary dysfunctions: Lifelong/Acquire Type, Generalized/Situational Type, due to Psychological Factors/Combine Factors)*

SEXUAL DESIRE DISORDERS	302.71	Hypoactive Sexual Desire Disorder
	302.79	Sexual Aversion Disorder
SEXUAL AROUSAL DISORDERS	302.72	Female Sexual Arousal Disorder
	302.72	Male Erectile Disorder
ORGASMIC DISORDERS	302.73	Female Orgasmic Disorder
	302.74	Male Orgasmic Disorder
	302.75	Premature Ejaculation
SEXUAL PAIN DISORDERS	302.76	Dyspareunia (Not Due to a General Medical Condition)
	306.51	Vaginismus (Not Due to a General Medical Condition)

continues

SEXUAL DYSFUNCTION DUE TO GENERAL MEDICAL CONDITION		
(Specify General Medical Condition)	625.8	Female Hypoactive Sexual Desire Disorder
	608.89	Male Hypoactive Sexual Disorder
	607.84	Male Erectile Disorder
	625.0	Female Dyspareunia
	608.89	Male Dyspareunia
	625.8	Other Female Sexual Dysfunction
	608.89	Other Male Sexual Dysfunction
	—.—	Substance-Induced Sexual Dysfunction
	302.70	Sexual Dysfunction NOS
PARAPHILIA	302.4	Exhibitionism
	302.81	Fetishism
	302.89	Frotteurism
	302.2	Pedophilia *(Sexually Attracted to Males, Females, or Both/ Limited to Incest/Exclusive or Nonexclusive)*
	302.83	Sexual Masochism
	302.84	Sexual Sadism
	302.3	Transvestic Fetishism *(Specify if With Gender Dysphoria)*
	302.82	Voyeurism
	302.9	Paraphilia
GENDER IDENTITY DISORDER	302.xx	Gender Identity Disorder
	.6	In Children
	.85	In Adolescent or Adult
	302.6	Gender Identity Disorder NOS
	302.9	Sexual Disorder NOS

Eating Disorders

	307.1	Anorexia Nervosa *(Restricting Type, Binge-Eating/Purging Type)*
	307.51	Bulimia Nervosa *(Purging Type/Nonpurging Type)*
	307.50	Eating Disorder NOS

Sleep Disorders

PRIMARY SLEEP DISORDERS		
Dyssomnias	307.42	Primary Insomnia
	307.44	Primary Hypersomnia *(Specify if Recurrent)*
	347	Narcolepsy
	780.59	Breathing-Related Sleep Disorder
	307.45	Circadian Rhythm Sleep Disorder
	307.47	Dyssomnia NOS
Parasomnias	307.47	Nightmare Disorder
	307.46	Sleep Terror Disorder
	307.46	Sleepwalking Disorder
	307.47	Parasomnia NOS

continues

| SLEEP DISORDERS RELATED TO ANOTHER MENTAL DISORDER | 307.42 | Insomnia Related to *(Specify Mental Disorder)* |
| | 307.44 | Hypersomnia Related to *(Specify Mental Disorder)* |

OTHER SLEEP DISORDERS	780.xx	Sleep Disorder *(Specify General Medical Condition)*
	.52	Insomnia Type
	.54	Hypersomnia Type
	.59	Parasomnia Type
	.59	Mixed Type
	—.—	Substance-Induced Sleep Disorder

Impulse-Control Disorders Not Elsewhere Classified

	312.34	Intermittent Explosive Disorder
	312.32	Kleptomania
	312.33	Pyromania
	312.31	Pathological Gambling
	312.39	Trichotillomania
	312.30	Impulse-Control Disorder NOS

Adjustment Disorders

	309.xx	Adjustment Disorder
	.0	With Depressed Mood
	.24	With Anxiety
	.28	With Mixed Anxiety and Depressed Mood
	.3	With Disturbance of Conduct
	.4	With Mixed Disturbance of Emotions and Conduct
	.9	Unspecified *(Acute or Chronic)*

Personality Disorders

	301.0	Paranoid Personality Disorder
	301.20	Schizoid Personality Disorder
	301.22	Schizotypal Personality Disorder
	301.7	Antisocial Personality Disorder
	301.83	Borderline Personality Disorder
	301.50	Histrionic Personality Disorder
	301.81	Narcissistic Personality Disorder
	301.82	Avoidant Personality Disorder
	301.6	Dependent Personality Disorder
	301.4	Obsessive-Compulsive Personality Disorder
	301.9	Personality Disorder NOS

Other Conditions That May Be a Focus of Clinical Attention

PSYCHOLOGICAL FACTORS AFFECTING MEDICAL CONDITION	316	Mental Disorder Affecting Medical Condition
		Psychological Symptoms Affecting Medical Condition
		Personality Traits or Coping Style Affecting Medical Condition

continues

		Maladaptive Health Behaviors Affecting Medical Condition
		Stress-Related Physiological Response Affecting Medical Condition
		Other or Unspecified Psychological Factors Affecting Medical Condition
MEDICATION-INDUCED MOVEMENT DISORDERS	332.1	Neuroleptic-Induced Parkinsonism
	333.92	Neuroleptic Malignant Syndrome
	333.7	Neuroleptic-Induced Acute Dystonia
	333.99	Neuroleptic-Induced Acute Akathisia
	333.82	Neuroleptic-Induced Tardive Dyskinesia
	333.1	Medication-Induced Postural Tremor
	333.90	Medication-Induced Movement Disorder NOS
OTHER MEDICATION-INDUCED DISORDER	995.2	Adverse Effects of Medication NOS
RELATIONAL PROBLEMS	V61.9	Relational Problem Related to a Mental Disorder or General Mental Disorder or General Medical Condition
	V61.20	Parent-Child Relational Problem
	V61.10	Partner Relational Problem
	V61.8	Sibling Relational Problem
	V62.81	Relational Problem NOS
PROBLEMS RELATED TO ABUSE OR NEGLECT	V61.21	Physical Abuse of Child
	V61.21	Sexual Abuse of Child
	V61.21	Neglect of Child
	—.—	Physical Abuse of Adult
	V61.12	(if by partner)
	V62.83	(if by person other than partner)
	—.—	Sexual Abuse of Adult
	V61.12	(if by partner)
	V62.83	(if by person other than partner)
ADDITIONAL CONDITIONS THAT MAY BE A FOCUS OF CLINICAL ATTENTION	V15.81	Noncompliance With Treatment
	V65.2	Malingering
	V71.01	Adult Antisocial Behavior
	V71.02	Child or Adolescent Antisocial Behavior
	V62.89	Borderline Intellectual Functioning
	780.9	Age-Related Cognitive Decline
	V62.82	Bereavement
	V62.3	Academic Problem
	V62.2	Occupational Problem
	313.82	Identity Problem
	V62.89	Religious or Spiritual Problem
	V52.4	Acculturation Problem
	V62.89	Phase of Life Problem

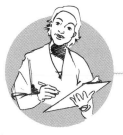

Mini-Mental Status Exam (Sample)

Orientation	Ask the year, season, date, day, month state, county, town, hospital, floor	5 _____ 5 _____	
Concentration	Repeat and ask person to remember three words	3 _____	
Attention and processing	Ask person to do serial 7s (5 times) or spell WORLD backward	5 _____	
Recall	Ask person to recall the above three items	3 _____	
Language	Ask person to name two common objects when shown (i.e., watch, clock, glasses)	2 _____	
	Ask person to repeat "No ifs and no buts"	1 _____	
Command	Give person a plain piece of paper with a three-step command—"Take this paper, fold it, place it on table"	3 _____	
Read and do	Show person **Close Your Eyes** in big letters. Observe if person does what is asked	1 _____	
Write a sentence	Ask person to write a sentence with proper grammar	1 _____	
Copy	Ask person to copy the overlapping pentagons below	1 _____	

Total

_____/30

Folstein, M. F., Folstein, S. E., McHugh, P. R. (1975). Mini-Mental State: a practical method for grading the cognitive state of patients for the clinician. *Journal of Psychiatric Research*, 12:189-198.

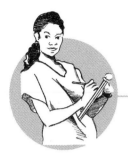

C

North American Nursing Diagnosis Association (NANDA) Nursing Diagnoses Most Frequently Used in Mental Health & Psychiatric Settings

- Activity intolerance (related to mental disorder)
- Activity intolerance, risk for
- Adjustment impaired
- Airway clearance, ineffective
- Anxiety
- Aspiration, risk for
- Attachment
- Body image disturbance
- Body temperature, risk for altered
- Bowel incontinence
- Breastfeeding, ineffective
- Breastfeeding, interrupted
- Breathing pattern, ineffective
- Cardiac output, decreased
- Caregiver role strain
- Caregiver role strain, risk for
- Communication, impaired verbal
- Community coping, ineffective
- Confusion (specify acute or chronic)
- Constipation, colonic
- Constipation, perceived
- Coping, defensive
- Coping, individual ineffective
- Decisional conflict
- Denial, ineffective
- Diarrhea
- Disorganized infant behavior
- Disuse syndrome (immobility associated with mental disorder)
- Diversional activity, deficit
- Dysreflexia
- Energy field, disturbance
- Environmental interpretation syndrome, impaired
- Failure to thrive
- Falls, risk for
- Family coping, ineffective, compromised
- Family coping, ineffective, disabling
- Family process, altered
- Fatigue
- Fear
- Fluid volume deficit
- Fluid volume excess
- Gas exchange, impaired
- Grieving, anticipatory
- Grieving, dysfunctional
- Growth and development, altered

- Health maintenance, altered
- Health-seeking behaviors
- Home maintenance management, impaired
- Hopelessness
- Hyperthermia
- Hypothermia
- Incontinence, functional
- Incontinence, stress
- Incontinence, total
- Incontinence, urge
- Infant behavior, disorganized
- Infant feeding pattern, ineffective
- Infection, risk for
- Injury, risk for
- Knowledge deficit
- Loneliness
- Memory, impaired
- Nausea
- Noncompliance
- Nutrition, altered, less than body requirements
- Nutrition, altered, more than body requirements
- Oral mucous membrane, altered
- Pain
- Pain, chronic
- Parent/infant attachment, altered
- Parental role conflict
- Parenting, altered
- Perioperative positioning injury, risk for
- Peripheral neurovascular dysfunction, risk for
- Personal identity disturbance
- Physical mobility, impaired
- Poisoning, risk for
- Post-trauma response
- Powerlessness (actual or risk for)
- Protection, altered
- Rape-trauma syndrome
- Relocation stress syndrome (actual or risk for)
- Role conflict
- Role performance, altered
- Self-care deficit (bathing, hygiene, feeding, dressing, grooming, toileting)
- Self-esteem, chronic low
- Self-esteem, situational low (actual or risk for)

- Self-mutilation, risk for
- Sensory/perceptual alteration (specify visual, auditory, tactile, kinesthetic, gustatory, olfactory)
- Sexual dysfunction
- Sexuality patterns, altered
- Skin integrity, impaired
- Sleep pattern disturbance
- Social interaction, impaired
- Social isolation
- Spiritual distress
- Spiritual well-being, potential for enhancement
- Spontaneous ventilation, inability to sustain

- Suffocation, risk for
- Suicide, risk for
- Swallowing, impaired
- Therapeutic regimen, family, ineffective management
- Therapeutic regimen, individual, ineffective
- Thermoregulation, ineffective
- Thought processes, altered
- Tissue integrity, impaired
- Tissue perfusion, altered
- Trauma, risk for
- Unilateral neglect
- Urinary elimination, altered
- Urinary retention
- Ventilatory weaning response, dysfunctional
- Violence, risk for, directed at self/others
- Wandering

*Adapted from North American Nursing Diagnosis Association (2001).
NANDA nursing diagnoses: Definitions and classification. Philadelphia.*

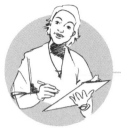

Anxiety Scale (Sample)

Anxiety scales are rating scales developed to quantify the severity of anxiety symptoms a person is feeling at the present time. There is no right or wrong answer to the questions. A 5-point scale is used for rating each item:

0 = Not present
1 = Rarely
2 = Some of the time
3 = Much of the time
4 = All or most of the time

1. **Anxious feelings**
   Worry _____
   Anticipate the worst _____
   Sudden panic _____

2. **Tension**
   Startle easily _____
   Cry easily _____
   Restless _____
   Tremors _____

3. **Fears**
   Fear of dark _____
   Fear of strangers _____
   Fear of being alone _____
   Fear of animals _____
   Fear of closed spaces _____
   Fear of public places _____
   Fear of crowds _____
   Fear with no real cause _____

4. **Insomnia**
   Difficulty falling asleep _____
   Difficulty staying asleep _____
   Uncomfortable dreams _____

5. **Thinking**
   Problems concentrating _____
   Memory blanks _____
   Lose train of thought _____

6. **Depressed mood**
   Decreased interest in _____
   previously enjoyed
   activities
   Reduced contact with _____
   friends and family

7. **Somatic complaints**
   Dizziness _____
   Nausea _____
   Constipation _____
   Chest pain _____
   Choking sensation _____
   Palpitations _____
   Shortness of breath _____

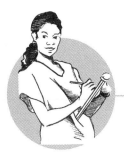

Beck's Depression Scale (Sample)

The questionnaire is completed by the individual or with the help of an examiner.

Directions:
Please read each group of statements carefully. Then pick out the one statement in each group, which best accounts for the way you have been feeling the PAST WEEK, INCLUDING TODAY! Circle the letter of the statement that best describes this feeling. If several statements in the group seem to apply equally, choose only one answer and circle the appropriate response.

(a) I do not feel sad. (b) I feel sad. (c) I am sad all the time and I can't snap out of it. (d) I am so sad or unhappy that I can't stand it.	(a) I don't feel disappointed in myself. (b) I am disappointed in myself. (c) I am disgusted with myself. (d) I hate myself.
(a) I am not particularly discouraged about the future. (b) I feel discouraged about the future. (c) I feel I have nothing to look forward to. (d) I feel that the future is hopeless and that things cannot improve.	(a) I do not feel like a failure. (b) I feel I have failed more than the average person. (c) As I look back on my life, all I can see are a lot of failures. (d) I feel I am a complete failure as a person.
(a) I don't have thoughts of killing myself. (b) I have thoughts of killing myself, but I would not carry it out. (c) I would like to kill myself. (d) I would kill myself if I had the chance.	(a) I don't cry any more than usual. (b) I cry more now than I used to. (c) I cry all the time now. (d) I used to be able to cry, but now I can't cry even though I want to.
(a) I get as much satisfaction out of things as I used to. (b) I don't enjoy things the way I used to. (c) I don't get real satisfaction out of anything anymore. (d) I am dissatisfied or bored with everything.	(a) I am no more irritated now than I ever am. (b) I get annoyed or irritated more easily than I used to. (c) I feel irritated all the time now. (d) I don't get irritated at all by the things that used to irritate me.
(a) I don't feel particularly guilty. (b) I feel guilty some of the time. (c) I feel guilty most of the time. (d) I feel guilty all of the time.	(a) I don't feel I am being punished. (b) I feel I may be punished. (c) I expect to be punished. (d) I feel I am being punished.
(a) I make decisions about as well as I ever could. (b) I put off making decisions more than I used to. (c) I have lost most of my interest in other people. (d) I have lost all of my interest in other people.	(a) I don't get more tired than usual. (b) I get tired more easily than I used to. (c) I get tired from doing almost anything. (d) I am too tired to do anything.
(a) I can work as well as before. (b) It takes an extra effort to get started at doing something. (c) I have to push myself very hard to do anything. (d) I can't do any work at all.	(a) I don't feel I look any worse than I used to. (b) I am worried that I am looking old and/or unattractive. (c) I feel that there are permanent changes in my appearance that make me look unattractive. (d) I believe that I look ugly.

(a) I don't feel I am any worse than anybody else.
(b) I am critical of myself for my weakness or mistake.
(c) I blame myself all the time for my faults.
(d) I blame myself for everything bad that happens.

(a) I have not lost interest in other people.
(b) I am less interested in other people than I used to be.
(c) I have lost most of my interest in other people.
(d) I have lost all of my interest in other people.

(a) My appetite is no worse than usual.
(b) My appetite is not as good as it used to be.
(c) My appetite is much worse now.
(d) I have no appetite at all anymore.

(a) I haven't lost much weight, if any, lately.
(b) I have lost more than 5 pounds.
(c) I have lost more than 10 pounds.
(d) I have lost more than 15 pounds.

(a) I have not noticed any recent change in my interest in sex.
(b) I am less interested in sex than I used to be.
(c) I am much less interested in sex now.
(d) I have lost interest in sex completely.

(a) I can sleep as well as usual.
(b) I don't sleep as well as I used to.
(c) I wake up 1–2 hours earlier than usual and find it hard to get back to sleep.
(d) I wake up several hours earlier than I used to and cannot get back to sleep.

(a) I am no more worried about my health than usual.
(b) I am worried about physical problems such as aches and pains, or upset stomach, or constipation.
(c) I am very worried about physical problems, and it's hard to think of much else.
(d) I am so worried about my physical problems that I cannot think about anything else.

SCORING:
  (1) = 1 point
  (2) = 2 points
  (3) = 3 points
  (4) = 4 points
Score is totaled to determine evidence of depression symptoms.

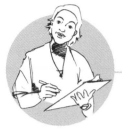

Answers to Worksheets

Chapter 1
Fill in the Blank
1. asylums
2. antipsychotic/psychotropic
3. Linda Richards

Matching
1. C
2. D
3. B
4. E
5. A

Multiple Choice
1. A
2. C

Chapter 2
Fill in the Blank
1. ethics
2. informed consent
3. confidentiality

Matching
1. D
2. F
3. E
4. B
5. A
6. C

Multiple Choice
1. C
2. D

Chapter 3
Fill in the Blank
1. problem solving
2. therapeutic milieu
3. subjective
4. objective
5. contributing factor
6. collaboratively

Matching
1. C
2. D
3. A
4. E
5. F
6. B

Multiple Choice
1. A
2. D
3. B
4. C
5. D

Scenario
1. Subjective data may include: (a) What are you feeling at this time? (b) Can you tell me what happened before you came here? (c) What type of work do you do? (d) Are you involved in a relationship? (e) Are you blaming yourself for what happened in your life? (f) Have you been using any drugs or alcohol?
2. Objective data may include: (a) his behavior prior to current incident, (b) his immediate reaction following his recent losses, (c) any unusual statements or gestures, (d) any present or past substance use, (e) past or present medical illness, (e) previous mental problems.
3. Life situation, statement of "not knowing where he should go."
4. Multiple loss, disoriented with dissociation ("lost").
5. Temporary loss of identity, unable to state who he is or why he is in parking lot at 2:00 a.m.

Chapter 4
Fill in the Blank
1. fight or flight
2. stress reaction
3. overreaction
4. perception; reaction
5. unpredictability

Matching
1. D
2. H
3. B
4. F
5. C
6. G
7. E
8. A

Multiple Choice
1. B
2. C
3. A
4. B

Seek and Find
1. Think of a way to deal with the problem (first step is assess if it really is what it seems to be).
2. Adaptive (palliative).
3. Mental escape (reframing).
4. Fight the anxiety with our body defenses (accept the anxiety rather than fight it).

Chapter 5
Fill in the Blank
1. empathy
2. self-awareness
3. situation; needs
4. congruent
5. independence
6. boundaries

Matching
1. E
2. C
3. A
4. B
5. D

Multiple Choice
1. B
2. A
3. D
4. C
5. A
6. B

Seek and Find
1. reflection (open-ended question)
2. validation (restating)
3. clarification (focusing)
4. closed-ended question (false reassurance)
5. giving advice (false reassurance)

Chapter 6
Fill in the Blank
1. personality traits
2. temperament
3. equilibration
4. assimilation
5. accommodation
6. B. F. Skinner
7. Lawrence Kohlberg
8. reinforcement
9. level; differentiation
10. solid

Matching
1. C
2. G
3. B
4. D
5. H
6. A
7. F
8. E

Multiple Choice
1. C
2. A
3. B
4. C
5. D
6. A
7. B

Seek and Find
1. behaviorism (humanistic theory)
2. superego (ego)
3. latency stage (phallic stage)
4. preschool years during the stage of initiative vs guilt (toddler years during the stage of autonomy vs shame and doubt)
5. identity vs role confusion (intimacy vs isolation)

Chapter 7
Fill in the Blank
1. grief
2. anticipatory
3. bereavement
4. empty clichés
5. loss
6. magical
7. dysfunctional grief

Matching
1. B
2. E
3. C
4. A
5. D

Multiple Choice
1. B
2. D
3. C
4. A

Scenario
1. sense of sadness, despondence, loss
2. empathy, reassurance this common reaction to grief
3. depression
4. grief support group, spiritual support

Chapter 8
Fill in the Blank
1. connect; stimulus
2. automatic relief
3. avoid
4. specific phobia
5. embarrassment
6. obsessions
7. compulsions

Matching
1. E
2. F
3. D
4. G
5. C
6. B
7. A

Multiple Choice
1. C
2. D
3. A
4. B
5. C
6. C
7. D
8. C
9. D
10. B

Seek and Find
1. to provide a secondary gain (serve no prupose but to relieve the anxiety)
2. immediately before (well in advance of)
3. excessive display of emotions (expression of little or no emotion)
4. reassuring (may pose a threat)

Scenario # 1
1. Calm and supportive to decrease level of anxiety
2. Coping tool to decrease her overwhelming anxiety in feared situations
3. Anxiety, high level; coping ineffective; social isolation

Scenario # 2
1. Subjective: "I could not concentrate . . ." "I was afraid to make decisions . . ." "I just don't know what I'm going to do . . ." "I can't sleep . . ."
2. Objective: tearful, jumpy, on edge, rapid speech, fidgeting, dark suborbital circles
3. Calm, unhurried supportive approach
4. Ventilates anxiety appropriately; identifies effective coping methods; demonstrates anxiety-reducing strategies

Chapter 9
Fill in the Blank
1. suicidal erosion
2. suicidal ideation
3. unipolar
4. dysthymia
5. 4
6. persecution
7. cyclothymic
8. lithium carbonate
9. 3
10. random

Matching
1. J
2. F
3. D
4. G
5. A
6. B
7. H
8. I
9. E
10. C

Multiple Choice
1. C
2. A
3. D
4. C
5. C
6. C
7. B
8. A
9. C

Scenario
1. Ascertain if she is thinking of killing herself; if yes, does she have a plan?
2. Scarves, belts, shoelaces, nail files, scissors, electric cords.
3. Helps client to feel safe and secure— shared responsibility and support for their decisions.
4. "Tell me more about your plans . . ." Recognize that increased energy as depression lifts can provide mental capacity to carry out suicidal plan.

Chapter 10
Fill in the Blank
1. consistent; stable
2. ambivalent
3. withdrawn
4. magical thinking
5. ideas of reference
6. antisocial
7. self-mutilating
8. no-win
9. entitlement
10. histrionic

Matching
1. F
2. E
3. I
4. G
5. A
6. D
7. H
8. B
9. C

Multiple Choice
1. B
2. D
3. B
4. A
5. C
6. D
7. A

Seek and Find
1. power (powerlessness)
2. able to excel (inferior)
3. personal gain (failure)
4. very concerned (unconcerned)

Scenario
1. Matter-of-fact approach that behavior is inappropriate; reinforce nurse–client relationship
2. Antisocial
3. Require him to take responsibility for the behavior
4. Explosive anger with verbal acting-out; projection of blame; cold and insensitive
5. Unlikely

Chapter 11
Fill in the Blank
1. disorganization
2. illusions
3. half
4. water intoxication
5. commanding
6. grandeur
7. blunted or flat
8. prodromal
9. undifferentiated
10. extrapyrimidal

Matching
1. F
2. G
3. E
4. B
5. D
6. C
7. A

Multiple Choice
1. B
2. D
3. A
4. C
5. D

Seek and Find
1. responsive and nonreactive (unresponsive and nonreactive)
2. negative (positive)
3. insertion (withdrawal)

Scenario
1. Reinforce reality such as, "I understand this is threatening to you, but there is no evidence of the machine."
2. Somatic, persecution.
3. Provide foods in sealed containers or plastic wrappers; monitor I /O; monitor weight.

Chapter 12
Fill in the Blank
1. somatization
2. secondary gain
3. primary gain
4. "la belle"
5. physician-shopping

Matching
1. D
2. E
3. A
4. B
5. C

Multiple Choice
1. C
2. A
3. B
4. D
5. A

Seek and Find
1. consciously (person is unaware of connection)
2. primary (secondary)
3. typical of actual neurologic pathway disorder (typical pattern does not show a dysfunction of neurologic disorder)
4. migrate from one body location to another (location and description of pain does not change)

Scenario
1. When did the symptoms begin? What was happening about the time they started? What are vital signs and current and past health status? Have symptoms occurred before? Note inconsistencies in description of symptoms; attitude toward symptoms; level of anxiety; previous coping methods. What, if any, limitations are imposed by the symptoms?
2. Anxiety, depression, worthlessness, guilt
3. Wife and family worry about his condition, provide sympathy, and wait on him
4. Self-esteem disturbance, related to unmet dependency needs and job loss
5. Denial, ineffective, related to avoidance of psychologic cause for his symptoms

Chapter 13
Fill in the Blank
1. dissociation
2. repressed
3. host
4. switching
5. depersonalization

Matching
1. D
2. A
3. E
4. B
5. C

Multiple Choice
1. C
2. B
3. A
4. C
5. C

Scenario # 1
1. Guilt, shame, regret, helplessness
2. To slowly reintroduce his identity in a safe environment
3. Allow him to remember past without risk of precipitating increased trauma
4. May cause him to regress further into dissociative state that is protecting him from the emotional pain

Scenario # 2
1. Trauma, mental anguish over events of war-related activity
2. Assists in stimulating memory of past without trauma and further emotional pain
3. Can cause further regression into dissociative state

Chapter 14
Fill in the Blank
1. substance
2. inhalants
3. craving
4. tolerance
5. withdrawal
6. codependent
7. use to relax; preoccupation with drugs; occasional blackouts; avoids situations where drug not available; personality change with substance use
8. several hours to days of last use
9. alcohol-induced delirium
10. Wernicke-Korsakoff syndrome

Matching
1. K
2. G
3. A
4. H
5. B
6. J
7. D
8. F
9. E
10. C
11. I

Multiple Choice
1. D
2. A
3. A
4. D
5. B
6. D
7. C
8. B
9. C
10. A

Scenario
1. Accepting, nonjudgmental attitude
2. Type of substance use; amount and frequency of use; when last used; method of administration; length of time substance has been used; any suicidal ideation
3. Unable to predict outcome of use; engages in behaviors to support habit; loss of insight into substance problem
4. Sensory-perceptual alteration, related to withdrawal symptoms
5. To prevent symptoms of heroin withdrawal and decrease craving for the drug
6. Anxiety, dysphoric, abdominal cramping, hallucinating
7. Calm reassuring approach; remove hazardous articles; seizure precautions; reorient; provide safe environment; vital signs and neuro checks; observe for respiratory depression, arrhythmias
8. Determine presence of suicidal ideation and whether plan has been devised; reflect statement to allow him to talk about his feelings of despondency

Chapter 15
Fill in the Blank
1. perception
2. calories; nutrients
3. success; failure
4. controlling, overprotective
5. calories
6. purging
7. weight
8. privileges; restrictions
9. 30 minutes
10. role-model

Matching
1. C
2. E
3. B
4. A
5. D

Multiple Choice
1. C
2. A
3. B
4. C

Scenario
1. Attitude of objectivity, nonjudgmental, caring, compassion, and concern
2. Decrease in pituitary and ovarian hormone production; decrease in thyroid functioning; impaired kidney function; anemia
3. Identify her strengths and positive attributes; help her set realistic self-expectations; avoid discussions that focus on food and weight; explore ways for her to increase autonomy and assertiveness

Chapter 16
Fill in the Blank
1. sexual dysfunction
2. diabetes mellitus
3. paraphilia
4. inhibition to arousal
5. cross-gender
6. traumatic
7. personality
8. thinking

Matching
1. E
2. G
3. D
4. A
5. B
6. C
7. F

Multiple Choice
1. C
2. B
3. A
4. D
5. C

Scenario #1
1. Evaluate own feelings; empathetic and nonjudgmental attitude
2. Concern, protective, confidential
3. Transvestic fetishism
4. Any suicidal ideation
5. Card game; puzzles; art projects
6. Confront and resolve traumatic developmental issues; confront distorted sexual fantasies and thought processes; develop more adaptive and effective coping skills

Scenario # 2
1. Report incident to the daycare administration
2. Frotteurism

Chapter 17
Fill in the Blank
1. genetic component
2. dyslexia
3. low self-esteem; impaired interaction
4. sixth grade
5. eye contact; facial expression; gestures
6. stuttering
7. attention
8. echopraxia
9. encopresis
10. impaired social interaction

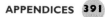

Matching
1. F
2. E
3. D
4. A
5. B
6. G
7. I
8. H
9. C

Multiple Choice
1. C
2. B
3. B
4. A
5. D
6. A
7. C
8. C
9. A
10. B

Seek and Find
1. more (less)
2. urine (feces)
3. does not usually involve (usually involves)
4. aware (unaware)
5. 6 months (3 years)

Scenario
1. Lack of role model; embarrassment; low self-esteem; shame; lack of maternal support
2. Inability to concentrate; easily distracted; inability to complete goal-oriented task; inability to follow instructions
3. Self-doubt; worthlessness; hopelessness
4. Educate about disorder; refer to support group and help networks; encourage her to set boundaries for Anthony's behavior; maintain consistent approach to behavior; role-model acceptable ways to express feelings; teach ways for her to assist Anthony to think about the consequences of his behavior

Chapter 18
Fill in the Blank
1. primary
2. secondary
3. delirium; dementia; amnesic disorders
4. consciousness; short
5. metabolize and excrete the drug
6. irreversible; progressive
7. pneumonia; urinary tract infections; infected decubitus ulcers
8. catastrophic events

Matching
1. D
2. B
3. E
4. F
5. A
6. H
7. G
8. C

Multiple-Choice
1. C
2. A
3. C
4. B
5. D
6. B
7. C
8. A

Seek and Find
1. progressive (steplike)
2. insidious (acute)
3. depressed (demented)
4. amnesic disorder (Alzheimer's disease)

Scenario # 1
1. Driving, confusion, spoiled food items
2. Reminisce with her, reassure her the children are fed
3. Redirect her; provide food items or packages in a basket to divert her from taking food from other clients
4. Find activity for her to do; reminisce with her about Katy, her students; provide jewelry items to divert her attention

Scenario # 2

1. Fear of unfamiliar persons or environment; inability to process and comprehend incoming stimuli; privacy with personal hygiene; dependence on caregiver
2. Leave him alone and allow him time to regain control; approach at a later time; calm soft voice; routine schedule; one-step commands.
3. Reassurance of caregiver's presence
4. Inability to communicate pain may be responsible for his aggression.
5. Observe for nonverbal clues of pain; provide analgesia for pain relief when agitation is noted; frequent rest periods; provide diversional activity that allows him to be seated—distraction from pacing behavior
6. Caregiver role strain, related to dependency of client
7. Refer to support group; encourage her to find diversional activity or hobby; encourage family support; spiritual support

Chapter 19
Fill in the Blank

1. neurotransmitter systems
2. posture, muscle tone, and voluntary smooth muscle activity
3. rapid; onset of symptom relief
4. the neurotransmitter; balance the deficit
5. side effects of sedation, orthostatic hypotension, photosensitivity
6. interaction and communication with others, participation in self-care and other activities
7. aged cheese, alcoholic beverages, caffeine, chocolate, bananas, avocados, smoked and processed meat, caviar, pickled herring, meat tenderizer, raisins, figs, sour cream, yogurt, soy sauce, chicken livers, corned beef
8. fatigue, nausea, dry mouth, flatulence, dizziness, insomnia, tremors
9. anticholinergic; extrapyramidal
10. AIMS Assessment Scale

Matching

1. B
2. A
3. C
4. D
5. A
6. A
7. B
8. D
9. B
10. A
11. D
12. E

Multiple Choice

1. A
2. B
3. C
4. A
5. D
6. B
7. D

Seek and Find

1. lows than the highs (highs than the lows)
2. low (high)—absorbed slowly (rapidly absorbed)
3. decrease (increase)—no more than 1000 mL (2000–3000 mL)
4. several days (several weeks)
5. decreased (increased)
6. extrapyramidal (anticholinergic)— anticholinergic (extrapyrimidal)
7. increase (decrease)

Scenario

1. Possibility of suicidal ideation and intent—safety is primary concern
2. Potentiates the CNS depressant activity
3. Effect will not be immediate—requires about 3 weeks for effects to be realized, sedating effects
4. Apathy, confusion, drowsiness, weight changes, altered taste, nausea, cough, agitation, decreased libido or sexual functioning, weakness, dry mouth
5. Bianca is able to go back to her job at the store, becomes involved in care of her children, improved coping strategies; reduced substance use

Chapter 20

Fill in the Blank

1. social; therapeutic
2. therapeutic process
3. consistency
4. psychotherapy
5. play therapy
6. caregiver

Matching

1. J
2. E
3. I
4. A
5. G
6. D
7. H
8. F
9. C
10. B

Multiple Choice

1. C
2. B
3. A
4. D
5. B

Chapter 21

Fill in the Blank

1. empowerment
2. powerlessness
3. exacerbation; delayed
4. consistency
5. thinking
6. hepatitis B and C
7. firm

Matching

1. D
2. C
3. A
4. E
5. B

Multiple Choice

1. C
2. B
3. A
4. C

Seek and Find

1. reasonable (unreasonable)
2. does not usually interfere (may interfere)
3. usually are able to cope with crisis situations without a threat (may at times experience periods of psychologic disarray and instability)

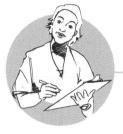

Glossary

Accommodation: process of responding to cognitively unbalancing information about the environment by modifying relevant schemas, thereby adapting the schemas to fit the new information and reestablishing cognitive balance.

Acetylcholine: neurotransmitter found in various organs and tissues of the body, thought to play an important role in the transmission of nerve impulses at synapses and myoneural junctions. It is quickly destroyed by an enzyme, cholinesterase.

Adaptation: manner in which individuals manage their anxiety.

Addiction: physiological and psychological dependence upon alcohol or certain drugs of abuse noted for their effects on the central nervous system that is characterized by withdrawal symptoms when the substance is discontinued.

Affect: describes facial expression that is displayed in association with the mood.

Ageism: discrimination against aged persons.

Agnosia: loss of comprehension of auditory, visual, or other sensations although the sensory sphere is intact.

Agoraphobia: fear of being in a place from which escape might be difficult or embarrassing.

Akathisia: motor restlessness, inability to sit still.

Alzheimer's dementia: chronic, organic mental disorder or dementia due to atrophy of frontal and occipital lobes that involves a progressive, irreversible loss of memory, deterioration of intellectual functions, apathy, speech and gait disturbances, and disorientation.

Amnesia: loss of memory applied to episodes during which individuals forget their identity, though they conduct themselves properly and following which no memory of the period exists.

Anergia: marked decrease in energy level that may slow a person to a dependency on others for even basic needs.

Anhedonia: lack of interest in previously enjoyed activities.

Anomia: inability to remember the names of objects.

Anorexia nervosa: disorder characterized by extreme concern with body weight, an intense fear of becoming fat, and maintenance of body weight below expected levels for height and age. Individuals often perceive themselves as heavier than they are, or place unrealistic value on body weight and shape.

Antianxiety: central nervous system depressant that is shown to be effective in treating anxiety disorders by reducing overactivity in the CNS.

Anticipatory anxiety: anxiety that is experienced for some time prior to an event or happening.

Anticipatory grief: grief experienced prior to the impending death of a loved one.

Antidepressant: central nervous system depressant that acts to prevent, cure, or alleviate mental depression.

Antipsychotic: drug agents, also referred to as neuroleptics, that are used to treat serious mental illness such as bipolar affective disorder, depressive and drug-induced psychosis, schizophrenia, and autism. They may be used in some cases of movement disorders (Tourette's syndrome) and nausea or intractable hiccups.

Anxiety: built-in part of our basic instinct to respond in the event we are confronted with a threat to our well-being.

Anxiolytic: drug agent used to counteract or diminish anxiety.

Aphasia: absence or impairment of the ability to communicate through speech, writing, or signs, due to dysfunction of brain centers.

Apraxia: inability to perform purposeful movements although there is no sensory or motor impairment.

Assimilation: absorption of newly perceived information into the existing subjective conscious schema structure.

Avolition: lack of motivation.

Behaviorism: theory of conduct that regards normal and abnormal behaviors as the result of conditioned reflexes separate from the concept of will or choice.

Bereavement: expected reactions of grief and sadness after learning of the loss of a loved one.

Binge eating: recurrent eating of an amount in excess of 1000 calories in a short period of time with a lack of control over eating during the episode.

Biofeedback: training program designed to develop one's ability to control the autonomic or involuntary nervous system using monitoring devices, followed by an attempt by the individual to reproduce the conditions that caused the desired change.

Biomedical: application of biological and natural sciences to the study of medicine.

Bipolar: brain dysfunction that causes abnormal and erratic shifts in mood, energy, and functional ability.

Blackout: sudden loss of consciousness; an episode of forgetting all or part of what occurred during or following a period of alcohol intake.

Blocking: unconscious block that results in loss of thought process and person stops speaking.

Bulimia nervosa: eating disorder characterized by periods of significant overeating (binge-eating) and inappropriate methods of compensating for the overeating to prevent weight gain such as self-induced vomiting, use of laxatives or diuretics, and excessive exercise.

Catastrophic event: overwhelming state of anxiety or panic experienced by a demented individual in response to any type of new situation related to an inability to process environmental observations accurately.

Catatonic: phase of schizophrenia in which there is a tendency to assume and remain in a fixed position with inability to move or talk.

Chemical restraint: use of a drug to control behavior.

Circumstantiality: cannot be selective when speaking and describes in lengthy, great detail.

Clang association: words strung together in rhyming phrases that have no connected meaning.

Cocopraxia: sudden tic-like obscene gesture.

Co-dependent: term used to describe addiction or dysfunctional dependence in which the individual denies self while living and doing for another in either a passive or contentious way.

Cognitive therapy: based on the cognitive model of how individuals respond in stressful situations to their subjective perception of the event. Therapy strives to assist the individual to reduce anxiety responses by altering the cognitive distortions.

Compulsion: uncontrolled impulse to perform an action or ritual repeatedly to decrease anxiety.

Concrete operations: stage of cognitive development in Piaget's theory of development, in which the individual engages in mental manipulations of internal images of tangible objects.

Confabulation: behavioral reaction to memory loss in which the person fills in memory gaps with inappropriate words.

Confrontation: communication technique in which a client's behavior and feelings are exposed in order to facilitate client understanding of behavior.

Conscious: being aware and having perception of the environment; having the ability to filter that information through the mind with the awareness of doing so.

Contracting: implied agreement between two parties (i.e., health professional and client) that imposes conditions that if breached, will result in a loss of privileges or other compensation.

Conventional grief: feelings of sadness expected or experienced after a loss.

Conversion: process by which a psychological thought, event, or memory is transferred to a physical or sensory symptom.

Craving: strong inner drive to use a substance in situations of substance dependence.

Crisis: a state of disorganization and disarray that occurs when usual coping strategies fail or are not available.

Defense mechanism: methods for protecting the ego from anxiety associated with conflicting urges and restrictions of the id and superego.

Delirium: state of mental confusion and excitement that happens in a short period of time and is characterized by disorientation for time and place, usually with illusions and hallucinations.

Delirium tremens: dramatic complication of alcoholism following a period of abstinence after a prolonged drinking spree, or in the chronic alcoholic who is admitted for treatment; characterized by visual, auditory, and tactile hallucinations, incessant and incoherent talking, disorientation, tremors, jerky restless movements, and overactivity of the autonomic nervous system.

Delusion: fixed, false belief without appropriate external stimuli that is inconsistent with reality and the person's own knowledge or experience.

Delusion of reference: false belief that the behavior of others in the environment refers to oneself.

Dementia: broad impairment of intellectual function that usually is progressive and that interferes with normal social and occupational activities.

Depersonalization: belief that one's awareness of reality is temporarily lost or altered with a feeling of estrangement or detachment from thoughts or body.

Depression: persistent and prolonged mood of sadness that extends beyond two weeks duration.

Derailment: gradual or sudden change in thought process without thought blocking.

Derealization: feelings of being unreal.

Disorientation: inability to be cognizant of time, direction or location, and person.

Dopamine: catecholamine neurotransmitter; a precursor in the synthesis of norepinephrine important in understanding the pathology of schizophrenia and parkinsonism.

Dyslexia: learning disorder in the reading domain.

Dystonia: muscle rigidity that affects posture, gait, eye movements.

Echolalia: involuntary parrot-like repetition of words spoken by others, often accompanied by twitching of muscles.

Echopraxia: repetitive tic-like movements.

Eclectic: selecting from various sources what seems to be the best.

ECT: Electroconvulsive therapy.

Ego: in Freudian theory, one of the three major divisions in the model of the psychic apparatus that possesses consciousness and memory, and serves to mediate between the id and the superego or conscience.

Emotional numbing: expression of little or no emotion soon after an event as an attempt to prevent future mental pain.

Enabler: person who displays dysfunctional defensive actions that tend to normalize or excuse the behavior of a drug or alcohol user.

Encopresis: involuntary passage of feces in inappropriate places after age of voluntary control has been established.

Enuresis: involuntary passage of urine after age of voluntary control has been established.

Entitlement: narcissistic claim of being superior and owed by others.

Equilibration: process of cognitive development in which a person seeks to balance between information and experiences encountered in the environment with existing modes of thought and schemas.

Euphoria: excessive feeling of happiness or elation.

Eustress: positive and motivating stress shown by one's confidence in the ability to master a challenge or stressor.

Exhibitionism: tendency to attract attention to oneself by any means; psychosexual disorder manifesting an abnormal impulse that causes one to expose the genitals to a member of the opposite sex.

Extrapyramidal: outside the pyramidal tracts of the central nervous system; coordinates involuntary movements; side effects caused by drugs that block dopamine.

Fetishism: erotic stimulation or sexually arousing fantasies involving contact with nonliving objects, such as articles of dress or a braid of hair.

Flight of ideas: rapid shift between topics that are unrelated to each other.

Focusing: communication technique that helps client concentrate on a specific issue.

Formal operations: stage of cognitive development in Piaget's theory in which the individual can engage in mental manipulation of abstract ideas or symbols that may not have a specific concrete basis.

Free-floating anxiety: occurs when a person is unable to connect the anxiety to a stimulus.

Frotteurism: recurrent intense sexual urges and fantasies involving touching and rubbing against a nonconsenting person, usually in crowded places where arrest is unlikely.

Fugue: dissociative disorder in which there is an inability to recall one's past or identity accompanied by sudden and unexpected travel away from home.

Generalized amnesia: inability to recall important personal information usually of a traumatic or stressful nature that is too extensive to be explained by ordinary forgetfulness.

Grandiose: unrealistic or exaggerated sense of self-worth, importance, wealth, or ability.

Grief: emotional process of coping with a loss.

Group therapy: process of helping clients to develop an understanding of and insight into their feelings, behaviors, and roles in relationships through involvement and interaction with others who have similar problems.

Hallucination: false sensory perceptions unrelated to actual external stimuli.

Hierarchy: ordering or classification of anything in descending order of importance or value.

Holistic: philosophy that individuals are complete organisms and function as complete units that cannot be reduced to the sum of their parts.

Hypnosis: subconscious condition in which the objective manifestations of the mind are essentially inactive, accompanied by an unusual response to suggestions made by the hypnotist.

Hypochondriasis: persistent abnormal anxiety that one has a disease although medical evidence has proven otherwise.

Id: one of three divisions of the psyche that is the obscure, inaccessible part of our personality that serves as a collection of instinctual drives continually striving for satisfaction in accordance with the pleasure principle.

Ideas of reference: belief that some events have a special personal meaning.

Illusions: mental misperception of actual sensory stimuli.

Inhalant: psychoactive substance of volatile solvent, aerosol, gas, or nitrite used for sniffing/inhaling to achieve a quick high; may cause serious respiratory problems, permanent brain damage, and death.

Interpersonal: concerning the relations and interactions between persons.

Involuntary commitment: occurs when a person is admitted to a psychiatric unit against his or her will.

La belle indifference: unrealistic degree of complacency about physical symptoms as a result of psychological conversion.

Level of differentiation: degree to which a person's intellect or emotions control his or her functioning.

Localized amnesia: acute inability to recall important personal information that usually occurs within a few hours following the event or traumatic incident, most commonly seen in response to war combat, natural disaster, or severe trauma.

Logoconia: repetitious, continuous, and excessive monosyllabic utterances.

Loose associations: vague, unfocused, illogical collection of thoughts seen in psychosis.

Magical thinking: belief that thoughts, words, and actions can cause or prevent an occurrence by extraordinary means.

Malingering: factitious illness assumed usually to arouse sympathy, to escape work or arrest, or to receive compensation.

Mania: frenzied unstable mood in which the person may be out of touch with reality.

Manipulation: conscious or unconscious process by which one person attempts to influence another person in order to get his or her own needs or desires met.

Mental retardation: intellectual functioning significantly below average with IQ of 70 or below.

Milieu: environment or setting.

Monoamine inhibitor: group of drugs that inhibit monoamine oxidase; effective in treating depression.

Mood: emotion that is prolonged to the point that it colors a person's entire psychological thinking.

Necrophilia: abnormal concern or sexual intercourse with a dead body.

Neologism: meaningless new word created to which the person gives a special significance (seen in psychosis).

Neurotransmitter: substance released when the axon terminal of a presynaptic neuron is excited that travels across the synapse to act on the target cell to either inhibit or excite.

Norepinephrine: hormone produced by the adrenal medulla similar in chemical and pharmacological properties to adrenaline (epinephrine), but primarily a vasoconstrictor with little effect on cardiac output.

Obsession: reoccurrence of persistent unwanted thoughts or images that cause a person intense anxiety.

Panic attack: intense feeling of fear or terror that occurs suddenly and intermittently without warning.

Paralalia: repetitious, sometimes continuous repetition of one word.

Paraphilia: psychosexual disorder in which unusual or bizarre imagery or acts are necessary in order to achieve sexual excitement.

Passive-aggressive: anger expressed in an indirect and subtle way that acts on hostile feelings.

Pedophilia: unnatural desire for sexual relations with children.

Persecution: false belief that one is being threatened or in danger of being harmed.

Personality traits: defining characteristics that are unique to each individual.

Personality disorder: extreme pathological and maladaptive behavior patterns that are destructive to the person and others.

Postconventional: phase of moral development in which the individual recognizes the importance of societal rules as a basis for behavior but may also follow internal moral principles that supercede these rules.

Postsynaptic receptor: cell component that is distal to the synapse that combines with a drug, hormone, or chemical to alter the function of the cell.

Poverty of speech: little or no verbal speech.

Powerlessness: feeling of inability to control the outcome of one's actions or environmental situation.

Preconscious: level of the mind not present in consciousness, but able to be recalled at will.

Preconventional: phase of moral development in which moral reasoning is guided by punishments and rewards with a focus on avoiding punishment and obedience to authority without concern for the interests or feelings of others.

Primary gain: relief that is felt when anxiety is converted into physical symptoms of a disorder.

Preoperational: second stage of cognitive development, according to Piaget, that is characterized by the development of internal mental representations (schema) and verbal communication.

Presynaptic compartment: location before the nerve synapse that stores and receives neurotransmitters from the reuptake process.

Pseudo self: self a person presents to the world.

Psychiatrist: physician who specializes in the study, treatment, and prevention of mental disorders.

Psychodynamics: scientific study of mental actions or forces and motivations and the causes of these mental phenomena.

Psychological crisis: state of reaction within a person who is responding to a threatening event.

Psychologist: one who is trained in methods of psychological analysis, therapy, and research.

Psychosis: mental state in which there is mental disorganization and loss of contact with reality.

Psychosocial: related to both psychological and social factors.

Psychotherapy: method of treating disease by mental means rather than physical.

Psychotropic: drugs that affect psychic function, behavior, or experience.

Purging: evacuation of the digestive tract by means of induced vomiting or a cathartic laxative.

Reflection: communication technique that paraphrases message client has conveyed to nurse.

Reframing: way of restructuring our thinking about a stressful event into one that is less disturbing and over which we can have some control.

Reinforcement: stimulus used in operant conditioning that increases the probability that a given behavior associated with the stimulus will be repeated.

Relapse: recurrence of a disorder or symptoms after apparent recovery.

Reuptake: deactivation of neurotransmitters by their entry into the presynaptic compartment from the synaptic cleft.

Seclusion: refers to the placement of a patient in a controlled environment in order to treat a clinical emergency.

Secondary gain: attention that is received from others as a result of physical symptoms.

Secondary trait: personality traits that have some bearing on a person's behavior but that are not particularly central to what the person does.

Self-mutilation: harmful acts toward oneself such as burning, cutting, or overdosing that are not meant to be lethal, but in a distorted way reestablish a sense of realism.

Sensorimotor: first stage of cognitive development in Piaget's theory in which individuals largely develop in terms of sensory input and motor output abilities with reflexive responses and gradually expanding to schema and purposeful actions.

Serotonin: potent vasoconstrictor thought to be involved in neural mechanisms related to arousal, sleep, dreams, mood, appetite, and sensitivity to pain.

Sexuality: feelings and life of an individual as related to sex including the physical, chemical, and psychological functioning characterized by gender and sexual behavior.

Sexual dysfunction: degree of persistent or recurrent symptoms, subjective distress, or decrease in the quality of sexual stimulation during any phase of the sexual response cycle.

Sexual masochism: actual beating, binding, humiliating, or otherwise causing the victim to suffer.

Sexual orientation: individual preference or sexual attraction.

Sexual sadism: individual receives sexual excitement from observing psychological or physical suffering by the victim, while receiving additional satisfaction from the feelings of complete control over the victim.

Social Phobia: excessive and persistent irrational fear of specific objects or situations that actually pose little threat of danger.

Solid self: self which includes the beliefs a person has about themselves and their environment as a result of life experiences.

Splitting: extreme view of an all or none relationship with the world.

SSRIs: serotonin-specific reuptake inhibitors; used in the treatment of depression.

Stress: condition that results when a threat or challenge to one's well-being requires a person to adjust or adapt to the environment.

Stuttering: repetitive or prolonged sounds or syllables with pauses and monosyllabic broken words.

Substance: refers to any drug, medication, or toxins that share the potential for abuse.

Substance abuse: maladaptive recurring use of a substance accompanied by repeated detrimental effects as a result of continued use.

Substance dependence: maladaptive pattern of substance use leading to clinically significant impairment or distress with continuance in using the substance regardless of the adverse substance-related problems they may be experiencing.

Substance intoxication: overindulgence or being poisoned by a drug or toxic substance.

Suicidal erosion: long-term accumulation of negative experiences throughout a person's lifetime that leads to suicidal thoughts.

Sundowning syndrome: increase in psychiatric symptoms of psychomotor restlessness and confusion at night or during evening hours.

Superego: one of three psychodynamic concepts which includes all internal norms and values of society acquired during early development through interactions with parents as figures of societal authority.

Synaptic cleft: point of junction between two neurons in a neural pathway where neurotransmitters trigger receptor response.

Tardive dyskinesia: extrapyrimidal syndrome after long-term use of antipsychotic drugs (grimacing; slow, rhythmic, stereotyped movements; and tongue movements)

Temperament: individual differences in the intensity and duration of emotions including the characteristics of one's disposition.

Thought broadcasting: false belief that one's thoughts can be heard by others.

Thought insertion: false belief that thoughts of others can be implanted in one's mind.

Thought withdrawal: false belief that others can remove thoughts from one's mind.

Tic: sudden, repetitive, arrhythmic, stereotyped motor movement or verbal speech.

Tolerance: condition that develops through continued use of a substance as the brain adapts to repeated doses of the drug with a declining effect as it is taken repeatedly over time.

Tricyclic (TCA): drugs with three hydrocarbon rings that inhibit reuptake of norepinephrine and serotonin in the treatment of clinical depression.

Unconscious: level of consciousness at which thoughts, wishes, and feelings are not retrievable to conscious awareness.

Unipolar: having depressive episodes but does not experience mania or hypomania.

Unresolved grief: process of grieving becomes prolonged and may be considered abnormal or maladaptive when symptoms are still present two months after the loss.

Validation: verify the nurse's perception of feeling conveyed by either verbal or non-verbal message of the client.

Vascular dementia: vascular disorder in which there are multiple large and small cerebral infarctions leading to symptoms of dementia. Symptoms of dementia appear within the first year of existing neurologic symptoms. (Also referred to as multi-infarct dementia.)

Verbigeration: repeating of words, phrases, or sentences several time.

Voyeurism: experiencing of sexual gratification by observing nude persons or the sexual activity of others.

Water intoxication: condition in which an excessive amount of water is consumed, leading to abdominal cramps, dizziness, lethargy, nausea and vomiting, convulsions and possible coma.

Waxy flexibility: posturing in which a person's body part can be moved and it will remain in that position until moved by another person.

Wernicke-Korsakoff syndrome: mental disorder characterized by amnesia, clouding of consciousness, confabulation, memory loss, and peripheral neuropathy. The disorder is associated with thiamine and niacin vitamin deficiency seen in chronic alcoholism.

Withdrawal: maladaptive change in behavior accompanied by physiological and psychological alterations that occur as the blood or tissue concentrations of a substance decline in a person who has engaged in heavy prolonged use of a substance.

Word salad: meaningless and incoherent mixture of words or phrases.

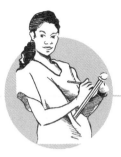

Index